FIRST AID
HANDBOOK

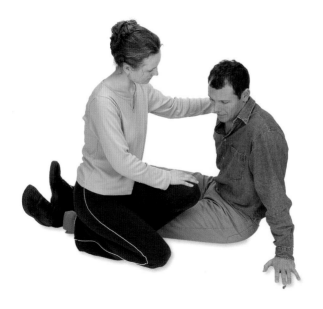

D1511761

FIRST AID
HANDBOOK

FAST AND EFFECTIVE EMERGENCY CARE

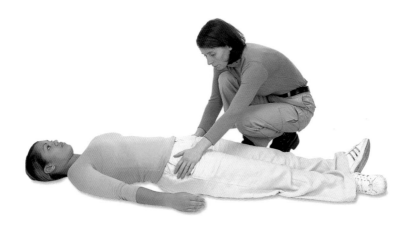

DR PIPPA KEECH MB ChB MRCGP
EDITORIAL CONSULTANT: ANNE CHARLISH

southwater

This edition is published by Southwater

Southwater is an imprint of Anness Publishing Ltd
Hermes House, 88–89 Blackfriars Road, London SE1 8HA
tel. 020 7401 2077; fax 020 7633 9499
www.southwaterbooks.com; info@anness.com

UK agent: The Manning Partnership Ltd, 6 The Old Dairy, Melcombe Road, Bath BA2 3LR;
tel. 01225 478444; fax 01225 478440; sales@manning-partnership.co.uk

UK distributor: Grantham Book Services Ltd, Isaac Newton Way, Alma Park Industrial Estate, Grantham, Lincs NG31 9SD;
tel. 01476 541080; fax 01476 541061; orders@gbs.tbs-ltd.co.uk

North American agent/distributor: National Book Network, 4501 Forbes Boulevard, Suite 200, Lanham, MD 20706;
tel. 301 459 3366; fax 301 429 5746; www.nbnbooks.com

Australian agent/distributor: Pan Macmillan Australia, Level 18, St Martins Tower, 31 Market St, Sydney, NSW 2000;
tel. 1300 135 113; fax 1300 135 103; customer.service@macmillan.com.au

New Zealand agent/distributor: David Bateman Ltd, 30 Tarndale Grove, Off Bush Road, Albany, Auckland;
tel. (09) 415 7664; fax (09) 415 8892

A CIP catalogue record for this book is available from the British Library.

Publisher: Joanna Lorenz
Managing Editor: Helen Sudell
Project Editors: Melanie Halton, Ann Kay
Editorial Consultant/Additional Text: Anne Charlish
Text Editors: Sue Barraclough, Kim Davies, Tracey Kelly, Mary Lindsay, Nikki Sims
Designer: Lisa Tai
Photographer: Mark Wood
Special effects make-up: Dauphine's of Bristol
Illustrations: Samantha Elmhurst
Production Controller: Steve Lang
Editorial Reader: Penelope Goodare

Previously published as *Practical Guide to First Aid*

1 3 5 7 9 10 8 6 4 2

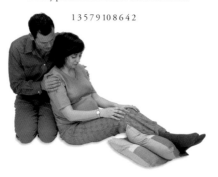

Publisher's Note:

Author's Foreword

The very first point to make is that you have done a highly worthwhile thing in picking up this book. Understanding first aid is a vital life skill – if only many more people knew even the basics. Such knowledge is indispensable for finding the most effective way to deal with the array of problems that face us and our families – from minor everyday problems such as headaches and cut fingers to more serious emergencies.

What saves lives?

So, what is it that really saves lives? Well, it certainly isn't a perfectly equipped first-aid kit, although a good kit always helps. It is *you* that will save a life – using whatever resources are at hand, your first-aid knowledge and a large dose of practical common sense. In fact, first aid is largely about common sense: putting pressure on a nasty wound to stop it bleeding, making sure a casualty's airway is clear, keeping them warm…

Common sense comes in handy in preventing accidents too. We can't cocoon ourselves against all danger, and life would be dull without adventure, but it is worth recalling the mountain-hiker who suffered from hypothermia because "the guide book said it never rains in the mountains". The value of being aware of danger and taking sensible safety precautions cannot be overestimated – remember that most accidents take place in our homes, where we like to think we are safest.

Help at hand

What follows has been designed to be your personal guide through the many first-aid scenarios you might encounter, highlighting all kinds of preventative tips along the way. Even so, I must stress that nothing replaces a really good practical first-aid course, which should give you the confidence and skills to deal with most situations. This book is the perfect companion to such a course. Good luck!

Dr Pippa Keech
MB ChB MRCGP

Contents

Author's Foreword 5
Introduction 8
How to use this book 10

Chapter 1
Action at an Emergency 11
What is first aid? 12–13
Making your assessment 14–15
Examining the casualty 16–17
Removing clothing and helmets 18–19
Moving and handling safely 1 20–21
Moving and handling safely 2 22–23
Skills checklist 24

Chapter 2
Life-saving Priorities 25
Understanding resuscitation 26–27
Responsiveness and the airway 28–29
Rescue breathing 30–31
Cardiac compressions 32–33
Full resuscitation sequence 34–35
The recovery position 36–37
Coping with choking 1 38–39
Coping with choking 2 40–41
Skills checklist 42

Chapter 3
Children's Life Support 43
Basic life support 44–45
Resuscitating a baby or child 46–47
The recovery position 48–49
Choking in babies and children 50–51
Skills checklist 52

Chapter 4
Lungs and Breathing 53
Understanding the respiratory system 54–55
Dealing with breathing difficulties 56–57
Tackling fume inhalation 58–59
Drowning: what to do 60–61
Hanging and strangling: what to do 62–63
Skills checklist 64

Chapter 5
Heart and Circulation 65
Understanding the cardiovascular system
  66–67
Dealing with shock 68–69
Managing anaphylactic shock 70–71
Coping with a heart attack 72–73
Dealing with an abnormal heart rate 74–75
Skills checklist 76

Chapter 6
Brain and Nervous System 77
Understanding the nervous system 78–79
Dealing with head injury 80–81
Coping with epilepsy 82–83
Recognizing a stroke 84–85
Coping with headache 86–87
Managing dizziness and fainting 88–89
Skills checklist 90

Chapter 7
Other Medical Emergencies 91
Coping with antenatal emergencies 92–93
Helping with emergency childbirth 94–95
Managing diabetic conditions 96–97
Dealing with nausea and vomiting 98
Tackling diarrhoea, fever and cramp 99
Dealing with abdominal pain 100–101
Coping with allergy 102–103
Dealing with bites and stings 104–105
Managing heat and cold disorders 106–107
Skills checklist 108

Chapter 8
Childhood Problems 109
Recognizing childhood illness 110–111
Dealing with problems in babies 112–113
Coping with fever 114
Dealing with vomiting and diarrhoea 115
Managing abdominal pain 116–117
Coughs and breathing difficulty 118–119
Tackling headaches 120–121
Managing other problems 122–123
Skills checklist 124

Chapter 9
Wounds and Bleeding 125
Types of wound 126–127
Wounds and wound healing 128–129
Tackling embedded objects 130–131
Treating infected wounds 132–133
Dealing with major wounds 134–135
Coping with severed body parts 136
Managing crush injuries 137
Controlling severe bleeding 138–139
Recognizing internal bleeding 140–141
Bleeding from orifices 142–143
Miscellaneous foreign bodies 144–145
Skills checklist 146

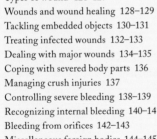

Chapter 10
Bone and Muscle Injuries 147
Understanding the skeleton 148–149
Dealing with broken bones 150–151
Tackling skull and facial fractures 152–153
Managing spinal injuries 154–155
Coping with neck injuries 156–157
Tackling upper limb fractures 158–159
Managing rib fractures 160–161
Coping with pelvic and upper-leg injuries 162–163
Handling knee and lower-leg injuries 164–165
Coping with dislocations 166–167
Managing sprains and strains 168–169
Controlling back pain 170–171
Skills checklist 172

Chapter 11
Burns and Scalds 173
Understanding and assessing burns 1 174–175
Understanding and assessing burns 2 176–177
Managing burns 178–179
Chemical, electrical and inhalation burns 180–181
Coping with facial burns 182
Tackling sunburn 183
Skills checklist 184

Chapter 12
Action on Poisoning 185
Understanding poisoning 186–187
Managing drug poisoning 188–189
Tackling alcohol and illicit drug poisoning 190–191
Dealing with food and plant poisoning 192–193
Managing poisoning in children 194–195
Skills checklist 196

Chapter 13
First-Aid Kit 197
Assembling a first-aid kit 198–199
Applying dressings and bandages 200–201
Applying bandages 1 202–203
Applying bandages 2 204–205
Fixing slings 206–207
Skills checklist 208

Chapter 14
Complementary Therapies 209
Understanding complementary therapies 210-211
Complementary first-aid kit 212-213
Using complementary therapies 1 214-215
Using complementary therapies 2 216-217
Skills checklist 218

Chapter 15
Keeping Safe 219
Keeping yourself safe 220–221
Safety on the road 222–223
Safety in the home 224–225
Safety in the kitchen 226–227
Safety in the bathroom 228–229
Safety in the garden 230–231
Dealing with fire 232
Avoiding electrical accidents 233
Safe home for infants 234
Avoiding cot death 235
Skills checklist 236

Chapter 16
Outdoor Safety 237
Safety in sport 238–239
Safety in land sports 240–241
Safety in water sports 242–243
Safety in snow sports 244–245
Travelling safely 246–247
Skills checklist 248

Useful Information 249
Useful addresses 250–252
Index 253–256
Acknowledgements 256

Introduction

Understanding the basics of first aid will help you to stay calm and in control in an emergency. This is vital in a crisis, regardless of the level of your specific knowledge. It is also enormously reassuring to the casualty, whatever the eventual outcome, and will often inspire bystanders to offer assistance. Remember, even those with no training can do something really useful, such as phoning for help or comforting the casualty.

FIRST PRINCIPLES

Here are a few first principles that anyone attempting to help out in an emergency must be aware of; many of them are elaborated upon throughout the book:
- Do not delay in calling for emergency help, it may take some time to arrive.
- Do not put yourself in any danger – if you get hurt, you won't be helping anyone.
- Remember that you may make matters worse if you act too impulsively.

WHAT TO EXPECT AT THE ACCIDENT AND EMERGENCY DEPARTMENT

You may well end up going to hospital with a casualty. If you know what to expect in an accident and emergency department, you will cope more calmly when you get there. You will also be able to talk to the casualty about what to expect, which should in turn help to reduce their anxiety.

A nurse should greet you almost as soon as you register at the accident and emergency desk. The nurse's job is to assess what immediate treatment is needed and how urgently the casualty needs to be seen. This is called "triaging". Casualties who need immediate care are often moved to a room called the "resuscitation room". Cases such as

possible heart attacks and asthmatics will be classed as urgent. After this the triage nurse will deal with people who need a bed to lie on, usually classified as a major casualty; the more minor casualties will need to wait a little longer to be treated. Unless the wound or problem is very minor, the nurse will usually ask the casualty to undress and put a hospital gown on. This makes it much easier for medical personnel to examine the patient.

In some hospitals, there may be a separate area for children in A and E, and this spares them the distressing scenes that are often played out in a hospital's emergency department.

- If you find yourself in charge, try to formulate an overall plan of action.
- Look around the accident site for hazards such as flammable substances, but leave dangerous situations to be dealt with by professionals.
  - Be aware of your limitations. Do not try clambering up a rock face to help someone if you are terrified of heights. Do not attempt mouth-to-mouth if you have no idea what to do – summon help as an urgent priority.
    - Tackle aggressive casualties cautiously – get trained help as fast as possible.
    - Protect yourself in whatever way you can from body fluids, especially blood.

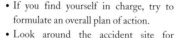

◁ Improvising a dressing for an injured hand.

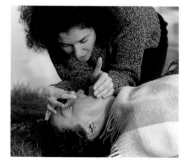

△ Carrying out resuscitation procedures on a victim of drowning at the water's edge.

- If you were the first to turn up at an incident, but other helpers come to your aid and seem better qualified to help, then forgo your pride and defer to them. That in itself will have been an immensely helpful thing to do.
- If you are in charge and a large crowd gathers, try to get everyone out of the way except for close friends or relatives and those who are giving actual aid.
- Remember that it is often a good idea to

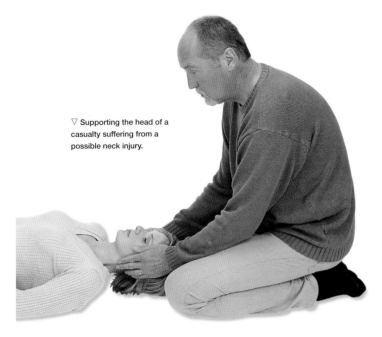

▽ Supporting the head of a casualty suffering from a possible neck injury.

FIRST-AID PRIORITIES

➤ Don't panic.

➤ Assess the situation quickly and calmly and try to identify the problem.

➤ Waste no time in summoning any professional help.

➤ Give medical aid if you feel you can; do nothing if in doubt.

➤ Comfort a conscious casualty.

➤ Stay with the casualty until help arrives.

"debrief" after an emergency event – talking to family and friends, or to a counsellor if necessary. You may be more shaken up than you realize.

WHEN YOU SHOULD DO NOTHING

You should always remember that it is sometimes better to do nothing than to risk doing the wrong thing. In one particular example, a man dealt with an elderly lady who had collapsed in the street by kneeling beside her and gathering her up so that he was cradling her slumped against his chest. In this position, her head was lolling forwards, her breathing tortuous. He meant well, but he was actually compromising her breathing – and her chances of survival.

BE PREPARED

Another important part of being a potential first-aider, especially when helping people within your circle of family and friends, is thinking through in advance what would need to be done in an emergency. This means, for example, that if a crisis arises,

you don't end up having to take four children and the family dog to the accident and emergency department.

Advance preparation means that you will be able to cope with whatever happens more confidently. It might mean thinking about which family members or friends are close enough to look after the children at

▽ With children, it can be hard to distinguish mild from serious problems. Learning to recognize tell-tale symptoms is a vital skill.

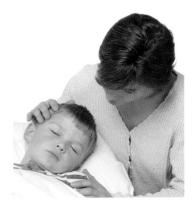

short notice, having a list of medication to hand that you or a potential casualty needs, or discussing with a neighbour whether they would feed your animals in a crisis.

Keeping the following two lists by the telephone will help enormously if sudden emergencies arise:

1 A list of important telephone numbers – neighbours, friends and relatives who live close by, plus your doctor and the emergency services.

2 A list of medication taken by any members of the household (this may be quite extensive in the case of an elderly person). Also make sure you have a record of any allergies – this might be invaluable to a doctor or paramedic.

▽ It is important to understand the kinds of substances that may trigger adverse reactions, from certain foods and drinks to dust and pollen.

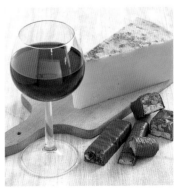

How to use this book

This essential guide has been specially arranged to help readers target the precise kind of information they need at any one time. The introductory chapters offer special guides explaining how to cope with emergencies and how to formulate a life-saving action plan. Other chapters highlight a vast range of vital topics – from children's health to sports injuries – while some deal with a specific body system, placing problems in their proper anatomical context. Each chapter closes with a helpful Skills Checklist – handy summaries that can be ticked off by the reader.

First-aid procedures are presented throughout in a clear step-by-step style, featuring helpful colour photographs and straightforward, jargon-free text, supported where necessary by fully annotated colour artworks. A range of special features, from flow charts to symptoms boxes, has also been used, in order to help readers access vital facts as readily as possible – these are explained below.

See Also boxes
These refer readers to related topics in the book. Cross-references may be to whole chapters (in capital letters), or to specific pages.

Flow charts
Lilac-coloured flow charts appear regularly throughout, summarizing the essential steps to follow in all kinds of situations.

Step-by-step sequences
Wherever relevant, procedures are broken down into numbered steps, where techniques can be seen clearly in full-colour photographs.

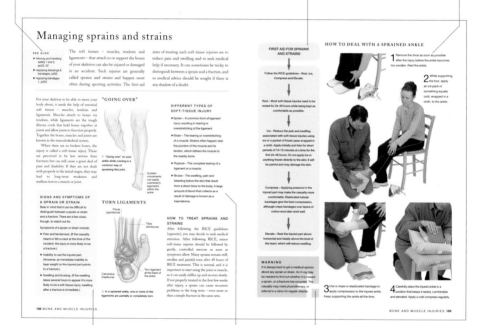

Signs and Symptoms boxes
These blue boxes pick out the major symptoms of each condition, making them easily accessible to first-aiders.

Information boxes
Beige-tinted boxes contain a range of valuable supporting information, from prevention advice and action checklists to useful facts and figures.

Warning boxes
These green-tinted boxes with white crosses alert readers to matters of particular importance. *Always* pay good attention to this advice.

1

ACTION AT AN EMERGENCY

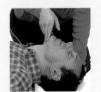

The action that you take at an emergency may have a lasting effect on the casualty. You will need to think quickly and make the correct decisions. Your assessment and examination of the casualty are all-important. This chapter takes you through those initial stages and shows you how to move and handle a casualty who may be badly injured and/or unconscious safely without causing further injury. If you are in any doubt at all about what to do or how to do it, it may be best to do nothing: simply call the emergency services and do what you can to reassure the casualty and keep them warm and safe from further injury.

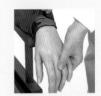

CONTENTS What is first aid? 12–13

Making your assessment 14–15

Examining the casualty 16–17

Removing clothing and helmets 18–19

Moving and handling safely 1 20–21

Moving and handling safely 2 22–23

Skills checklist 24

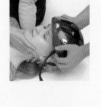

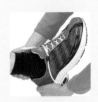

What is first aid?

SEE ALSO

➤ Responsiveness
and the airway, p28

➤ Cardiac
compressions, p32

➤ Full resuscitation
sequence, p34

First aid is literally the very FIRST assistance you give someone who has been injured. All of us should know basic first-aid techniques, in the home, at the office or when out and about. One in three of all accidents takes place in our homes, the majority involving children and the elderly.

Knowing what to do first and recognizing how potentially serious a casualty's condition is may speed recovery and even prove vital to saving a life. Please note that the text on these two pages is a summary and is expanded in detail over subsequent chapters.

First aid help can cover an extremely varied range of scenarios – from simple reassurance after a small accident to dealing with a life-threatening emergency. A speedy response is crucial. Emergency workers refer to the first hour after an accident as the golden hour: the more help given within this hour, the better the outcome for the casualty.

THE GOALS OF FIRST AID

• To keep the casualty alive. The ABC of life support – Airway, Breathing and Circulation – constitutes the absolute top priority of first aid.
• To stop the casualty getting worse.
• To promote their recovery.
• To provide reassurance and comfort to the casualty.

THE DRSABC CODE

Remembering and acting on these can save lives:

D for DANGER
R for RESPONSE
S for SHOUT
A for AIRWAY
B for BREATHING
C for CIRCULATION

WHAT TO DO IN AN EMERGENCY

First, STAY CALM. Secondly, ASSESS THE SITUATION promptly. Now carry out the "DRSABC" sequence, as follows:

1 DANGER

Your assessment should have alerted you to any potential hazards. Now you should:
• Keep yourself out of any danger.
• Keep passers-by out of danger.
• Make safe any hazards, if you can do so without endangering yourself or others. Only move the casualty away from danger in extreme circumstances.

2 RESPONSE

Try to establish the responsiveness level.
• If the casualty appears unconscious or semi-conscious, speak loudly to them – as in "Can you hear me?".
• If this fails to get a response, tap them firmly on the shoulders.

3 SHOUT

If step 2 fails to raise any response:
• Shout out loudly to passers-by for help with the situation.

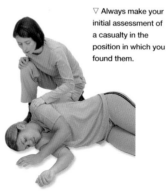

▽ Always make your initial assessment of a casualty in the position in which you found them.

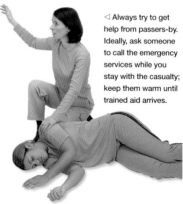

◁ Always try to get help from passers-by. Ideally, ask someone to call the emergency services while you stay with the casualty; keep them warm until trained aid arrives.

4 AIRWAY

Now determine whether the airway (the passage from the mouth to the lungs) is clear enough to allow proper breathing.
• Check the mouth and remove any visible obvious obstructions, such as food, that are at the front of the mouth only.
• Tilt the casualty's head back gently to prevent the tongue from falling back and blocking the airway. Place a hand on the forehead/top of head and two fingers under the jaw. Tilt back gently until a natural stop is reached.

▷ Tilt the head using a hand on the forehead/top of head and two fingers under the jaw. This casualty was found on his back. Avoid moving a casualty on to their back unless you need to start rescue breaths or chest compressions (see steps 5 and 6).

5 BREATHING

Is the casualty breathing?

- LOOK to see if the chest is moving.
- LISTEN for breathing sounds – put your ear against their mouth.
- FEEL for expired air by placing your cheek or ear close to their face.
- CHECK for other signs of life (e.g. body warmth, good colour, ability to swallow).
- If these checks are negative, the casualty is probably not breathing. You must now CALL AN AMBULANCE; ideally, get someone else to go.
- Without delay, start artificial respiration procedures (giving 2 breaths).

6 CIRCULATION

Look for signs of a working circulation.

- Check for breathing, coughing or any movement.
- Never waste time trying to find a pulse unless you are highly experienced in medicine.
- If there are no signs of a circulation, start cardiac massage (chest compressions) – but only if you are trained to do so.

GETTING HELP

Phoning the emergency services is free on all kinds of phone. If the casualty is inside a building and other people are present, ask someone to stand outside the building in order to guide the emergency services. If you are at a house and it's dark outside, switch on any outside lights.

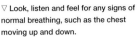
▽ Look, listen and feel for any signs of normal breathing, such as the chest moving up and down.

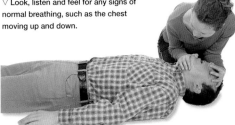

▽ If there are no signs of breathing, give 2 normal-force breaths by means of mouth-to-mouth resuscitation.

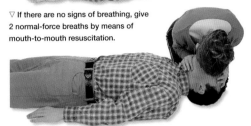

INFORMATION FOR THE EMERGENCY SERVICES

- ➤ Whether the casualty is conscious and breathing – information you will have if you have followed DRSABC.
- ➤ Your location (a landmark will do if you know no more) and phone number.
- ➤ Your name.
- ➤ What the problem is and what time it happened.
- ➤ If it is relevant, how many casualties there are, and their sex and age.
- ➤ Report any hazards, such as ice on the road or hazardous substances.
- ➤ Don't hang up the telephone until the authorities tell you to do so.

◁ Tell the emergency services useful information such as the presence of a medical alert/ID tag.

▷ If someone falls from a height, keep them warm and do not move them – unless it is necessary for resuscitation.

VITAL NUMBERS

Some national emergency services numbers:

- ➤ UK: 999
- ➤ US: 911
- ➤ Australia: 000

On mobile phones, use these numbers or 112 (but check with your network).

DON'T MOVE THEM!

There are good reasons for leaving a casualty in place until more skilled personnel arrive. Injuries to the spine, especially to the neck, are possible after accidents and falls, and further movement can cause serious damage to the spinal cord. You may have to use some movement to deal with an injury, but the golden rule after an accident is not to move an injured person unless they are in danger, need to be resuscitated, or are unconscious and should be put into the recovery position. If moving a casualty is unavoidable, you should be very careful with their neck.

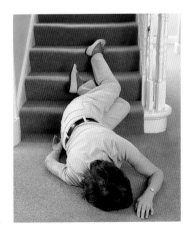

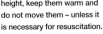

Making your assessment

SEE ALSO
➤ What is first aid?, p12
➤ Examining the casualty, p16
➤ Moving and handling safely 1 and 2, pp20, 22

Your initial assessment may be of major importance to the outcome of an accident. Remember DRS (Danger, Response, Shout) and ABC (Airway, Breathing, Circulation). Together these form DRSABC, which you can also remember as "the doctors' ABC". Once you know a casualty is conscious and breathing, you can start to identify the nature of the problem. Ask if they can remember what happened. Look around for clues to the accident. Appearing as calm as possible will help to give vital reassurance to the casualty.

Once you have checked DRSABC and established that breathing and circulation are functioning, you have more time to address the casualty's specific problems. They may be simple and the remedy straightforward. If the situation is less clear, however, the "Signs and Symptoms" box indicates what you should look out for.

In general, after completing DRSABC, a first-aider should gather basic initial information (what has happened, plus vital medical facts such as whether the casualty is diabetic), call for any emergency aid, and locate and treat – as far as possible – any obvious physical injury. They may then go on to gather further information from the casualty about the incident and their medical history, and carry out a more thorough examination – by looking, feeling, and questioning the casualty.

TAKING A HISTORY

This involves gathering information by asking questions and listening. Remember that it is very reassuring for everyone concerned to see that something is being done for a friend or relative, and this information may be vital for the ambulance and medical staff later on. Begin by questioning the casualty; if their answers are vague or unhelpful, ask anyone else who may know something useful.

1 Ask their name. It is very comforting to be called by name, and useful to use if the casualty starts to lose consciousness.

2 Ask children their age and, if they are old enough to have the information, ask them how you can contact a parent or carer.

3 What is the problem? Let the casualty talk for a while. They may end up telling you not only what their current problem is, but also useful details about previous similar episodes and what their causes were. If they are still vague, you may find it useful to ask about possible symptoms relating to different systems of the body such as the:

• **Nervous system** – Headache, dizziness, weakness of arms or legs, tingling, pins and needles, loss of movement or sensation.
• **Chest** – Cough, shortness of breath, wheeze, pains in the chest – especially on taking a deep breath.
• **Heart** – Chest pains, swollen ankles.
• **Gut** – Vomiting, diarrhoea, stomach or pelvic pain.

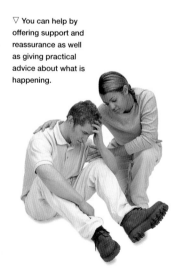

▽ You can help by offering support and reassurance as well as giving practical advice about what is happening.

△ Note the casualty's name, age and address, and the phone number of anyone they would like you to ring.

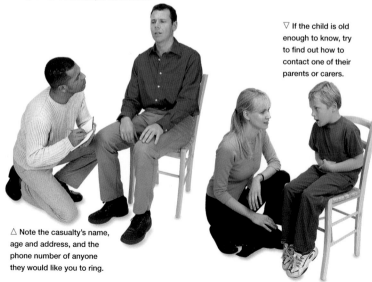

▽ If the child is old enough to know, try to find out how to contact one of their parents or carers.

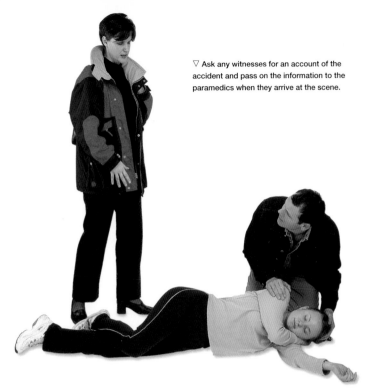

▽ Ask any witnesses for an account of the accident and pass on the information to the paramedics when they arrive at the scene.

SIGNS AND SYMPTOMS

➤ **Symptoms** – What can the casualty tell you about their injury or illness? Are they in pain or stiff, feeling anxious, hot, cold, dizzy, nauseous, faint or thirsty? Is there a sensation of tingling, weakness or memory loss?

➤ **Visual signs** – What can you see in relation to the casualty's condition? Anxious or painful expression, unusual chest movement, burns, sweating, bleeding, bruising, abnormal skin colour, swelling, deformity, vomiting or incontinence? Look for foreign bodies and objects related to substance abuse, such as aerosol cans and small plastic bags. Check for a medical ID tag.

➤ **Other signs** – What can you feel, hear or smell in relation to the casualty? Dampness, abnormal temperature, groaning, sucking sound, alcohol, acetone, solvents or glue, gas or fumes, vomit, urine or faeces?

➤ **Vital signs** – In what state are the casualty's pulse, respiration, colour and temperature? Sum up their general condition.

4 Ask about known medical problems such as diabetes, heart attacks or strokes, which may give you a clue as to what has happened this time.

5 Ask for information about any medication they are currently taking and whether they have any known allergies.

6 Ask when they last ate. If they are going to need emergency surgery, this is a very important question, and it may also be vital if they have diabetes.

GATHERING INFORMATION

Never underestimate how useful bystanders' information can be. People often become ill when they are out by themselves, and passers-by may see what has happened but don't accompany the casualty to hospital; the information is then lost. Exact sequences of events are vitally useful to the medical staff, because they often give big clues about the cause of a collapse or illness.

Sick or injured people may be very vague about what has happened to them, and will not know if, for example, they had a convulsion while they were unconscious. They may not know that one side of their face drooped for a short time, or that they lost their speech. These events will determine what investigations are carried out at the hospital. Ultimately, long-term outcomes – such as whether they will be allowed to drive home or not – depend very much on what actually happened. Any information you can gather and relay to the emergency services is very useful.

IDENTIFICATION DEVICES

If a casualty is alone and collapses, medical ID tags, which are worn as a necklace or bracelet, can be life-saving. One side often features a staff-and-snake emblem (an international medical symbol), and the other will have useful information about the casualty, for example if they suffer from diabetes or epilepsy. Tell the emergency services about the information on the tag.

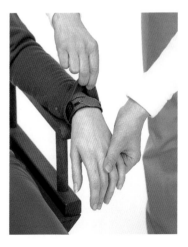

△ Always check a casualty's neck, wrists and ankles for a medical ID tag and pass on the information it carries to the paramedics.

Examining the casualty

SEE ALSO

➤ What is first aid?, p12

➤ Removing clothing and helmets, p18

➤ Responsiveness and the airway, p28

➤ The recovery position, p36

Once you are happy that a casualty is conscious and breathing, try to identify the problem by carrying out an examination. One of the first steps is to look at their face – are they very pale, for example? Don't move them at this stage, especially the neck or back. Now check the body for injury. Start with the head and finish with the arms and legs. Always try to gain a casualty's consent before starting an examination ("I just need to examine you to check for injuries; is that OK?") and keep the casualty and any friends or relatives informed as you go along.

You can tell a lot from looking at people, even before you touch them. Are they grey and anxious? Are they breathing easily, or is breathing laboured, painful or noisy, with wheezing or choking sounds? Remember that ensuring that a casualty's airway is clear is a top priority before any physical check. The feel and colour of skin is another hint. People in shock have pale, cold, clammy skin; a fever makes skin hot, dry and often flushed. Blue skin and lips suggest a heart that is not pumping well, or breathing problems that are preventing enough oxygen from reaching the blood.

Examine people in a systematic, gentle but businesslike way. Place unconscious but breathing casualties in the recovery position (on one side; explained elsewhere) before examining them. If you suspect any injuries that may worsen with movement, especially spinal injuries, examine them first. Always ensure that you protect the casualty's spine.

WHAT TO CHECK FOR

➤ Bruising, swelling, puncture wounds, burns and tender or painful areas.

➤ Changes in the casualty's appearance, breathing or state of consciousness.

➤ The presence of a medical ID tag.

➤ Any medication carried by the casualty, such as an inhaler.

VITAL NOTE: Anyone with a suspected spinal injury (see Step 5) must be kept as still as possible (especially the head) as you check. Ideally, hold them still while a helper checks areas other than the back.

HEAD-TO-TOE EXAMINATION

1 HEAD
Check the scalp for injury – swelling, depressions, cuts and bleeding. Also look out for blood or clear fluids in the nose or ears. Check the mouth for any objects or fluids (such

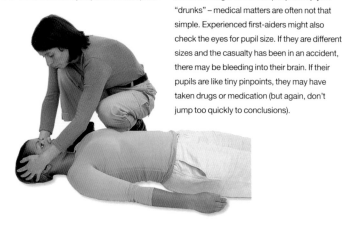

as vomit) that could obstruct breathing and remove if very easy to do (only remove dentures that are loose or broken and easy to extract). Smell the casualty's breath for alcohol, but do not be too eager to dismiss people simply as "drunks" – medical matters are often not that simple. Experienced first-aiders might also check the eyes for pupil size. If they are different sizes and the casualty has been in an accident, there may be bleeding into their brain. If their pupils are like tiny pinpoints, they may have taken drugs or medication (but again, don't jump too quickly to conclusions).

2 NECK
Make sure clothing is not tight, and check for a medical ID tag. Working very gently, feel along the back of the neck, without moving the head, for swelling or tenderness. Some people who have undergone a tracheotomy have a surgical opening called a stoma at the front of the neck that acts as an airway, so make sure that nothing obvious is blocking it.

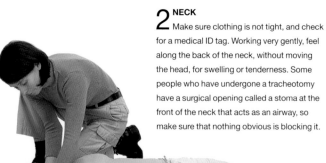

3 CHEST

Is the chest moving normally? Are there very tender places over the ribs (these may be rib fractures)? If there is an object stuck in the chest, leave it there. Feel the collarbones for swelling and tenderness. In some cases, it may be necessary to remove clothing to look at the chest, to check for obvious lacerations or bruises, for example. Typically, you might do this if the emergency services are delayed, but always proceed with sensitivity.

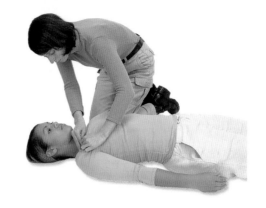

4 ABDOMEN

Feel the stomach gently for any large swellings or tender places. If the casualty is conscious, they will flinch, moan or cry out if you touch an area that is painful.

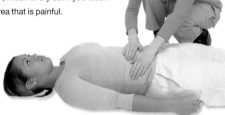

5 LOWER BACK

If you suspect a spinal injury, from the circumstances of the accident or from what the casualty says, do not try examining the back – even the tiniest amount of movement could risk further damage (see also What to Check For box). If you do not suspect spinal injury, gently feel the back for any tender areas.

6 PELVIS

Note any tender places over the hips. Maintain a very light touch because a pelvic injury can be excruciatingly painful.

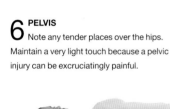

7 ARMS AND LEGS

Look for injuries. Now test the limbs' function by asking whether the casualty can feel you touching their arms and legs. Ask them to grip your hand with theirs and to try tensing their leg muscles.

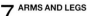

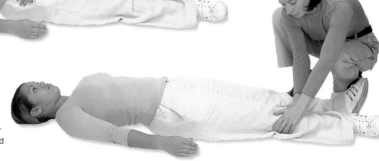

Removing clothing and helmets

SEE ALSO
➤ Examining the casualty, p16
➤ Moving and handling safely 1 and 2, pp20, 22

Removing a casualty's clothing should not be an automatic reaction. It is often unnecessary, especially if the casualty will soon be seen at a hospital, and can make people feel anxious and vulnerable, as well as exposing them to the elements. The movement required may also cause further injury. Only remove clothing if the emergency services are delayed and you feel it is absolutely essential in order to treat the casualty effectively. Do not attempt it if you are unpractised, as you may cause harm, and always seek consent and respect people's privacy.

You may need to look at a wounded site that is hidden by clothing in order to assess and deal with the injury. It may be possible to undress the casualty by unfastening and sliding off clothing but often it is necessary to cut the garments before removing them.

POINTS TO CONSIDER

➤ People can get upset at having their clothes removed by a stranger. Unless it is absolutely necessary, it is usually best to wait until they reach hospital. Remember, you can often feel injuries adequately through clothing.

➤ If you are in any doubt about removing an item of clothing or footwear, or if you are causing the casualty increased pain, it is best to wait for the paramedics.

➤ Try to seek the casualty's consent for your actions and explain what you are doing, so that they are not alarmed.

➤ Remove clothes and shoes with the minimum of movement, to avoid further injury and pain – never pull at clothing.

➤ The injured area will be very sensitive, so try to keep clothing away from it.

➤ Cutting clothes may injure the skin, especially if you are not using scissors designed for this job.

➤ The easiest route for cutting is along the seams.

➤ With leg and foot injuries, try to take off shoes or boots before the leg and ankle become so swollen that it is more painful to remove the footwear.

SWEATERS AND T–SHIRTS

If the injury is in the upper part of the body, then you may need to remove the casualty's top garment. Make sure that you do not attempt to do this if there is any chance that the casualty may have sustained a spinal injury.

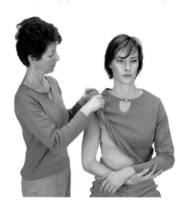

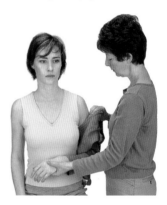

1 Release the uninjured arm carefully, before trying to undress the injured arm. Roll the garment up to the shoulder.

2 Pull the garment over the head, then slowly and very gently pull it down over the injured arm and smoothly off the hand.

SHOES

Removing shoes can be tricky because the foot or ankle may have become swollen. Undo the shoe entirely and support the foot under the ankle with one hand, while gently sliding the shoe off the heel and then over the toes with the other hand.

▽ Make sure that the laces are loose before you attempt to remove shoes.

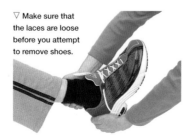

SOCKS

The tight fit of socks causes problems for removal. If there is no swelling or pain you can try rolling the sock down over the foot. If the ankle or foot is very swollen, it is easier to cut off the sock. Pull the material away from the skin as you cut.

▽ You should cut the sock off an injured foot rather than trying to pull it off.

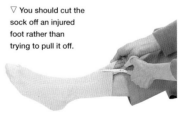

TROUSERS

If trousers are too tight to pull up from the ankle to reach a leg wound, you may need to cut them along the seam.

▽ Hold the trousers clear of a leg injury while pulling them up.

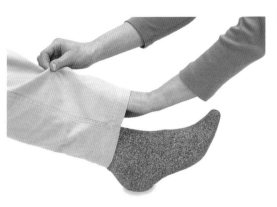

▽ You may have to cut the trousers and socks off the injured leg in order to avoid causing any further pain.

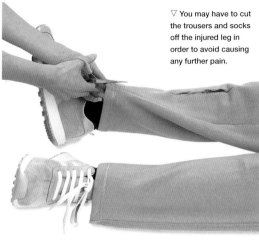

HELMETS

Only remove helmets as a last resort – as a rule of thumb, do so only if they are impeding a casualty's breathing. If the casualty is breathing and has an unrestricted airway, leave removal to the experts. If you have to proceed urgently, try to get someone to assist you so that the neck is supported, in a straight line with the head and spine if possible, while the helmet is taken off.

Full-face helmets

Ideally, two people are needed to remove a full-face helmet. One person is in charge of supporting the casualty's neck and holding on to the lower jaw; the second person undoes (or cuts) the straps and places their fingers under the helmet's rim. Sitting behind the casualty's head, the second person starts to ease off the helmet. The first person must keep the head still. The helmet may have to be tilted back to get it over the chin, and then forwards in order to lift it over the back of the head.

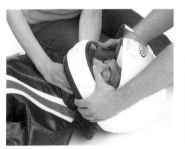

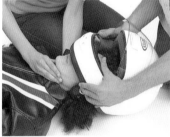

1 One helper firmly supports the casualty's neck and jaw while the other carefully undoes the straps and eases the helmet up.

2 The first helper maintains neck and jaw support while the other helper slowly lifts the helmet over the chin and over the head.

Open-face helmets

These helmets should also be removed by two people, if possible. One person supports the neck and jaw while the second person undoes (or cuts) the chin strap. The second person then grips the sides of the helmet from the inside and pulls the straps apart. The helmet can then be lifted off without causing pain or further injury.

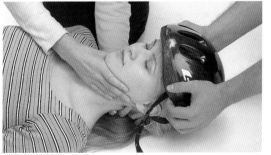

◁ To remove this type of open-face helmet, often used by cyclists, one helper supports the jaw and neck and the other releases or cuts the strap and then gently lifts the helmet away from the head.

Moving and handling safely 1

SEE ALSO
➤ Moving and handling safely 2, p22
➤ WOUNDS AND BLEEDING, p125
➤ BONE AND MUSCLE INJURIES, p147

Never move a casualty if there is any chance that they could have a spinal injury, especially in the neck area. Sometimes, however, you will have no choice in the matter – the injured person may not be breathing and the airway must always take first priority, although there are ways of protecting the neck during resuscitation. Very rarely, it may be vital to move the casualty away from danger into a safer environment, perhaps because of fire or danger of explosion, or because there is a risk of hypothermia or sunstroke.

There are various reasons for having to move a casualty, such as needing to get to water if someone has serious chemical burns, or to reach other injured people. You must know how to move people without causing further injury or endangering yourself. And never forget: if someone is a stretcher case, they need an ambulance.

Causing further injury is always a risk with moving people, so doing nothing may be wise – it is a question of weighing up the relative perils. Always observe the rules of safe lifting, listed below. Also, think laterally and don't automatically rush to drag people all over the place. It may be easier to remove the danger from the casualty than the other way around. So, if a casualty is lying in a busy road, you might be able to park your car so that others will drive around the incident area.

SAFE MOVING

If moving another adult, you must be certain that this is necessary and that you are strong enough to do so. It is vital to protect your own back, so always remember to:

• Lift or move someone only if you are trained or if it is a dire emergency.
• Get the casualty to move himself or herself if possible.
• Keep your feet slightly apart.
• Use your legs to lift, not your back.
• Do not twist or turn as you lift.
• Keep your back straight and locked.
• Keep the weight that is being lifted close to your body.

MOVING A CASUALTY SINGLE-HANDEDLY

The moving techniques shown below and on the opposite page are for when there is just one rescuer at the accident scene. Here the options for moving a casualty are more limited than if there are two or more rescuers. Careful thought must be given to the technique you choose: consider your strength and fitness, the weight of the casualty, whether they are conscious and whether there could be a spinal injury.

Unconscious casualty

An unconscious person is unable to protect their airway so you must ensure there is no danger of their head flopping forwards and blocking their airway when you move them. Dragging is the best way to move the casualty in this instance.

Dragging can also be used when the casualty is too heavy to lift.

Mobile casualty

If the casualty can still walk in a limited way you can try the human crutch. This helps to stabilize their walking.

Immobile casualty

If the casualty cannot move, they may have a spinal injury. If there is any risk of this, never move a casualty – call the emergency services immediately.

DRAGGING

You may have to drag a casualty away from the risk of further injury, such as in a fire. Bend down at the knees, lock your arms around the casualty's chest and keep them as close to you as possible as you move back. Do not drag the casualty sideways.

THE HUMAN CRUTCH

If the casualty is still at all mobile, this highly useful "assisted walk" technique allows the casualty to use your body as a crutch, to give them greater stability. Place a supporting arm firmly around their waist and grasp their nearest hand in your other hand. Make sure that you tell them about any obstacles in their path or changes in floor level, and take only small steps.

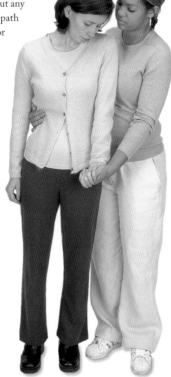

CRADLE CARRY

This method works particularly well with children and helps them to feel reassured and safe. Never attempt this lift on someone unless they are a great deal lighter than you, as you may damage your back; there is also the danger of dropping the casualty and causing further injury.

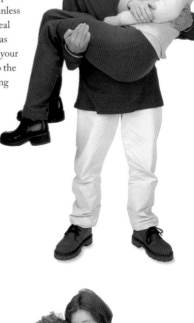

PIGGYBACK

Use this only in a severe emergency and if confident of your strength. Your approach will vary depending on how tall, heavy and strong you are in relation to the casualty. With your back to the casualty, bend forward and get the casualty to put both arms over your shoulders. Pull them on to your back and grasp their thighs. If you can, take hold of their hands. Try to keep your knees slightly bent. If lifting a small, light casualty, you may choose to crouch down in front of them and grasp their thighs before coming up gradually with your back kept straight.

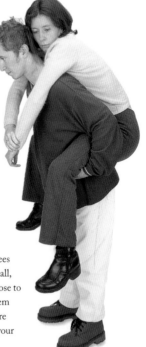

WHICH SINGLE-HANDED CARRY TO USE

➤ Try to use the human crutch wherever possible, especially if you are small and light. This excellent technique poses minimum risk to the rescuer, and little risk of damaging the casualty's internal organs. Ideally, the cradle and piggyback carries are usually best left for lifting someone about half your weight or less, making them particularly suitable for children.

➤ Avoid the "fireman's lift" (where the casualty is carried over the rescuer's shoulder), as this is tricky to do well and safely and could potentially cause severe damage to the casualty.

▷

Moving and handling safely 2

MOVING A CASUALTY WITH TWO OR MORE HELPERS

It is much easier and less likely to cause further injury if you can move or lift a casualty with two or more people helping. This is because you have more control over the move, and your combined strength means you are sharing the burden of weight. At the scene of an accident, always try to enlist help from any bystanders before attempting to move the casualty single-handedly. Explain step-by-step exactly what you intend to do and ensure they understand the importance of coordinating every move.

Unconscious casualty

If the casualty is unconscious or is immobilized as a result of their injuries, you can attempt a fore and aft carry. This can also be used if the person is conscious, but it should be avoided if the arms, shoulders or ribs are injured. If four helpers are available and you have a blanket or piece of cloth handy, a blanket lift provides a safe, supportive method of transporting an injured person – except when spinal injury is suspected, in which case, avoid it. If there is an immediate risk to life, such as fire or water, that outweighs the danger of movement, very carefully roll the victim away from the danger with as many helpers as possible supporting and controlling the body to minimize damage. All helpers must act in sync when rolling the casualty.

Conscious casualty

The two-hand seat carry can be used if the casualty is conscious and able to move into a sitting position. If the casualty is extremely heavy, then do not try to lift them – leave this to the experts.

FORE AND AFT CARRY

With an unconscious or immobile casualty and two helpers, the stronger should take the upper body and the other the legs. Make sure you synchronize your actions and move in the same direction. Move slowly and carefully and watch out for any obstacles such as steps or stairs.

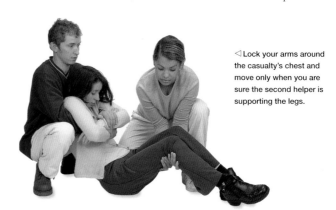

◁ Lock your arms around the casualty's chest and move only when you are sure the second helper is supporting the legs.

TWO-HAND SEAT

This move should be used when the casualty is conscious. Squat one on each side of the casualty and cross arms across their back. Hold on to the casualty's clothes, then pass your other hands under the casualty's knees and grip each other's wrists. Keep close to the casualty and lift together, keeping knees bent.

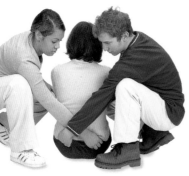

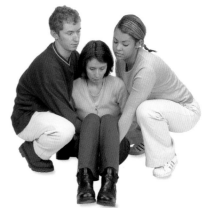

1 Get as close to the casualty as you possibly can in order to reduce strain on your own back. Bend at the knees and take hold of the casualty's clothes, on or just above the buttocks, with your hands crossed.

△ Detail of hand grip.

2 With your other hands, support the casualty's legs. Lock wrists with the other helper and lift, keeping your back straight.

BLANKET LIFT

This rudimentary "stretcher" is the safest, easiest way of moving an unconscious or immobile casualty if there are at least four helpers – doing it with fewer risks further injury. You need a blanket, sheet, rug or any large piece of fabric such as a coat, opened out. Use this to carry the casualty a short way or to transfer them to a proper stretcher. All helpers must move the casualty in a synchronized action. Note that you should never attempt to improvise any kind of stretcher if you are uncertain what to do.

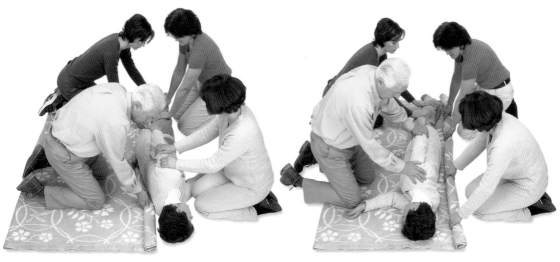

1 With the casualty placed on their side, and the blanket edge rolled up lengthways, position the roll against the casualty's back.

2 Move the casualty over the rolled edge, on to their other side. Make sure the casualty's head isn't close to the edge.

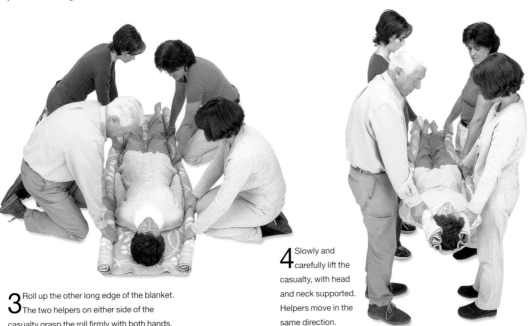

3 Roll up the other long edge of the blanket. The two helpers on either side of the casualty grasp the roll firmly with both hands.

4 Slowly and carefully lift the casualty, with head and neck supported. Helpers move in the same direction.

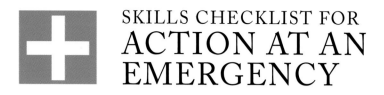

SKILLS CHECKLIST FOR
ACTION AT AN EMERGENCY

KEY POINTS

- Always do the DRSABC ☐

- Assess the situation promptly but with thought – do not rush in impulsively ☐

- Do not move the casualty before the paramedics arrive unless it is absolutely necessary ☐

- Always treat casualties with respect; seek permission for actions of a personal nature where possible, and keep them well informed of what you are doing ☐

SKILLS LEARNED

- The principal rules of approaching and dealing with emergencies safely and effectively ☐

- The basics of life-saving: what the DRSABC of Danger, Response, Shout, Airway, Breathing, Circulation is all about ☐

- Assessing the nature of the problem ☐

- When and how to remove clothing and helmets, without causing further injury ☐

- Handling and moving a casualty safely ☐

LIFE-SAVING PRIORITIES

For the best possible outcome, it is essential that life-saving techniques are carried out in the correct order. Once you have assessed DRSABC (see the previous chapter), you need to concentrate on issues such as continuing resuscitation, possibly moving the casualty into the recovery position, or deciding which technique is best to use for choking, depending on whether the casualty is conscious or unconscious. You must also consider the impact of shock on any casualty and do your best to calm and reassure them at every stage of the emergency.

CONTENTS Understanding resuscitation 26–27

Responsiveness and the airway 28–29

Rescue breathing 30–31

Cardiac compressions 32–33

Full resuscitation sequence 34–35

The recovery position 36–37

Coping with choking 1 38–39

Coping with choking 2 40–41

Skills checklist 42

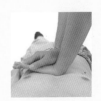

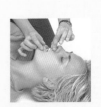

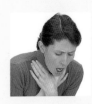

Understanding resuscitation

SEE ALSO

➤ Responsiveness and
  the airway, p28
➤ Rescue breathing, p30
➤ Cardiac
  compressions, p32
➤ The recovery
  position, p36

You could save someone's life by applying basic resuscitation skills. Equipped with these, you should be able to maintain a person's breathing and circulation, and this greatly increases their chances of survival once the emergency services arrive. The key elements of resuscitation are ensuring that oxygen gets into the lungs and that oxygenated blood gets to the brain. Resuscitation should only be attempted by those who have received proper training and practice in these techniques, which are explained in full detail in this chapter.

WHAT IS CARDIOPULMONARY RESUSCITATION (CPR)?

CPR is the technique of providing basic life support using chest compressions and artificial ventilation. The latter is also called "the kiss of life", mouth-to-mouth resuscitation, or rescue breathing. Although the technique has been used for over 50 years, it was not until the 1970s that the idea of training the public in these skills began.

CPR is needed after a cardiac arrest, that is, when the heart suddenly stops beating and circulation of the blood around the body ceases. A person who has had a cardiac arrest is unresponsive to voice or touch, is not breathing and has no pulse. Since two-thirds of cardiac arrests occur unexpectedly and not in hospitals, it makes sense for members of the public to be able to carry out resuscitation.

After only 3–4 minutes without oxygen, the brain can suffer irreversible damage, and this can be fatal, so you should act swiftly.

(There have been some instances of successful resuscitation up to 40 minutes after cardiac arrest when it occurred in cold water, but this is the exception as most incidents occur on dry land.) In most cases, a little knowledge and training can definitely save lives. If CPR is started within seconds of the cardiac arrest, the victim has a significantly improved chance of surviving.

NORMAL CIRCULATION

Blood flows through the blood vessels in one direction at a fairly constant rate. The heart is at the centre of the circulatory system, pumping blood around the body. The heart pumps blood to the lungs where it absorbs oxygen and gives up the carbon dioxide collected as it travels around the body. The blood then returns to the heart, and the oxygenated blood is sent to all parts of the body including the brain. The

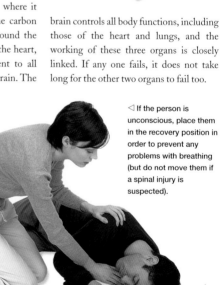

◁ Unless unconsciousness in an adult is the result of injury or choking, summon the emergency services first and then carry out resuscitation.

brain controls all body functions, including those of the heart and lungs, and the working of these three organs is closely linked. If any one fails, it does not take long for the other two organs to fail too.

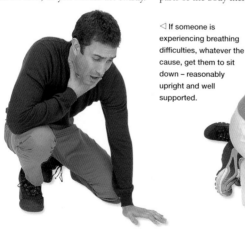

◁ If someone is experiencing breathing difficulties, whatever the cause, get them to sit down – reasonably upright and well supported.

◁ If the person is unconscious, place them in the recovery position in order to prevent any problems with breathing (but do not move them if a spinal injury is suspected).

THE "CHAIN OF SURVIVAL"

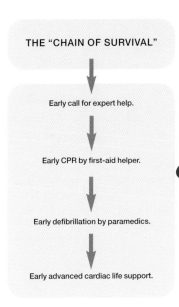

Early call for expert help.

Early CPR by first-aid helper.

Early defibrillation by paramedics.

Early advanced cardiac life support.

HOW CPR WORKS

Keeping the casualty's airway open, breathing for them and doing chest compressions means that an oxygenated blood supply continues to reach their brain. This "buys" really valuable time for the casualty by keeping their brain alive until more specialized help is available.

ARTIFICIAL VENTILATION

If someone has stopped breathing, their brain will soon be deprived of oxygen, and there will be a build-up of toxic carbon dioxide in the blood. You can breathe for them by artificial ventilation, but if the heart has stopped as well, you must give chest compressions to help move the oxygenated blood around the body.

CHEST COMPRESSIONS

The blood is kept circulating by the use of external chest compressions. By pressing down on the breastbone, blood is forced out of the heart and forced into the rest of the casualty's body. When pressure is released, the heart fills up with more blood, ready for the next compression, and so on. This is done at a rate of 100 compressions per minute.

BASIC LIFE SUPPORT PRINCIPLES FOR AN UNRESPONSIVE CASUALTY

1 Follow the "ABC" of DRSABC by ensuring that the casualty's AIRWAY is clear: check their mouth for obvious obstructions such as vomit and remove them if you can. Tilt the head back and look, listen and feel for BREATHING for up to 10 seconds. If they are not breathing, call an ambulance and give 2 rescue breaths.

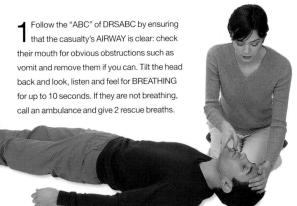

2 Check for any signs of a working CIRCULATION for up to 10 seconds. If there are none, then begin chest compressions – do 15 of these.

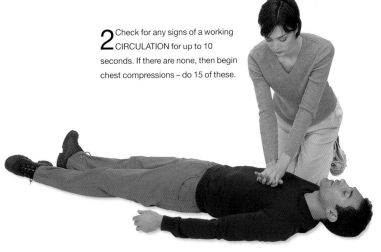

3 Now give 2 rescue breaths and then continue a cycle of 2 rescue breaths and 15 chest compressions until the paramedics arrive.

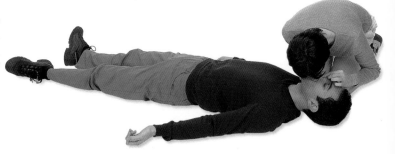

Responsiveness and the airway

SEE ALSO

➤ What is first aid?, p12

➤ Moving and handling safely 1 and 2, pp20, 22

➤ Coping with neck injuries, p156 (for log roll technique)

You must assess a casualty's responsiveness before acting. In the first instance, obtain basic responsiveness information that will tell you whether or not a casualty is conscious – look for signs of life and try for a verbal response – before dealing with any urgent breathing issues and assessing injuries. After performing these essential steps, you might consider a casualty's precise level of consciousness, as explained below. Other issues you need to understand are whether you should move an unresponsive casualty and how to keep their airway open.

If a casualty has any level of response, then they don't need to be resuscitated, but it is very important that the first-aider maintains a vigilant watch on their ABC (Airway, Breathing, Circulation). Offer reassurance while you wait for the paramedics to arrive.

People who have collapsed have different levels of consciousness, from fully alert to a deep coma. Once you have dealt with the immediate dangers (DRSABC and assessing the extent of any injuries), you might try to determine this level (experienced first-aiders only may be able to run through this checklist very rapidly at an early stage) – such additional responsiveness information may be useful, and you can pass it on to the paramedics when they arrive. Professionals use the letters AVPU for the levels of consciousness – Alert, Verbal, Painful and Unresponsive.

RESPONSIVENESS ASSESSMENT IN DETAIL – THE AVPU CODE

ALERT

An alert casualty is awake and will be able to talk to you spontaneously. Reassure them that help is on the way and that you will do all you can to make them comfortable. Then try and find out exactly what happened.

VERBAL

The casualty may seem to be unconscious but will respond to a verbal prompt. Shout "Are you OK?" close to their ear, and they will respond as if being roused from sleep. You could also try tapping them on the shoulder, or even giving them a gentle shake (but not if there is any possibility of a spinal injury).

PAINFUL

If shouting and gentle tapping or shaking does not wake the casualty, they might respond to a painful stimulus such as rubbing hard on their breastbone with your knuckles or giving a gentle pinch. Do not do anything that could draw blood, such as pricking them with a pin or sharp object.

UNRESPONSIVE

This is when the casualty does not respond at all, in any way – you may well have decided this when going through DRSABC initially. If you run through A, V and P, and none of these techniques works, then the casualty is considered unresponsive.

SHOULD YOU MOVE AN UNRESPONSIVE CASUALTY?

If, while following the DRSABC procedure, your initial conclusion is that a casualty is unresponsive, then you must assess their breathing and circulation. Always make your first assessment of a casualty in the position in which you find them. Only move them if absolutely necessary – if this is the only way you can check their vital signs and keep their airway unobstructed, or if you have to get them into a position where you are able to perform resuscitation.

If there is any likelihood at all of injury, take great care to protect the injured person's spine if you move them. Ideally, move them by using the log-roll technique – although at least three helpers are needed to do this safely.

1 If it is essential to move an unresponsive casualty on to their back (most notably, to perform resuscitation), first straighten the casualty's legs and put their arms as close to their sides as possible. Make sure their airway is always kept clear by ensuring the head does not drop down towards their chest.

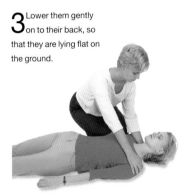

2 Cradle the head and neck with one hand, while holding the lower shoulder with your other hand.

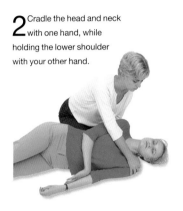

3 Lower them gently on to their back, so that they are lying flat on the ground.

KEEPING THE AIRWAY CLEAR

The airway is just that – a passage through which air passes. This passage stretches from the nose and mouth, through the throat (pharynx), then into the windpipe (trachea), and down to the lungs. Food also passes through the upper part of this tube – the mouth and throat. The airway must be clear for the casualty to be able to breathe, either alone or by means of rescue breaths.

The most common things that block a casualty's airway are the tongue, blood and vomit. When checking an airway, look in the mouth. Do not sweep your finger around blindly, don't risk getting your fingers bitten, and avoid the throat area altogether; never risk pushing something further in. Scoop out objects such as sweets and food with two fingers. If an obstruction is likely to slip further down, or if there is liquid in the mouth, turn the person on their side in order to remove it.

Opening the airway

In an unconscious casualty, the tongue flops to the back of the throat and blocks the airway. To prevent this, put your hand on their forehead and tilt the head back; with two fingers under the chin and thumb on top, lift the jaw. If the casualty is upright, you can support their neck and tilt their head back to open the airway.

If there is a possibility of spinal injury, you must adapt your manoeuvre. Your priority is to get a person breathing, so if they cannot breathe and have a possible neck injury, it is important to open the airway without further injury. Instead of tilting the head back, lift the jaw forwards by pushing upwards at the angle of the jaw.

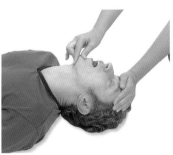

△ Carrying out the simple move of opening the airway can be enough to save someone's life.

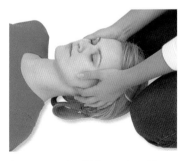

△ In a suspected neck injury, push up at the sides of the jaw, as shown, to open the airway.

Rescue breathing

SEE ALSO

➤ What is first aid?, p12
➤ Cardiac compressions, p32
➤ Full resuscitation sequence, p34
➤ The recovery position, p36

Rescue breathing (also called "kiss of life", mouth-to-mouth respiration and artificial ventilation) is a technique that supplies oxygen to the lungs of a person who is not breathing. Usually performed mouth to mouth, it may be done mouth to nose (if the mouth is damaged), mouth to mouth and nose (for babies) or mouth to stoma (a hole in the neck seen in people who have had a tracheotomy). Never let hygiene fears hold you back – infection is unlikely. There are special masks available, but these should be used only by those who are trained in their use.

MOUTH-TO-MOUTH RESCUE BREATHING

1 Following the DRSABC procedure, assess the casualty's airway and breathing. Kneeling beside the casualty, ensure that obstructions are removed from the mouth, and tilt the head back. Keeping the airway open, look, listen and feel for breathing for up to 10 seconds. If you decide that breathing is absent, call an ambulance and prepare to give rescue breaths as follows.

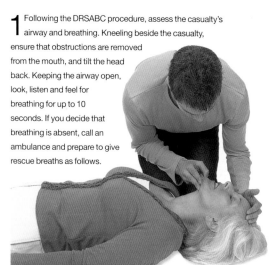

2 If the casualty is not already on their back, you will need to move them on to their back in order to give rescue breaths. Pinch the nose closed by squeezing the nostrils together with your index finger and thumb.

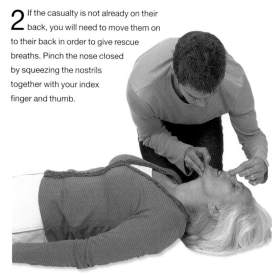

3 Maintaining the head tilt and pinching the nose, open your mouth wide and take a deep breath. Put your mouth against the casualty's mouth and make a tight seal with your lips around their mouth, so that when you breathe out no air escapes around the sides.

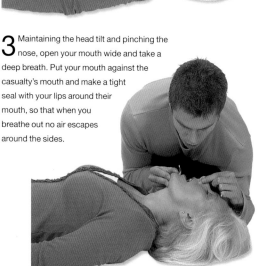

4 Breathe out into the casualty's mouth, making this breath last for approximately 2 seconds. If you are in the correct position, you will see their chest rising as you breathe out. If you do not think you are getting air into their lungs on this first attempt, reposition the head, keeping the airway open, and try again.

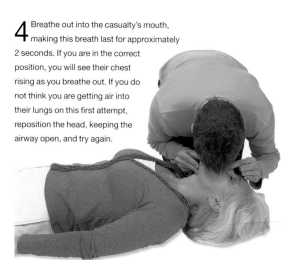

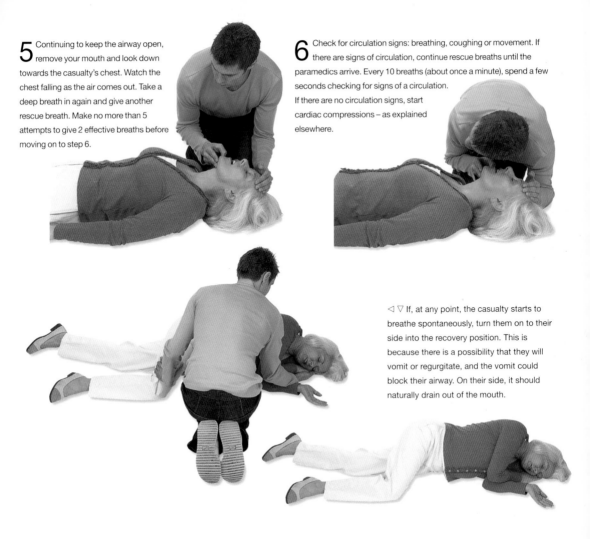

5 Continuing to keep the airway open, remove your mouth and look down towards the casualty's chest. Watch the chest falling as the air comes out. Take a deep breath in again and give another rescue breath. Make no more than 5 attempts to give 2 effective breaths before moving on to step 6.

6 Check for circulation signs: breathing, coughing or movement. If there are signs of circulation, continue rescue breaths until the paramedics arrive. Every 10 breaths (about once a minute), spend a few seconds checking for signs of a circulation. If there are no circulation signs, start cardiac compressions – as explained elsewhere.

◁ ▽ If, at any point, the casualty starts to breathe spontaneously, turn them on to their side into the recovery position. This is because there is a possibility that they will vomit or regurgitate, and the vomit could block their airway. On their side, it should naturally drain out of the mouth.

MOUTH-TO-MOUTH PROBLEM-SOLVING

If the chest is not rising after each rescue breath:

➤ Check the position of the casualty's head and neck – is the airway open? Often people do not tilt the head back far enough.

➤ Check their mouth for any obvious obstructions.

➤ Check that there is a good mouth-to-mouth seal and the nostrils are completely closed.

If air is filling the stomach:

➤ You may be blowing in too much air, or blowing it in too fast. Stop breathing into their chest when it stops rising. Do not press on their distended abdomen – they might vomit and there is a danger that they might inhale the vomit.

If the mouth is bruised or battered:

➤ Use the mouth-to-nose resuscitation technique if the casualty's mouth is so badly injured that you cannot form an effective seal.

1 Open the airway by tilting the casualty's head back and lifting their chin.

2 Keeping the casualty's mouth closed, take a deep breath and form a seal around their nose with your lips – the seal should be good but do not squeeze the nose shut.

3 Let the air come out of the casualty's mouth by allowing the mouth to open as the chest deflates.

Cardiac compressions

SEE ALSO

➤ What is first aid?, p12

➤ Understanding resuscitation, p26

➤ Full resuscitation sequence, p34

Cardiac compressions are also known as chest compressions, or as cardiac/chest/heart massage. These compressions form part of the CIRCULATION stage of DRSABC. If you are faced with a casualty who is not breathing and who appears to have no obvious signs of a circulation, then you must start to give compressions along with rescue breaths – a combination known as cardiopulmonary resuscitation (CPR). However, you should never carry out cardiac compressions if you have not been trained to do so.

For cardiac compressions to be effective, the casualty should be lying flat on their back on a firm surface such as the floor – or the ground if they are outside. If your hands are in the wrong place, or if you use the wrong technique, the heart massage may not work, and you might also cause some unnecessary damage to surrounding structures, such as the ribs or the liver. Although it is a good idea to practise finding the CPR compression site, never carry out practice compressions on conscious volunteers, as you may cause harm. Always use a first aid dummy.

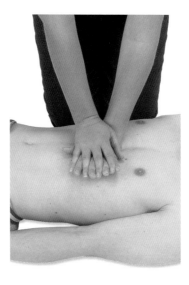

▷ When carrying out cardiac compressions, the heel of only one of your hands should come into contact with the compression site.

WARNING

In general, do not check for a pulse when assessing a person unless you are highly trained and can check it rapidly, without wasting vital seconds. It is not easy to find a pulse, even for trained people, especially in the recommended 10 seconds. The UK and US resuscitation councils have agreed that it is safer if the average first-aider does not check for a pulse before beginning CPR. People die when first-aiders mistakenly feel a non-existent pulse, and fail to resuscitate. Instead of checking for a pulse, look for signs of circulation such as movement, coughing or breathing. Do this for no more than 10 seconds before taking appropriate action.

HOW TO FIND THE COMPRESSION SITE

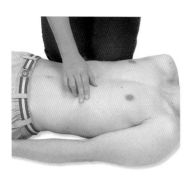

1 Kneel beside the casualty and run the fingers of your hand nearest the waist along the lower ribs until they meet the breastbone at the center of the ribcage.

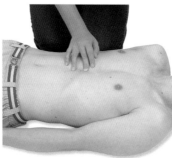

2 Keeping your middle finger at this notch, place the index finger of the same hand over the lower end of the breastbone.

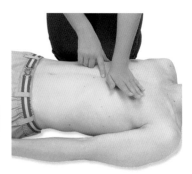

3 Place the heel of the other hand on the breastbone, and slide it down to lie beside the index finger already there. The heel of your hand is now on the compression site.

HOW TO GIVE CARDIAC MASSAGE

1 Kneel down at right angles to the person, so that you are positioned roughly halfway between their shoulders and waist.

2 Locate the compression site, and place the heel of one hand over this area. Place the heel of the other hand on top with both sets of fingers interlaced. Do not let the fingers touch the chest. Keep your elbows locked and arms straight all the time.

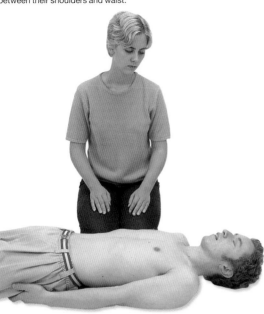

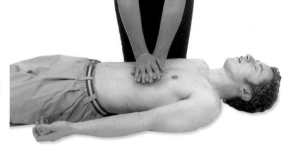

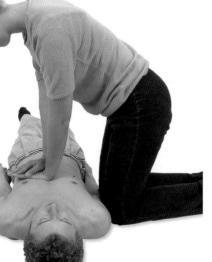

3 Place your shoulders directly over your hands so you are leaning over the person. This will concentrate pressure at the compression site. Compress the chest wall down by about 1½–2in. Release the pressure without taking your hands off the chest or bending your elbows.

4 Compress the chest at a rate of 80–100 compressions per minute. After 15 compressions, you must give 2 rescue breaths. Continue the cycle of compressions and rescue breaths until help arrives. Try to keep going until someone else, or the paramedics, can take over.

Full resuscitation sequence

SEE ALSO
➤ Understanding resuscitation, p26
➤ Rescue breathing, p30
➤ Cardiac compressions, p32
➤ The recovery position, p36

Here, all the component skills of cardiopulmonary resuscitation are shown in action together, to give the complete CPR sequence. Remember that CPR can buy valuable time for an unconscious person before paramedics arrive. You are keeping the person's brain alive by breathing for them and performing chest compressions to keep the blood circulating. Perform 2 rescue breaths for every 15 chest compressions at a rate of 80–100 compressions per minute. Practice on a dummy will help you remember the correct sequence.

HOW TO RESUSCITATE

The DRSABC resuscitation sequence should be followed exactly, with no short-cuts or changes of order. Each step has been described in detail separately, but this sequence shows how all the individual elements fit together.

Breathing check
To check for breathing:
• Look for chest movement.
• Listen at the mouth for breath sounds.
• Feel for breath on your cheek.

When to get emergency help
In general:
• If you have a helper: get them to go for help as you start rescue breaths. Continue resuscitation until paramedics arrive.
• If you are alone with an unconscious adult call the emergency services, then begin resuscitation. However, if you are treating a victim of injury, drowning, choking, drug or alcohol intoxication, or an infant or child, give CPR for about 1 minute before you go for help.

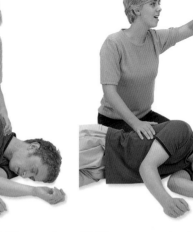

1 Check for responsiveness. If the person is responsive and breathing, they do not need to be resuscitated, and should be left in the position they were found in. Tap them firmly on the shoulder and ask if they are all right.

2 If they are unresponsive, shout for help from passers-by. Check the mouth for obstructions and get rid of them if you can do so easily. Tilt the head back gently, to keep the airway open. Look, listen and feel for breathing.

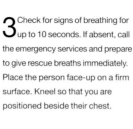

3 Check for signs of breathing for up to 10 seconds. If absent, call the emergency services and prepare to give rescue breaths immediately. Place the person face-up on a firm surface. Kneel so that you are positioned beside their chest.

4 To open up the airway, tilt the head back gently by placing one hand on their forehead and the other on their chin.

5 Now give your 2 effective rescue breaths via mouth-to-mouth: pinching the person's nose, keeping their airway open and sealing your lips around their mouth. Breathe with normal force – do not blow air forcefully. You should see their chest rise. Make up to 5 attempts to give 2 effective rescue breaths.

6 Check for a circulation by looking for breathing, coughing or movement. If there are no signs of circulation, perform 15 chest compressions and then give 2 breaths via mouth-to-mouth. (For when there are signs of a circulation, see box below, Tackling Different Situations.)

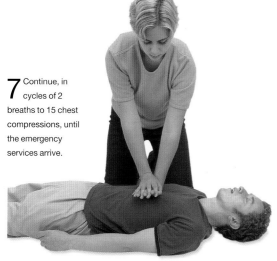

7 Continue, in cycles of 2 breaths to 15 chest compressions, until the emergency services arrive.

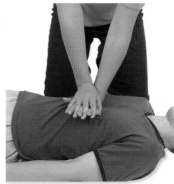

8 You must continue until aid arrives because the person's circulation is very unlikely to resume functioning without advanced techniques such as defibrillation – you are just keeping things going until help arrives with specialized equipment.

TACKLING DIFFERENT SITUATIONS

If the person is unconscious but breathing:

➤ Turn them into the recovery position.

You should be able to see the chest rising visibly as you give rescue breaths. If it is not rising:

➤ Recheck the mouth for any obvious obstructions in the airway and use your fingers to hook or sweep them out carefully, but try not to put your fingers past the teeth and don't risk pushing objects down the throat.

➤ Recheck that the head is tilted back and the chin lifted up so that the airway is clear.

➤ Check that there is a good mouth-to-mouth seal, and pinch the nostrils together.

If the person has signs of a circulation:

➤ If you notice movement suggesting that they have a circulation but they are not breathing, continue with rescue breathing until they start breathing again or the emergency services arrive.

➤ Check for signs of a circulation every 10 breaths. If the person resumes breathing spontaneously, turn them into the recovery position and continue to monitor and record their breathing, circulation and level of response.

The recovery position

SEE ALSO

➤ What is first aid?, p12
➤ Understanding resuscitation, p26
➤ Responsiveness and the airway, p28

This is for those who are unconscious but breathing. An unconscious person is not in control of their airway and, because of this, it can easily become blocked. If the airway remains blocked for more than a few minutes, the lack of oxygen will quickly lead to a cardiac arrest. To ensure that this does not happen, it is best to place the person on their side, so that their tongue falls forward and any fluids, such as vomit or blood, drain out of their mouth instead of down their airway. This is known in first aid as the recovery position.

PLACING SOMEONE IN THE RECOVERY POSITION

Placing an injured person in the recovery position means that they are in a secure pose that ensures an open airway for easier breathing, and also allows any fluid to drain out of their mouth. Plan the direction in which you will roll them in such a way that they remain accessible to help and are not exposed to potential further injury.

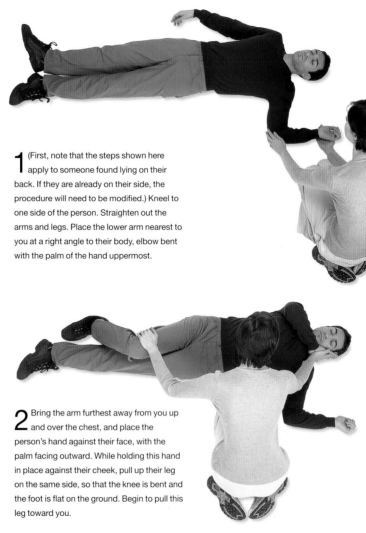

MODIFIED RECOVERY POSITION

In the following situations, you may have to alter the recovery position:

➤ If you feel that there is any possibility at all that the person has sustained a spinal injury, then keep them in the position in which you found them, if they are breathing. However, if you think they are in danger of inhaling vomit, then you must roll them onto their side, making sure that their head is kept in alignment with the rest of their body and not twisted or bent at the neck.

➤ If the limbs have been injured and cannot be bent, use rolled-up blankets or similar rolls of material, or even paper, in order to support them in a secure position.

➤ If the person's condition suggests multiple injuries and you have extra helpers available, use them to support the victim and prevent them from toppling over.

1 (First, note that the steps shown here apply to someone found lying on their back. If they are already on their side, the procedure will need to be modified.) Kneel to one side of the person. Straighten out the arms and legs. Place the lower arm nearest to you at a right angle to their body, elbow bent with the palm of the hand uppermost.

2 Bring the arm furthest away from you up and over the chest, and place the person's hand against their face, with the palm facing outward. While holding this hand in place against their cheek, pull up their leg on the same side, so that the knee is bent and the foot is flat on the ground. Begin to pull this leg toward you.

3 Continuing to support their hand against their face, pull them by the leg toward you, until their bent knee touches the ground. You can use your knees to stop them rolling all the way over onto their front.

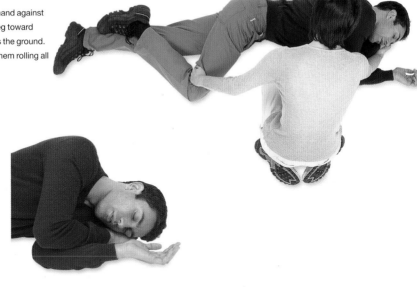

4 Check the airway, tilting their head back to keep the airway open. You may need to adjust the hand under their cheek, so that it is in the correct position to keep their airway open.

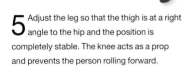

5 Adjust the leg so that the thigh is at a right angle to the hip and the position is completely stable. The knee acts as a prop and prevents the person rolling forward.

6 This is the recovery position. Note that you may need to separate out the arms if you feel that they are in a position where the circulation might be impeded. You should, ideally, have called the emergency services by now. However, if you are alone and need to leave the person for this reason, the recovery position is a safe and secure one in which to leave them. On your return, continue to check and record their breathing, circulation and level of response every few minutes until expert help arrives.

Coping with choking 1

SEE ALSO
➤ Rescue breathing, p30
➤ Cardiac compressions, p32
➤ Coping with choking 2, p40

This common hazard can cause death if prompt action is not taken. The brain can suffer irreversible damage if it is deprived of oxygen for as little as 3–4 minutes. Choking is most likely when people are eating, particularly if they are talking or laughing at the same time. In the elderly, poor teeth or dentures may make proper chewing difficult, or a stroke might have affected their swallowing abilities. Choking victims of all ages are best checked out in the hospital even if the object has been successfully expelled, as it may have harmed the airway lining.

Although food is most often the culprit, any foreign body may partially or completely block the airway if it is stuck at the back of the throat. The airway may also be obstructed by the tongue dropping back, especially in people who are unconscious.

COMPLETE OBSTRUCTION

Someone with a completely blocked airway will be unable to speak or cough. They may clutch their neck, or point frantically at their throat, and open their mouth wide. Initially the victim will be red-faced as they struggle for air; then they will become pale and their lips will turn blue as oxygen fails to reach their lungs. Eventually they will lose consciousness, and all chest movements will stop as they cease breathing. An effective circulation will quickly stop unless the airway is cleared and air starts getting through to the lungs once again.

INCOMPLETE OBSTRUCTION

A person may be choking but still be able to get air past the obstruction and into their lungs – this is an incomplete or partial obstruction. Do not interfere with their breathing efforts in any way, apart from encouraging them to cough. If they can cough, there must be enough room around the foreign body for air to pass, and a sharp cough might dislodge and expel it. You may decide to keep the victim seated, in order to reduce the body's demand on an imperfect supply of oxygen.

Other signs of partial blockage include:
• Snoring, gurgling and wheezing.
• Blue or gray lips, earlobes and tongue, even though the person is breathing.
• Breathing that alternates between normal and difficult/labored.

CLEARING THE AIRWAY

There are three principal ways in which the first-aider should deal with a blocked airway, depending in the first instance on whether the person who is choking is conscious or unconscious:

IF THE VICTIM IS CONSCIOUS:
• Encouraging the victim to cough.
• Abdominal thrusts (the "Heimlich Maneuver").

IF THE VICTIM IS UNCONSCIOUS:
• Chest thrusts.

These techniques can be used singly or in combination, depending on the circumstances, and on how well a method seems to be working.

Whichever technique you need to use, keep reassuring the person who is choking and stay as calm as possible yourself, as people who are choking tend to panic, quite understandably, and this makes breathing difficulties much worse. If the victim loses consciousness, open the airway and check for breathing: as the muscles relax this may start spontaneously. If not, you will need to attempt rescue breaths and begin chest compressions.

CLEARING THE AIRWAY OF A CONSCIOUS PERSON

1. COUGHING

This simple method is the first technique you should try on a conscious person, and is an instinctive reaction. As soon as you see that they are having difficulty breathing, ask them "Are you choking?" If they can answer you should not interfere. Simply encourage them to cough sharply and deeply in order to help move the foreign body. If the person becomes unable to speak or cough, you must proceed to abdominal thrusts. Tell them what you intend to do and obtain their permission to proceed.

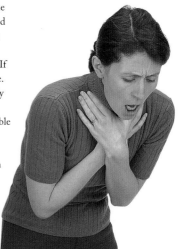

▷ People who think they are choking can panic very easily. Try to keep them calm.

2. ABDOMINAL THRUSTS

Known as the "Heimlich Maneuver", this technique relies on pressing forcefully into the abdomen to cause an artificial cough, which may force enough air against the blockage to shift it. This method can be used whether the victim is standing or sitting. It should never be used on a pregnant woman: chest thrusts should be used instead.

If someone is too large for you to get your arms around them, perform the thrusts with them standing up with their back against a wall. Kneel in front of them and, with one of your hands over the other, push upward and inward over the abdomen.

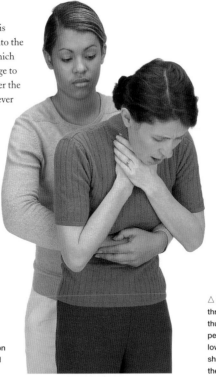

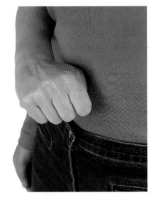

▷ Stand behind the person who is choking. Now slide your arms around the victim and wrap them around their trunk just below the bottom of the rib cage. Use the grip shown on the right. With your elbows out, press inward and upward in quick, sharp thrusts.

△ When holding someone for an abdominal thrust, one of your hands should form a fist. The thumb side of the fist is placed against the person's abdomen, between their navel and lower ribs, as shown above. Your other hand should be placed over the fist, grasping it, as in the picture on the left.

CLEARING THE AIRWAY OF AN UNCONSCIOUS PERSON

CHEST THRUSTS

These are similar to the chest compressions in cardiopulmonary resuscitation (CPR), but are sharper and slower, with each thrust attempting to relieve the obstruction.

Chest thrusts are sometimes used on conscious victims. For example, with a pregnant woman, it would be unsafe to perform abdominal thrusts. If a person is too large for you to fit your arms around them, you could use chest thrusts instead of doing abdominal thrusts from the front (see above). To perform chest thrusts on a conscious person, get them to stand or sit with their back firmly against a wall, and push against their chest with your hands from the front.

▷ To perform chest thrusts on an unconscious person, they should be lying on their back. Kneel to one side of them and make sharp cardiac compressions, but at a slower rate than for cardiac victim resuscitation. This should be done as part of a full emergency routine where the person's state of consciousness and breathing has been assessed, help has been called for and rescue breaths carried out (see Coping with Choking 2).

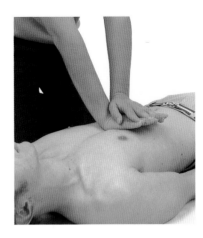

Coping with choking 2

PUTTING IT ALL TOGETHER

The individual techniques detailed in Coping with Choking 1 can now be slotted into full sequences. Time is vital when someone is choking – assess the situation and act as swiftly as possible. To recap: with conscious victims, try to calm them down – this will make your job much easier. Encourage them to dislodge the obstruction with a few deep coughs. If this fails, you will need to proceed to abdominal thrusts, if necessary. If a casualty is unconscious, or loses consciousness as you are helping them, call the emergency services and start resuscitation swiftly, as shown, using chest thrusts to shift the obstruction.

HELPING A CONSCIOUS PERSON

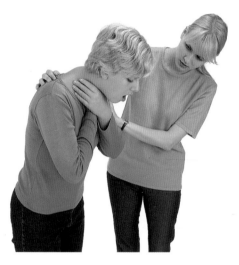

1 If the person who is choking is still managing to breathe, but feels that something is lodged in their airway, they will probably panic. Ask them to cough to try to dislodge the foreign body, but do not do anything else. Attempt to calm them, and summon emergency help.

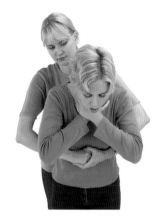

2 If coughing does not expel the object, give them abdominal thrusts. Continue until the foreign body has moved, or until the emergency services arrive.

HELPING AN UNCONSCIOUS PERSON

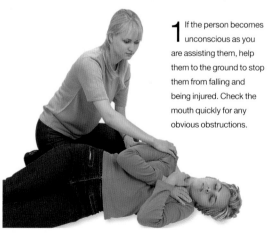

1 If the person becomes unconscious as you are assisting them, help them to the ground to stop them from falling and being injured. Check the mouth quickly for any obvious obstructions.

2 Lay the person flat on their back and place their arms at their sides.

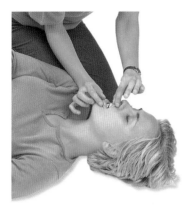

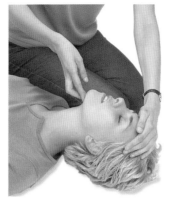

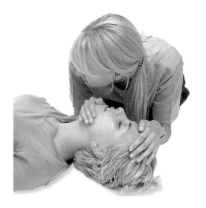

3 Recheck the victim's mouth for any visible obstructions and remove anything you can see very carefully; do not poke your finger blindly around the mouth.

4 Open the airway by placing one hand on the forehead and two fingers of your other hand under the chin, and tilting the head back gently, as far as possible.

5 Check for breathing by looking, listening and feeling – as muscles relax during unconsciousness the victim may now be breathing again.

6 If you decide that they are not breathing, get someone to call the emergency services. (If you are alone, give CPR for about 1 minute before going for help.) Give 2 rescue breaths. If unsuccessful, reposition the head and try again.

7 If the rescue breaths do not go in, start chest compressions in an attempt to dislodge the obstruction. Do not check for signs of circulation. After 15 compressions, check the mouth for the dislodged obstruction, remove anything you find and then attempt 2 further rescue breaths. Continue to give cycles of 15 compressions followed by 2 rescue breaths. If the breaths go in fairly easily, check for signs of a circulation and continue as for a non-choking person. If they do not, repeat the cycle of compressions and breaths until help arrives.

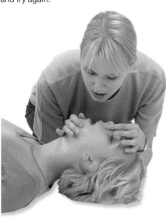

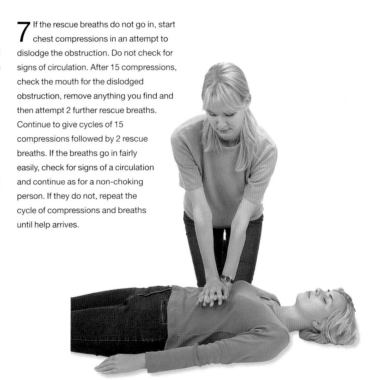

SKILLS CHECKLIST FOR
LIFESAVING PRIORITIES

KEY POINTS

- Every minute is vital ☐

- Don't waste time checking for a pulse unless you are highly trained in this technique ☐

- Always stick to DRSABC procedures when dealing with life-support situations ☐

- Don't attempt CPR unless you have had full training and practice ☐

- Pay plenty of attention to keeping the airway open ☐

- The technique for helping a choking victim depends on whether the person is conscious or unconscious ☐

SKILLS LEARNED

- Rescue breathing, also known as mouth-to-mouth resuscitation or artificial ventilation ☐

- Cardiac compression (heart massage) ☐

- The correct sequence of resuscitation ☐

- The recovery position ☐

- Abdominal thrusts to treat choking ☐

- Chest thrusts to treat choking ☐

3

CHILDREN'S LIFE SUPPORT

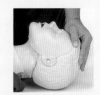

Children are notoriously accident-prone and both babies and children can get dangerously ill very rapidly, so every second counts and you must get help for a collapsed child as fast as possible. The whole story is not entirely depressing, however – children often have remarkable powers of recuperation. It is essential for first-aiders to appreciate the differences between dealing with an older child or adult and dealing with a baby or young child. Many of the basic principles remain the same as for adults, but the techniques used must be tailored to smaller, more fragile bodies.

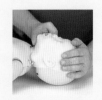

CONTENTS   Basic life support 44–45
Resuscitating a baby or child 46–47
The recovery position 48–49
Choking in babies and children 50–51
Skills checklist 52

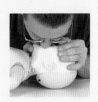

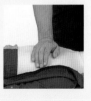

Basic life support

SEE ALSO

➤ What is first aid?, p12

➤ Resuscitating a baby or child, p46

➤ Choking in babies and children, p50

Young children are not mini-adults, but the basic life-support rules of checking airway, breathing and circulation still apply. Babies under 1 require different treatment than for older children. Children over 8 can be treated as adults. One important issue to bear in mind is that adult first-aiders may feel more emotionally affected when a young person is injured, and this can sometimes cloud their judgment – you must avoid this and act decisively. The elements of life support are shown below, and are then put together as a full routine on the following pages.

As in adults, basic life support in babies and children involves rescue breaths and chest massage, and is given to ensure that air continues to enter the lungs and blood to circulate around the body in an emergency. The techniques of rescue breathing and chest compressions are used, but the methods are slightly different depending on the age of the child.

The causes of cardiac arrest in children are very different from those in adults. Children rarely have problems with their hearts, but a healthy heart will stop if insufficient oxygen reaches other vital organs, such as the brain.

Children are anatomically different to adults, hence the need for different life-support techniques. They have narrower air passages and these are more prone to blockage. Their trachea is more flexible and, if the neck is bent back too far, the airway may become blocked. A child's tongue is bigger than an adult's relative to their mouth and throat, and it is more likely to block the airway, particularly if the child is unconscious.

MANAGING THE AIRWAY

Open the airway in the same way as in an adult. In children, be careful not to over-tilt the head and block off the airway. Children breathe mainly by using their diaphragms, rather than their chest muscles. Look for their stomach rising and falling when checking their breathing.

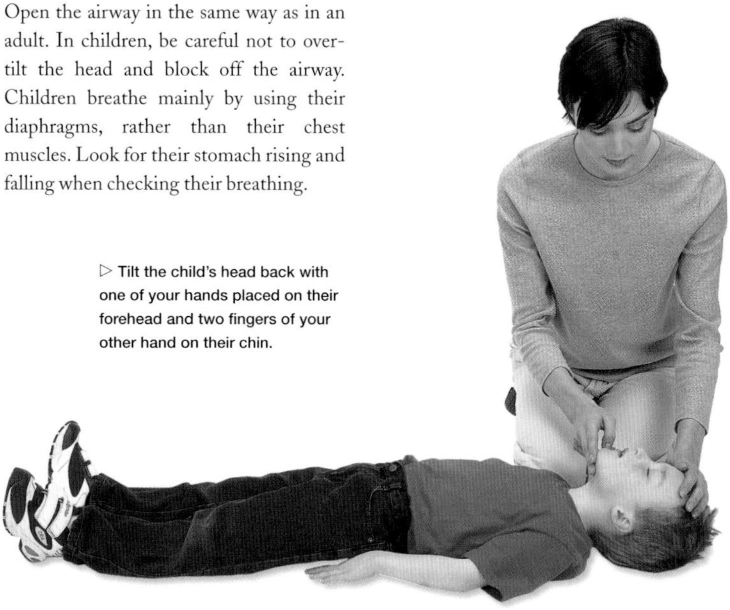

▷ Tilt the child's head back with one of your hands placed on their forehead and two fingers of your other hand on their chin.

REMEMBER DRSABC

Remembering and acting on these priorities will save lives:

D for DANGER
R for RESPONSE
S for SHOUT
A for AIRWAY
B for BREATHING
C for CIRCULATION

RESCUE BREATHING

If you are alone with a baby or child who is not breathing, give rescue breaths for 1 minute before calling the emergency service. Ideally, take the child with you when you go to make the call, but do not stop the rescue breathing. Don't blow an adult-sized breath – use just enough air to make their chest rise and then fall, as if they have taken a deep breath. In a baby, it is easier to put your mouth over both their nose and mouth. Use the following guidelines when you are administering CPR in children:

- Babies and children up to 8 years – 1 breath per 5 compressions.
- Older children (8+ years) – 2 breaths per 15 compressions.

It might be that you cannot get any air into their chest, even after trying to do so with their head in several different positions. In this case, they may have choked, and you must follow the appropriate choking procedure.

FINDING AND USING THE CPR COMPRESSION SITE IN A BABY (UNDER 1 YEAR)

1 Hold the index finger of one hand horizontally between the baby's nipples, in such a way that the center of your finger is at the sternum, or breastbone.

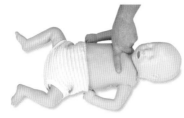

2 The correct compression site is located one finger's width beneath this line between the nipples. Position two fingertips over this site, ready to press down.

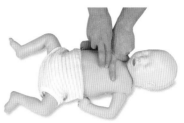

3 Using these two fingertips, compress the breastbone to a depth of ½–1 inch. Release. Give 5 compressions over a period of about 3 seconds (a little over 1 compression per second, or 100 per minute). For every 5 compressions performed, give 1 effective rescue breath. Continue to give the infant chest compressions and rescue breaths, at a ratio of 5:1.

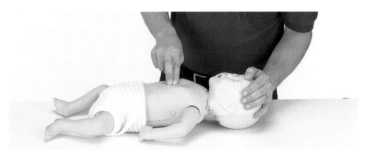

FINDING AND USING THE CPR COMPRESSION SITE IN A CHILD (1–8 YEARS)

1 First, find the child's xiphoid process – the small protrusions at the base of the breastbone, where the ribs join.

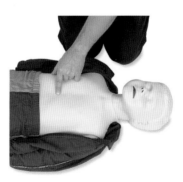

2 Place the heel of your other hand on the lower half of the child's breastbone. Make sure that you do not press on or below the xiphoid process.

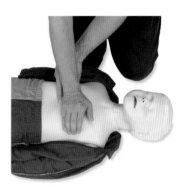

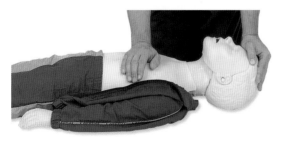

3 To give a chest compression, press down vertically with the heel of one hand to a depth of 1–1½ inches. Do this 5 times in about 3 seconds (a rate of 100 chest compressions per minute). After every 5 compressions, give 1 effective rescue breath. Continue with this ratio of 5 compressions followed by 1 effective rescue breath.

Resuscitating a baby or child

SEE ALSO

➤ Responsiveness and the airway, p28
➤ Rescue breathing, p30
➤ Basic life support, p44
➤ Recovery position, p48
➤ Choking, p50

Every second is vital when resuscitating a baby or child. If their heart stops, their chances of a full recovery are greatly reduced. Taking quick, effective action may prevent brain damage and save life. Resuscitation of a baby differs slightly from that of an older child, so familiarize yourself with both techniques. Also, your approach will vary depending on whether you are alone or have helpers. When checking for an initial response, remember that you cannot rely on a verbal response from babies and very young children, so look for other responsiveness clues.

RESUSCITATING A BABY (UNDER 1 YEAR)

DANGER, RESPONSE, SHOUT
• Make yourself and the baby safe.
• To test responsiveness, shout, tap the baby gently, or flick the soles of their feet. Never shake them – this can cause brain damage and may even prove fatal.
• Shout out to any passersby for help.

AIRWAY
• Open their airway: remove any obvious obstructions from the mouth and tilt the head back by lifting their chin with one finger, placing your other hand on their forehead, and tilting back gently.

BREATHING
• Look, listen and feel for breathing and for any signs of life, for up to 10 seconds.
• If they are unconscious but breathing, hold them in the recovery position and call the emergency services.

WHEN TO CALL THE EMERGENCY SERVICES

➤ If you are alone with a baby or child who is not breathing, perform resuscitation (breaths and compressions) for about 1 minute before going for help.

➤ Take the child with you if possible; if you can continue CPR as you go, so much the better.

➤ If you have help, one of you should start resuscitation while another goes to call the emergency services.

• If there are no signs of breathing after checking for up to 10 seconds, make up to 5 attempts to give 2 effective rescue breaths. Seal your lips tightly around the baby's mouth and nose, and breathe lightly into the lungs until the chest rises. If the airway is blocked and your breaths do not make the chest or stomach rise, you should treat as for choking.

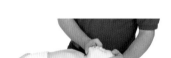

1 Having checked for a response and shouted for help, remove blood, vomit or other visible obstructions, as already explained. Tilt the head back to open up the baby's airway.

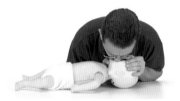

3 If breathing seems to be absent, place your mouth over the baby's mouth and nose. Make up to 5 attempts to give 2 effective breaths. If you have any helpers, send one to call the emergency services as you start the rescue breathing. If your rescue breaths aren't going in, then treat as for choking.

CIRCULATION
• **Look, listen and feel** for signs of circulation for up to 10 seconds.
• If there are no signs, give 5 chest compressions, using two fingers.
• Making sure that the chin is up and the head back, give 1 effective breath.
• Continue in cycles of 1 effective breath to 5 compressions.

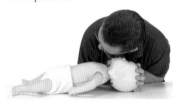

2 Look, listen and feel for signs of breathing, and vital signs such as warmth and color, for up to 10 seconds. If they are breathing, place in the recovery position and get help.

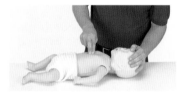

4 Check for a circulation. If absent, start chest compressions. Give 1 breath for every 5 compressions. If there is a circulation, continue rescue breaths at a rate of one breath every 3 seconds. If breathing starts, hold the baby in the recovery position and monitor and record their breathing, circulation and response.

RESUSCITATING A CHILD (1–8 YEARS)

Follow the same rules about when to call the emergency services (depending on whether you are alone or have helpers) as for a baby.

DANGER, RESPONSE, SHOUT
• Make yourself and the child safe.
• To test the child's responsiveness, shout or tap firmly on the shoulder.
• Shout out to any passersby for help.

AIRWAY
• Open the airway: remove any obvious obstructions and gently tilt back the head with two fingers under the chin and the other hand on the forehead.

BREATHING
• Look, listen and feel for breathing and for any signs of life, for up to 10 seconds.
• If the child is unconscious but breathing, place them in the recovery position and call the emergency services.
• If there are no signs of breathing after checking for up to 10 seconds, make up to 5 attempts to give 2 effective rescue breaths. If the child's airway is blocked and your breaths do not make the chest or stomach rise, treat as for choking.

CIRCULATION
• Check for signs of circulation: look, listen and feel for normal breathing, coughing and movement for up to 10 seconds.
• Give 5 chest compressions, using the heel of one hand, as previously explained.
• Making sure that the chin is up and the head back, give 1 effective breath.
• Continue in cycles of 1 effective breath to 5 compressions.

CHILDREN OVER 8 YEARS
For older children, it may be necessary to use two-handed compressions (as for an adult), to get sufficient depth of compression. Follow the same rules about going for help, whether you are acting alone or with helpers, as you would for a baby or younger child.

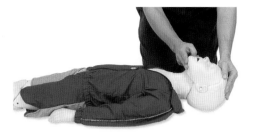

1 Having checked for a response and shouted for help, remove blood, vomit or any other visible obstruction, as already explained. Tilt the head back to open up the airway.

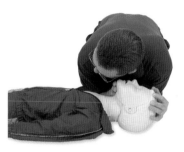 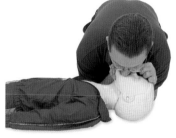

2 Look, listen and feel for signs of breathing, and vital signs such as warmth and color, for up to 10 seconds. If the child is breathing, place in the recovery position and get help.

3 If breathing seems to be absent, place your mouth over the child's mouth. Try up to 5 times to give 2 effective breaths. If you have help, send someone to call the emergency services as you start rescue breathing. If rescue breaths aren't going in, treat as for choking.

4 Check for a circulation. If absent, start chest compressions. Give 1 breath for every 5 compressions. If there is a circulation, continue rescue breaths at a rate of one breath every 3 seconds. If breathing starts, hold the baby in the recovery position and monitor and record their breathing, circulation and response.

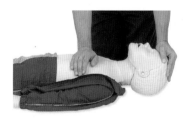

CONTINUE RESUSCITATING UNTIL:
➤ The baby/child shows basic signs of life (breathing or circulation).
➤ Someone else takes over.
➤ Qualified professionals arrive at the scene.
➤ You are completely exhausted.

The recovery position

SEE ALSO

➤ Rescue breathing, p30
➤ The recovery position, p36
➤ Basic life support, p44
➤ Choking in babies and children, p50

An unconscious child who is still breathing should be placed in the recovery position (essentially the same as for an adult). This simple procedure can be a life-saver. It keeps the airway open, allows the tongue to fall forward so it does not block the airway, and lets any fluids that could cause choking drain out of the mouth – most specifically lessening the likelihood of inhaling and choking on vomit while unconscious. This vital position should be learned by anyone who cares for or works with babies and children.

PLACING A CHILD IN THE RECOVERY POSITION

The purpose of the recovery position is to minimize the possibility of the child choking on their tongue or the contents of their stomach while you wait for professional help to arrive. The position is secure enough for you to leave the child for a short time to summon help. The sequence shown here starts with the child on their back; the technique is shorter if the child is found on their side or front.

1 Kneel near the head of the unconscious child. With one hand on their forehead and two fingers of the other hand under the chin, tilt the head back to keep the airway open.

TIPS FOR DEALING WITH UNCONSCIOUS CHILDREN

➤ A child's trachea is flexible, and it may close up if you over-extend their head when opening their airway.

➤ Keep an eye on their breathing and circulation and start resuscitating if either stops.

➤ Place the child in the recovery position before you go for help.

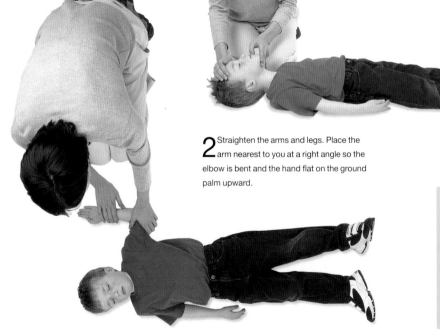

2 Straighten the arms and legs. Place the arm nearest to you at a right angle so the elbow is bent and the hand flat on the ground palm upward.

WARNING

If you suspect a spinal injury, move the child only if they are in danger. If you have to move them, modify the recovery position so the head and trunk are kept aligned at all times.

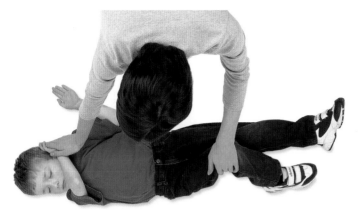

3 Move the other arm across the child's chest. Position the back of the hand against the cheek that is on the same side of the body as the bent arm. Bend the knee furthest from you and hold the leg at the thigh. Try to keep the foot of the bent leg on the ground as you do this.

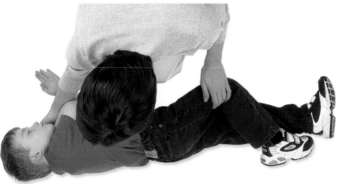

4 Hold the child's hand in position against their cheek. Pull them toward you using the bent leg to roll them over gently. The child should end up lying on their side.

PLACING A BABY IN THE RECOVERY POSITION

Infants under 1 year are too small to place in the conventional recovery position, but by keeping them on their side and with the head tilted down, the principles remain the same. Hold the baby with one hand under their head and the other under their lower back and buttocks. Place their head lower than the rest of their body. Try not to press against their stomach as this may make them vomit.

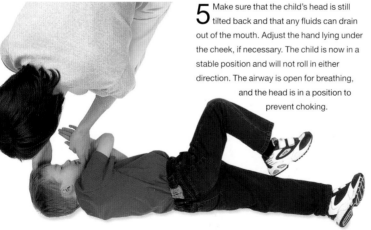

5 Make sure that the child's head is still tilted back and that any fluids can drain out of the mouth. Adjust the hand lying under the cheek, if necessary. The child is now in a stable position and will not roll in either direction. The airway is open for breathing, and the head is in a position to prevent choking.

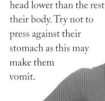

▷ Remember to keep the baby's head lower than their body. This is so that, if they vomit, they will not inhale it and choke.

Choking in babies and children

SEE ALSO
➤ Rescue breathing,
   p30
➤ Basic life support,
   p44
➤ Safety in the home,
   p224

A few common-sense measures will do much to prevent choking incidents in the young. These include avoiding foods such as nuts, boiled sweets and popcorn in children under the age of four, and making sure children don't run around with objects such as pens in their mouths.

However, if choking does occur, you must act decisively as there may not be enough time to wait for the emergency services. The sad fact is that significant numbers of small children die each year from choking, but the good news is that it is often easy to prevent.

SIGNS AND SYMPTOMS

➤ Unable to speak or cough.

➤ Blue lips.

➤ Pale/blue/ashen skin.

➤ Loss of consciousness/collapse.

TREATMENT FOR A CHOKING BABY (UNDER 1 YEAR)

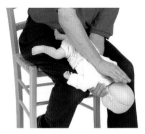

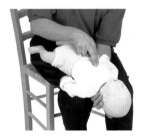

◁ Left and bottom left: to give a baby back slaps (top), lay the baby face down on your forearm, with their head down low. For chest thrusts (bottom), use two fingertips placed on the lower half of their breastbone, a finger's width below the nipples.

FIRST AID FOR A CHOKING CONSCIOUS BABY (UNDER 1 YEAR)

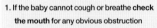

1. If the baby cannot cough or breathe **check the mouth** for any obvious obstruction

2. Place the baby face down on/along your arm and **give up to 5 back slaps.**

3. Carefully turn them face up and **re-check their mouth and breathing.** Remove any obvious obstruction.

4. If this is unsuccessful, use 2 fingers to **give up to 5 sharp chest compressions** (1 thrust per 3 seconds).

5. If alone, **repeat 1–4 for 1 minute** then call the emergency services. Repeat 1–4 until help arrives, the baby starts breathing spontaneously or becomes unconscious.

SOME BASIC ISSUES

There are certain differences between treating choking babies and choking children. There are also differences in their treatment depending on whether they are conscious or unconscious. One of the most important points to appreciate is that, whether you are dealing with a child or a baby, rescue breathing is started only if the child or baby becomes (or already is) unconscious. The airway may become clear of the obstruction as the muscles relax with loss of consciousness, in which case the rescue breathing will cause the chest to rise, and you should move on to basic life support measures.

FIRST AID FOR A CHOKING UNCONSCIOUS BABY (UNDER 1 YEAR)

1. **Check the baby's mouth**, remove obvious obstructions and open the airway.

2. **Give 2 rescue breaths.** If unsuccessful, reposition head and try again. If successful, check for circulation.

3. **If unsuccessful, give 5 back slaps.**

4. **Give 5 chest compressions.**

5. **Check the mouth**, remove any obvious obstructions and open the airway.

6. **If alone, repeat 2–5 for 1 minute before calling for help.**

TREATMENT FOR A CHOKING CHILD (1–8 YEARS)

△ Unconscious child – open airway.

△ Unconscious child – check for breathing.

△ Unconscious child – rescue breaths.

△ Unconscious child – chest compressions.

FIRST AID FOR A CHOKING CONSCIOUS CHILD (1–8 YEARS)

1. **Ask the child "Are you choking?"** If they can speak or cough, do not interfere, but be ready to take action if their condition worsens.

2. **Encourage the child to cough** to dislodge the obstruction.

3. If the child cannot cough or breathe, you will need to **give abdominal thrusts.** Explain to them what you are going to do and get their permission.

4. Stand behind the child, make a fist and place it against their abdomen, between the navel and lower ribs. Grasp the fist with your other hand and press sharply inward and upward up to five times. Check the mouth. Continue until the obstruction clears or the child loses consciousness.

5. Even if the obstruction is removed, **take the child to hospital** – the airway lining may be damaged.

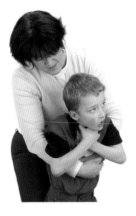

△ Abdominal thrusts on a conscious child who is choking are done from behind the victim, employing the same technique as for adults, but using less force.

IMPORTANT POINTS

➤ Never blindly sweep a finger inside anyone's mouth as it may make the obstruction worse.

➤ If the baby or child is still passing some air in and out of the lungs, and you know or suspect that an obstruction remains, do nothing but quickly call the emergency services.

➤ If a child has collapsed and is unconscious and not breathing they may have choked. Start the "ABC" of resuscitation, and if the chest does not move with up to 5 rescue breaths, treat for choking.

➤ Abdominal thrusts are not used at all in babies as they may damage their internal organs.

FIRST AID FOR A CHOKING UNCONSCIOUS CHILD (1–8 YEARS)

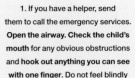

1. If you have a helper, send them to call the emergency services. **Open the airway. Check the child's mouth** for any obvious obstructions and **hook out anything you can see with one finger.** Do not feel blindly down the throat.

2. **Look, listen and feel for signs of breathing.** The throat muscles may relax with loss of consciousness, and the child may begin to breathe again. If so, place them in the **recovery position.**

3. If the child is not breathing, **begin rescue breathing.** Aim to give 2 effective breaths. If there are no chest movements, open the airway by tilting the head back further and try again.

4. If the child is still not breathing, **give 5 chest compressions.**

5. **Recheck the child's mouth** for the dislodged obstruction and remove anything you find.

6. If the child is still not breathing, repeat the sequence from 2 to 5 until the obstruction is ejected, help arrives or the chest starts rising, when you should move on to "C" in the ABC of the basic life support sequence. Start CPR if necessary.

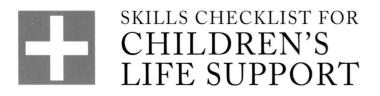

SKILLS CHECKLIST FOR
CHILDREN'S LIFE SUPPORT

KEY POINTS

- Resuscitation is carried out differently for babies and children than for adults ☐

- Following the correct sequence of resuscitation is of the utmost importance ☐

- Speedy action is particularly important where babies and children are concerned ☐

SKILLS LEARNED

- Basic techniques of life support for babies and children ☐

- Cardiac compressions for babies and children ☐

- The correct sequence of resuscitation techniques for babies and children ☐

- The recovery position for babies and children ☐

- Coping with a choking baby or child ☐

LUNGS AND BREATHING

Breathing is vital for each of us to stay alive, and two of the most important components of first aid are airway and breathing – the A and B of ABC (C being circulation). A basic knowledge of the parts of the respiratory system and how they work can help if you have to deal with an emergency involving breathing problems. While serious accidents can cause breathing to stop, a number of diseases and accidents directly affect the working of the breathing apparatus. These include certain respiratory conditions (such as asthma), inhalation of noxious fumes or smoke, drowning, hanging, and strangulation.

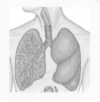

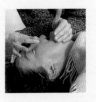

CONTENTS

Understanding the respiratory system 54–55

Dealing with breathing difficulties 56–57

Tackling fume inhalation 58–59

Drowning: what to do 60–61

Hanging and strangling: what to do 62–63

Skills checklist 64

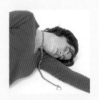

Understanding the respiratory system

SEE ALSO

➤ Understanding resuscitation, p26

➤ Responsiveness and the airway, p28

➤ Rescue breathing, p30

The technical term for breathing is respiration. With each breath, air enters the lungs and oxygen passes into the blood through the delicate tissues of the lung. Every cell in our bodies needs oxygen to work properly. Without oxygen, muscles cannot contract, nerves cannot send impulses, the heart stops, and the brain cannot function. The end product of respiration is carbon dioxide, which leaves the blood as oxygen enters it. If the lungs did not expel carbon dioxide as we breathe out, confusion, coma, and death would follow.

THE BREATHING APPARATUS

The lungs form the main part of the respiratory system – two spongy organs lying within the chest cavity. They are surrounded and protected by a bony cage comprising the ribs, spine, and sternum. The diaphragm is a dome-shaped muscle attached to the lower ribs lying under the lungs and is the main muscle of breathing control. Other muscles that help with breathing, especially during exercise, or in times of stress or illness, are the intercostal muscles lying between each rib. Together these structures form an airtight, protective cage around the lungs.

Air reaches the lungs through a series of branching airways, which become progressively more numerous and smaller, like the branches of a tree. Air enters the body through the nose and mouth, and down the throat. It then passes the larynx, or voice box, which contains the vocal chords. The epiglottis is a flap of cartilage that covers the larynx when we swallow food, in order to prevent food from entering the trachea.

The air then reaches the trachea, which soon divides into two branches called bronchi – one going to the left lung and the other to the right. These branch into smaller vessels called bronchioles. The bronchioles taper into smaller and smaller branches, until they end in tiny sacs of lung tissue called alveoli. This is where gas exchange takes place. Tiny branches of veins and arteries are wrapped around the alveoli, and through their walls, oxygen and carbon dioxide are transferred in and out of the blood.

THE RESPIRATORY SYSTEM

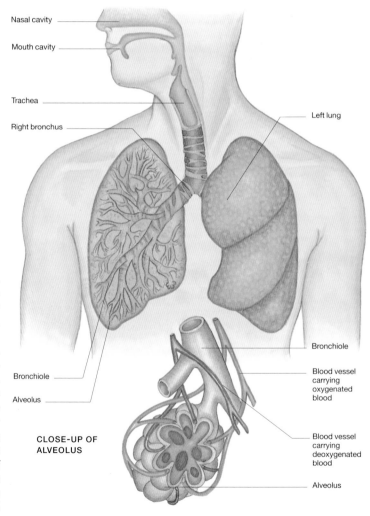

Nasal cavity

Mouth cavity

Trachea

Right bronchus

Left lung

Bronchiole

Alveolus

CLOSE-UP OF ALVEOLUS

Bronchiole

Blood vessel carrying oxygenated blood

Blood vessel carrying deoxygenated blood

Alveolus

HOW DO WE BREATHE?

We breathe automatically. Apart from being able to control how fast or deeply we breathe over a short period, our breathing is beyond our voluntary control. The respiratory center in the brain stem controls the basic rhythm of breathing. It is from here that messages are sent to and from the nerves supplying the diaphragm and intercostal muscles. This leads to a continuous cycle of relaxation and contraction of the breathing muscles.

As the diaphragm contracts and moves down, the intercostal muscles pull the ribs up and out. This causes an increase in chest volume, which in turn results in expansion of the lungs, and the reduced pressure causes air to be sucked in – this is called inspiration. In the reverse process, the diaphragm relaxes, the ribs move down and in, and air is pushed out – this is called expiration.

In an adult, the normal rate for breathing at rest is 13–17 breaths per minute. This rate increases during exercise, which is a normal response to the body's increased demand for oxygen. An increased rate at rest or during only mild exertion can be a sign of physical illness. Psychological problems, such as extreme anxiety and panic attacks, can also increase breathing rate.

In babies and young children, breathing rate is much higher, ranging from around 50 breaths a minute in a baby under 1 year to 30 breaths a minute in children over 5 years.

PROBLEMS WITH BREATHING

All kinds of different diseases and situations can adversely affect breathing. As soon as the delicate balance between air on one side and blood on the other is upset, problems start to arise. Part of a lung may fill with fluid from a tumor or infection. A lung may collapse or burst and then become squashed due to air escaping into the space between the lungs and the chest wall. The airways may go into temporary spasm, as in asthma, or become permanently narrowed, as in the chronic lung disease, emphysema.

Breathing problems may be caused by:
• Heart disease.

BREATHING IN AND OUT

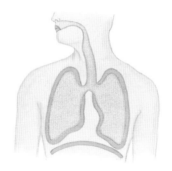

1 In between breathing in or out, the powerful diaphragm muscle found below the lungs rests in its relaxed position – in a pronounced dome shape.

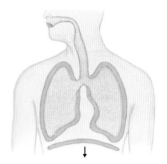

2 The diaphragm muscle now starts to contract, moving downward as it does so. The intercostal muscles also contract, expanding the rib cage.

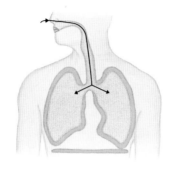

3 As the chest cavity and lungs expand, pressure in the cavity and lungs drops and air rushes in to equalize it – breathing in. At full contraction, the diaphragm lies flat.

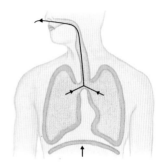

4 The diaphragm relaxes and moves up again. The intercostal muscles relax and the rib cage contracts. Pressure rises in the lungs, so air starts to rush out – breathing out.

• Chest infection.
• Lung tumor or lung disease.
• Collapsed or punctured lung.
• Asthma.
• Smoking.
• Fear, panic, and anxiety.
• Inhalation of fumes.
• Choking.
• Chest injury.
• Head injury.

A person who develops breathing problems suddenly must be seen by a doctor without delay. While you are waiting for help to arrive, give any necessary first aid.

SIGNS AND SYMPTOMS OF BREATHING PROBLEMS

➤ Pale or blue face and lips.

➤ A rapid respiratory rate (this will vary with age, but the rate should be less than 20 breaths per minute in a healthy adult).

➤ Noisy breathing.

➤ Cough.

➤ Shortness of breath.

➤ Confusion and aggression.

Dealing with breathing difficulties

SEE ALSO

➤ What is first aid?, p12
➤ Coping with choking 1 and 2, pp38, 40
➤ Coping with a heart attack, p72

Breathlessness occurs in healthy people as a normal response to exercising, but it can also be a symptom of many diseases, including chronic conditions such as asthma and emphysema. Breathing difficulty should always be taken seriously, especially if it starts suddenly. Even young, fit people can be affected by conditions that cause breathing difficulty, such as a collapsed lung (pneumothorax), or a clot in the lung (pulmonary embolus). These conditions can be life-threatening, so prompt recognition and medical treatment are very important.

ACTION FOR BREATHIING DIFFICULTY

Even if you do not know the cause of the breathing difficulty, act as follows:
• Sit the sufferer upright and supported.
• If they are on medication for breathing problems, get them to take it.
• Loosen clothing around the neck.
• Try to keep the sufferer calm.
• If the breathing does not return to normal, seek medical attention.

ASTHMA

At least 5 percent of people suffer from chronic, lifelong asthma. Asthma is a condition in which the airways become narrowed and blocked with secretions. Asthmatics typically suffer from repeated attacks of wheezing and breathlessness. People with diagnosed asthma may use a "rescue" or quick-relief inhaler (often blue) for immediate relief during an attack, and a "preventive" inhaler or other form of medication for longer-term treatment and prevention. The sufferer will know which medication they need during an attack: a preventive inhaler will not be effective.

Causes of asthma

Asthma tends to be triggered by factors that differ between individuals. Sufferers are often allergic to pollen, animals, dust, smoke, air pollution, foods or drugs. Asthma attacks may also be triggered by viral infections, exercise, certain chemicals, stress or intense emotions.

RECOGNIZING AN ASTHMA ATTACK

As asthma can be life-threatening, it is important that symptoms are recognized and action taken as early as possible.

Signs of worsening asthma that needs medical attention:

➤ Wheezing or coughing occurs during exercise and at night.

➤ Inhaled medications are less effective at controlling symptoms.

➤ Peak-flow measurements start dropping. (An instrument that many asthmatics have at home, a peak-flow device measures the maximum volume of air that a person can breathe out.)

Signs of a very serious attack (always call the emergency services for these):

➤ Inability to finish a sentence in one breath.

➤ Exhaustion from the effort of breathing.

➤ Confusion and irritability caused by lack of oxygen.

➤ Blue lips, and pale, clammy skin.

Signs of imminent respiratory arrest:

➤ Complete inability to talk.

➤ A silent chest (no wheezing) – the blocked airways cannot let air in.

➤ Weak, fast pulse.

FIRST AID FOR ASTHMA

People with long-term asthma usually carry medication – look for this first. Children and people having their first attack will probably need expert help. Never delay seeking help if in doubt, or if you can't find medication.

Most asthmatics will sit upright, often grasping the arms of a chair, to help them breathe. Leave them in whatever position is comfortable, as long as it is sitting up.

The sufferer should use an inhaler that will relieve symptoms, ideally with a spacer device so more drug reaches the lungs. Let them take the medication themselves. Help them only if necessary. If no spacer is available and they are not overly distressed, remind them to hold each inhaled puff for a few seconds. After the first dose, wait for 5 minutes then try again. If this does not relieve the wheezing, or there are signs of a serious attack, call the emergency services.

If hospital admission is necessary, more medication may be given, plus oxygen via a mask or tube. This treatment usually eases the attack within 12 to 24 hours.

DEALING WITH AN ASTHMA ATTACK

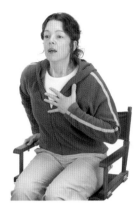

1 Make sure that a person having an asthma attack is sitting upright. They may be distressed and tense. Comfort them and let them choose the best position for themself, but try to encourage them to relax to conserve vital oxygen.

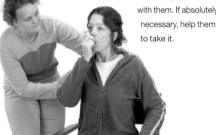

2 If the person carries a rescue inhaler, find it for them and get them to take the medication themself, ideally through a spacer device if they have one with them. If absolutely necessary, help them to take it.

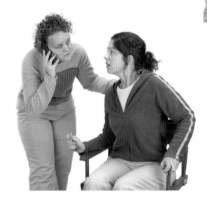

3 If the symptoms of wheezing persist or become worse, call for medical assistance. Keep reassuring the sufferer – panic always makes breathing difficulties worse – but be prepared to begin resuscitation if necessary.

DEALING WITH HYPERVENTILATION

Rapid breathing or over-breathing, also known as hyperventilation, is often caused by anxiety. It differs from breathing difficulty in that the sufferer has some control over the situation, although they may not feel this. Hyperventilation causes tingling in the extremities and around the mouth, dizziness, chest pains and cramps. These symptoms make the sufferer feel even more anxious, and so they over-breathe even more.

The symptoms are caused by a lack of carbon dioxide, which the sufferer is breathing out at a very fast rate. A vicious circle ensues, with more anxiety developing as the hyperventilation worsens. Eventually, if the sufferer does not stop over-breathing, they faint, and the body resumes a normal breathing pattern. Hyperventilation can be a feature of phobias and panic attacks, both of which can be treated by psychologists.

WHAT TO DO

Calm the sufferer and encourage them to slow their breathing. If possible, lead them away from the cause of anxiety and stay with them until they are calm. Advise them to seek medical attention.

PANIC ATTACKS

Hyperventilation may be a sign of a panic attack, a sudden and shortlived bout of exteme anxiety. The victim may also experience tension causing headache or pressure in the chest, trembling, sweating and palpitations.

➤ Try to identify the cause of the fear and escort the victim to a quiet place.

➤ Reassure them and stay with them until they are calm. Advise them to consult a doctor to address the underlying cause of the attack.

Tackling fume inhalation

SEE ALSO
➤ Dealing with
  breathing difficulties,
  p56
➤ Coping with
  headache, p86
➤ Managing dizziness
  and fainting, p88

Fumes inhaled into the lungs have the potential to do serious damage to the respiratory system. If you find a person you suspect has inhaled fumes, you must move them from the source, provided it does not put you at risk. Dangerous fumes include car exhaust, smoke, fumes emitted by faulty domestic appliances, such as boilers, or blocked chimneys, fumes from smoldering foam-filled upholstery, such as sofas, and tobacco smoke. Dry-cleaning solvents and some other chemicals also give off toxic fumes.

DAMAGE FROM FUMES

Accidental or deliberate inhalation of fumes – whether from a cigarette or the smoke in a burning building – is very damaging. The extent of the damage depends on the length of exposure and the type of fume. The likelihood of fume inhalation increases dramatically if the fire or leakage is in an enclosed space. It is important to know that people are usually overcome by the fumes of a fire well before the flames reach them.

Children and the elderly are the groups most vulnerable to fumes; children because of their size, and the elderly because they are generally less robust. Another problem is that this kind of injury may not be obvious until up to 36 hours after exposure to the fumes, by which time irreparable damage to the lung tissue may have occurred.

Why is smoke harmful?

Fire eats up oxygen, as do the materials that burn in a fire, which means little is left for someone to breathe. The burning materials give off toxic gases such as carbon monoxide and cyanide. These poison the victim as they breathe in and irritate the lining of their lungs, making them wheeze and cough. The heat of the fire burns the mouth, throat and upper airway, which then swells and obstructs entry of air even more.

What to do in an emergency

As serious damage can be done by fumes, always assess the situation before rushing in to a potentially lethal scene. You should not make a rescue attempt if it puts your own life at risk; do not go into a fume-filled building or room unless you are sure you are safe. Unless you are well protected yourself, you are likely to meet the same fate as the person you are rescuing. Never enter a room filled with smoke from a fire. If you are attempting a rescue, call the emergency services first.

If you can do so safely, get any trapped people away from the fumes as quickly as possible. Sit them upright, and if they are not too distressed, get them to take deep, slow breaths. If distressed people try to take deep breaths, they will simply become more distressed and breathless. Check for signs of fume inhalation, and also burns and any other injuries that may have been sustained in the accident. While waiting for the emergency services, check the victim's vital signs and begin resuscitation if necessary.

SIGNS AND SYMPTOMS OF SMOKE INHALATION

➤ A hoarse voice or no voice at all.

➤ Drooling or dribbling.

➤ Soot in the nostrils or phlegm.

➤ Singed hairs around the nostrils.

➤ Wheezing.

➤ Noisy breathing on inhaling.

➤ Burns around the mouth and neck.

➤ A large area of burns on any part of the body.

➤ Confusion.

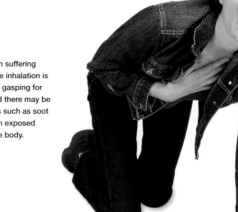

▷ A person suffering from smoke inhalation is likely to be gasping for breath, and there may be other signs such as soot or burns on exposed parts of the body.

IS YOUR HOME SAFE?

Many cases of fire and fume inhalation occur in the home, but with a few simple safety measures the risk of an accident can be greatly reduced. Follow these guidelines to safeguard your family, friends and home-based employees:

- Fit smoke detectors. These reduce the number of deaths from fires by 60 percent. They should be fitted on every floor of your home, including any areas, such as hallways, shared with other people. Check regularly that they work.
- Boilers and central heating systems should be serviced by a professional boiler engineer/plumber once a year.
- Gas appliances should be checked on a regular basis.
- Motor engines should not be left running in an enclosed space, for example a car engine in a garage or a gasoline-powered mower in a garage or garden shed.
- Tobacco smoke is a lethal cocktail containing over 4000 chemicals, all of which can injure the lungs in both the short term and the long term. Emphysema and lung cancer are the best-known conditions associated with smoking, but tobacco also causes many other disorders, such as chronic bronchitis. Giving up smoking is one of the most effective steps that you can take to improve your health. Passive smoking is also a health risk, so you should avoid smoky atmospheres. Smoking has been implicated as one of the causes of sudden infant death syndrome.
- A large proportion of modern upholstered furniture contains foam that can ingnite quickly if it has not been treated with fire-retardant chemicals, burning fiercely and giving off cyanide fumes. These fumes kill within 40 seconds of exposure and have caused many hundreds of deaths. Take extra care with old upholstered furniture, such as sofas and armchairs, as they are unlikely to have been made to the rigorous safety standards now adopted.
- Never use aerosol sprays and dry-cleaning products in a confined area.
- Solvents burn at low temperatures, and are easily ignited. Store them away from ignition sources, properly labeled, and never smoke near them.
- Purchase a carbon monoxide monitor and keep a regular check on emissions from heating appliances.

Outside the home, make sure that there are smoke detectors at your place of work and in your children's nursery or school buildings and anywhere else where they spend any length of time.

How to avoid fume damage

If you are in a situation where you have to escape from fumes, you need to employ a coordinated set of actions that, ideally, has been discussed previously with other members of the household. This should include a place for you to meet and be accounted for outside the building. If you are away from home during the day and your children are cared for by someone else, make sure that they know what to do in an emergency.

ESCAPING FROM FUMES

Leave as fast as possible. Do not stop too long to find the source of the smoke – you will put yourself and others at risk of inhaling a toxic level of fumes.

As you escape, lie low on the floor and crawl below the level of the heat and fumes. Otherwise, you may be overcome by fumes before you have time to act.

Smoke inhalation causes confusion and disorientation. If the smoke is so thick that you cannot see, work your way toward a safe exit by sticking to familiar walls. Always feel a door before you open it; if it is hot, leave it closed. It will provide a barrier to fire and fumes for as long as it is closed and standing.

CARBON MONOXIDE POISONING

Carbon monoxide is one of the most toxic fumes. It has no taste or smell so is hard to detect. It is present in exhaust fumes, most types of smoke and can escape from defective gas or kerosene heaters and blocked chimneys. A large amount of carbon monoxide is quickly fatal, but most cases occur more gradually as a result of a slow leakage from a faulty appliance. Simple detectors are available that indicate whether there is a leakage near a heater.

Symptoms of long-term exposure

➤ Irritability, confusion and bizarre behavior.

➤ Headache, nausea and vomiting.

Symptoms of sudden exposure

➤ Lips and tissues lining the mouth turn cherry red.

➤ Distressed breathing pattern leading very quickly to a loss of consciousness.

Action in suspected carbon monoxide poisoning

➤ Get the victim out into the fresh air without delay.

➤ Loosen any tight clothing worn by the person.

➤ Call the emergency services immediately. The victim may need special hyperbaric oxygen treatment, so you must act quickly to obtain professional help.

Drowning: what to do

SEE ALSO
- ➤ What is first aid?, p12
- ➤ Safety in the bathroom, p228
- ➤ Safety in the garden, p230

Drowning is the third most common cause of accidental death. It can happen not only in the ocean and rivers but also in swimming pools and backyard ponds, and even in the bathtub. Falling asleep in the bath through tiredness or being drunk can cause a fatal accident.

A toddler can drown in just a few inches of water, so you must never leave a young child alone in the bathroom or anywhere near water, even if it is very shallow. Knowing what to do in a drowning incident, and doing it as effectively and quickly as possible, can save someone's life.

Many of those who die through drowning are children and teenagers. It is not only non-swimmers who drown. Someone may have a heart attack while in the water, a boating accident may cause head injury, or a normally good swimmer may panic in a strong current or if they have cramp.

WHAT IS DROWNING?

Drowning is submersion in water causing death by suffocation. Most people die from "wet drowning", where water enters the lungs and rapidly causes respiratory failure and death. Sometimes a person may survive but deteriorate later from damage caused by fluid in the lungs ("secondary drowning"). "Dry drowning" occurs when a small amount of water makes the upper airways go into spasm, causing suffocation. Dry drowning can also cause cardiac arrest.

The effect of cold water

Cold water can be a blessing or a curse. Sometimes, especially in children, the cold water shuts the body down; the heart rate drops and blood vessels constrict in major organs and muscles, so that heart and brain function are prioritized. Hypothermia sets in and the body's demand for oxygen drops dramatically. In this state of "hibernation" people have survived for up to 40 minutes under water.

However, a more common reaction to cold water is for the victim to take an automatic and involuntary gasp as they hit the water, and then start hyperventilating. They may then drown before they have a chance to swim to safety. This is known as cold shock.

SIGNS AND SYMPTOMS OF NEAR DROWNING

- ➤ No breathing or labored breathing.
- ➤ Confusion, irritability or loss of consciousness.
- ➤ Cold, blue skin.
- ➤ Cough with frothy pink sputum.

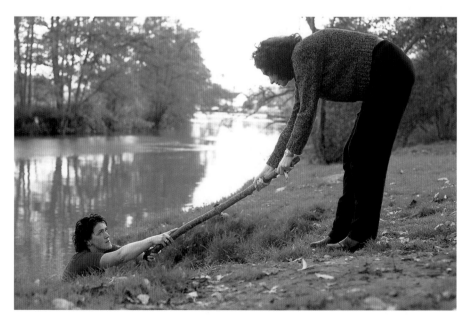

◁ Never jump into the water when dealing with a potential drowning. Hold out something for the person to hang onto, or throw a rope or float. If nothing is available, lie down and extend your arms so that they can haul themselves up to the safety of the bank.

FIRST AID FOR DROWNING

Remember that the victim may have swallowed a lot of water, as well as inhaling it. If they vomit, they may inhale the swallowed water into their lungs. To avoid this occurring, try to keep their head lower than the rest of their body when you take them out of the water.

If the victim is not breathing, do as follows. If the water is shallow enough for you to stand, start rescue breaths in the water. Never attempt rescue breaths in deeper water unless you are trained and practiced in lifeguard skills. If the victim's heart has stopped, remove them from the water and start CPR.

Follow DRSABC until help arrives.

Do not try to empty their lungs and stomach of water.

Keep them warm, as they may be suffering from hypothermia. Take off the wet clothes – but only if you have dry ones to use in their place. Cover the ground under them, as heat is lost via this route.

If they start breathing, place in the recovery position, protecting their neck and spine. As there is a risk of secondary drowning, they must go to the hospital even if they appear to have completely recovered.

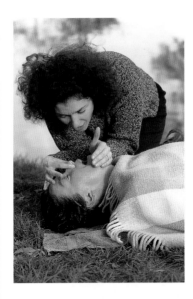

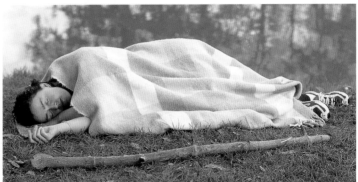

RESCUE SAFETY TIPS

➤ Do not enter the water if you can avoid it (never dive in). Water rescue is a skilled operation for which you need training.

➤ Throw the person a rope attached to a buoyancy aid and tow them ashore, or use a rowing boat to get them ashore.

➤ Remember that, in cold water, hypothermia may make it difficult to detect signs of a circulation.

◁ Lose no time in resuscitating. If you are alone, act as you would when resuscitating a child and perform CPR for 1 minute before going for help.

▽ If breathing, place the victim in the recovery position, keeping them warm and well covered until the emergency services arrive.

PREVENTION OF DROWNING

To minimize the chances of an accidental drowning, follow these guidelines:

➤ Children should be supervised when they are near water – at the beach, by a lake, river, or small pool. Even competent swimmers should be watched. Toddlers have drowned in minute amounts of water. Any water in the home should be kept covered – even fish tanks and toilets.

➤ Avoid alcohol if going for a swim. Many drownings are linked with excessive alcohol intake, especially in teenagers.

➤ Fence off swimming pools and ponds. Make sure the gate is self-shutting and the catch too high for a child to reach.

➤ Keep away from unfamiliar rivers, lakes or ponds, and never dive into unexplored or shallow waters.

➤ Ask the lifeguard on the beach about swimming conditions such as hidden currents or other hazards.

➤ Never swim outdoors if there is a storm brewing, as the risk of lightning striking the water is high and lethal.

Hanging and strangling: what to do

SEE ALSO
➤ What is first aid?, p12
➤ Responsiveness and the airway, p28
➤ The recovery position, p36

Both hanging and strangling involve compression of the trachea and major blood vessels in the neck, which eventually causes death. In hanging, when the body is suspended by a noose around the neck, the neck is often broken. Strangling is constriction around the neck. Babies and young children are very vulnerable to strangulation by items such as crib rails, banisters or railings. Such accidents occur with adults too, for example if clothing is caught in machinery. However, deliberate hanging as a form of suicide is also a possibility.

Although most cases of strangling in babies and children are accidents, hanging is a common method of suicide in men, and strangulation is often the method used in homicide. Death occurs because constriction of blood vessels in the neck stops oxygen reaching the brain, rather than because the airway is blocked. In hangings, the situation can be complicated because the neck is often broken.

It is essential to remove the constricting item and give first aid as quickly as possible to give the best chance of restoring breathing. If you are dealing with a victim of hanging you must handle them very carefully to avoid aggravating a spinal injury.

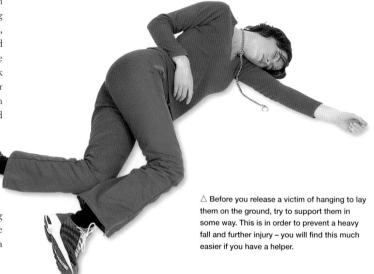

△ Before you release a victim of hanging to lay them on the ground, try to support them in some way. This is in order to prevent a heavy fall and further injury – you will find this much easier if you have a helper.

SIGNS OF HANGING OR STRANGLING

➤ Numerous tiny hemorrhages above the constriction line, including the whites of the eyes.

➤ Bruising, scratches and swelling around the neck – even finger marks may be obvious.

➤ If the victim is still conscious, their neck will be very tender.

➤ Very noisy breathing, due to the swelling around the airway, as well as a muffled voice and cough.

REDUCING THE RISKS

Babies under three months old are vulnerable to accidental strangling on crib rails, other railings or pacifiers on a string around their necks. They are not strong enough to physically push themselves out of trouble. Toddlers may lie with their neck over an object, and their body weight is enough to cause strangulation. Never leave babies and children alone in the house and be vigilant for hazards.

Older children, particularly boys, tend to take great risks when they are playing, and climbing trees and making dens are especially treacherous sources of potential danger. Children should always be made aware of the possible consequences – preferably without spoiling their fun and without making them terrified of anything and everything around them. Play with younger siblings should be supervised if at all possible.

Automatic doors in stores and public buildings, and electric vehicle windows, are responsible for significant numbers of accidental stranglings. Getting dangling clothing caught in escalators is another potential hazard. Always watch children very carefully whenever they are around such devices.

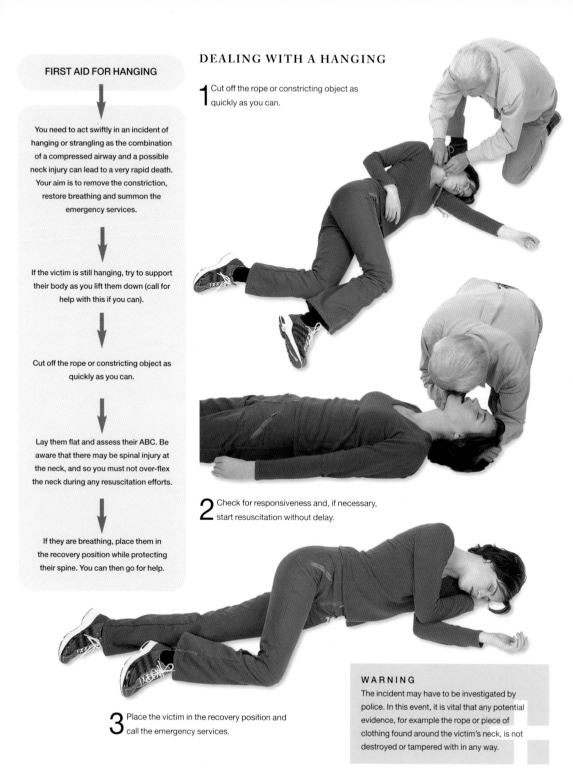

FIRST AID FOR HANGING

You need to act swiftly in an incident of hanging or strangling as the combination of a compressed airway and a possible neck injury can lead to a very rapid death. Your aim is to remove the constriction, restore breathing and summon the emergency services.

If the victim is still hanging, try to support their body as you lift them down (call for help with this if you can).

Cut off the rope or constricting object as quickly as you can.

Lay them flat and assess their ABC. Be aware that there may be spinal injury at the neck, and so you must not over-flex the neck during any resuscitation efforts.

If they are breathing, place them in the recovery position while protecting their spine. You can then go for help.

DEALING WITH A HANGING

1 Cut off the rope or constricting object as quickly as you can.

2 Check for responsiveness and, if necessary, start resuscitation without delay.

3 Place the victim in the recovery position and call the emergency services.

WARNING

The incident may have to be investigated by police. In this event, it is vital that any potential evidence, for example the rope or piece of clothing found around the victim's neck, is not destroyed or tampered with in any way.

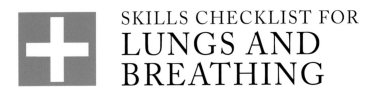

SKILLS CHECKLIST FOR
LUNGS AND BREATHING

KEY POINTS

- Always take any breathing difficulty seriously, and watch closely for deterioration ☐

- Swiftly follow basic guidelines for dealing with breathing difficulties, even if you don't know the root cause of the problem ☐

- Never put yourself at risk when dealing with noxious fume or drowning scenarios ☐

- Use common-sense vigilance to prevent all kinds of strangling and hanging accidents ☐

SKILLS LEARNED

- Recognizing the signs and symptoms of breathing problems ☐

- How to help an asthma sufferer during an attack ☐

- Recognizing the severity of an asthma attack ☐

- How to treat hyperventilation ☐

- How to help people who have inhaled toxic fumes ☐

- Preventing and dealing with drowning ☐

- Dealing with hanging and strangulation ☐

HEART AND CIRCULATION

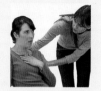

The heart and circulation are together responsible for providing every single cell in the body with blood – without blood there is no life. When things go wrong with this system, the outcome can quickly be catastrophic, so it is important to be prepared. This chapter describes the first aid to be given in conditions that affect the circulation, such as shock and anaphylaxis. Appropriate first-aid techniques are also given for heart attack and other abnormal heart conditions, including angina, heart failure and cardiac arrest. However, calling the emergency services is the single most important piece of action that can be taken to save life.

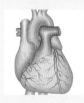

CONTENTS
Understanding the cardiovascular system 66–67
Dealing with shock 68–69
Managing anaphylactic shock 70–71
Coping with a heart attack 72–73
Dealing with an abnormal heart rate 74–75
Skills checklist 76

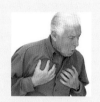

Understanding the cardiovascular system

SEE ALSO
➤ What is first aid?, p12
➤ Full resuscitation
  sequence, p34
➤ Cardiac
  compressions, p32

The cardiovascular system is made up of the heart ("cardio") and the blood vessels ("vascular"). The heart – which is essentially a large, powerful muscle about the size of your clenched fist – pumps blood at an average rate of 60–80 times a minute for a person's entire life span. The heart and the circulatory system can develop a range of disorders, due to the great demands placed on them. A number of these problems call for prompt emergency first-aid techniques in order to save the victim's life.

THE HEART

Situated between the lungs, the heart is slightly to the left side of the body. The hollow area inside the heart muscle is made up of two separate compartments: one on the left and one on the right.

In healthy people, these separate heart compartments have no communication with each other. However, some babies are born with a communication between the two – a condition known as having a "hole in the heart".

Each of the compartments has two chambers, an upper atrium and a lower ventricle, giving four compartments in total: the left ventricle and atrium, and the right ventricle and atrium.

THE BLOOD VESSELS

The ventricles send blood to all parts of the body through the arteries, which branch out all over the body into smaller vessels called arterioles. These then become minute vessels called capillaries, which form a network that bathes all body tissues, allowing easy exchange of oxygen, nutrients, carbon dioxide and other waste products. The capillaries then join with tiny vessels called venules, which form larger and larger veins, until the vena cavae arrive back at the right side of the heart.

THE CIRCULATION

The blood arriving at the right side of the heart has been around the body and therefore has a low oxygen content. This deoxygenated blood is a dark red color, rather than the bright red color it will turn when it has been through the lungs and has filled up with oxygen. This blood arrives back at the heart through the veins. The two veins that lead into the heart are the vena

STRUCTURE OF THE HEART

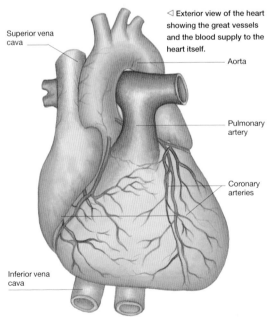

◁ Exterior view of the heart showing the great vessels and the blood supply to the heart itself.

Superior vena cava

Aorta

Pulmonary artery

Coronary arteries

Inferior vena cava

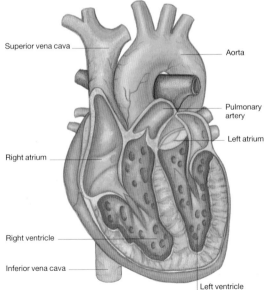

▽ Cross-section through the heart showing the four chambers surrounded by a thick muscular layer around the outside.

Superior vena cava

Aorta

Pulmonary artery

Left atrium

Right atrium

Right ventricle

Inferior vena cava

Left ventricle

CIRCULATING OXYGEN IN THE BLOOD

▷ The aorta supplies oxygenated blood (red areas) to all the arteries in the body, and the veins return deoxygenated blood (blue areas) back to the heart via the vena cavae.

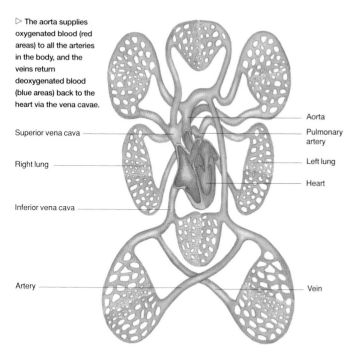

Superior vena cava

Right lung

Inferior vena cava

Artery

Aorta

Pulmonary artery

Left lung

Heart

Vein

ARTERIES AND VEINS

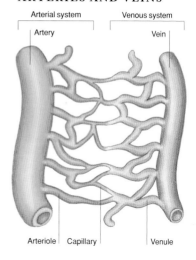

Arterial system

Venous system

Artery

Vein

Arteriole | Capillary | Venule

△ Close-up of a section of the circulatory system. The arterial system, which carries oxygenated blood (red), runs into smaller and smaller arteries until it reaches the tiny veins in the venous system, which carries deoxygenated blood (blue). The veins gradually enlarge until the blood reaches the vena cavae.

cavae. Deoxygenated venous blood arrives in the right atrium, moves down into the right ventricle, and is then pumped through the lungs and back into the left atrium. This fresh, oxygenated blood passes into the left ventricle and then exits the heart via the aorta (the body's biggest vessel), starting its journey round the body. The whole process – including the time taken for the chambers to fill with blood and then contract and circulate the blood – takes about 0.8 seconds at rest, or less when the pulse is rapid.

THE BLOOD

Blood carries nutrients around the body, as well as taking oxygen from, and carbon dioxide to, the lungs. It protects against blood loss through its clotting ability, and infection through its white blood cells.

Fifty-five percent of blood is made up of a straw-colored clear fluid called plasma, which is also rich in proteins. When bleeding occurs, we lose plasma, and the blood volume drops. Eventually, there is not

enough blood for the heart to pump, and the circulatory system collapses. Death swiftly follows. Within the plasma float red and white blood cells, plus substances (such as platelets) that are needed for clot-forming. White cells are mainly involved in fighting infection, while red cells carry oxygen.

WHAT IS THE PULSE?

The pulse is caused by the aorta springing back down to its normal size, having been filled with blood from the heart. This drives

▽ The "carotid" pulse in the neck is often a good one to find. Use two fingers to feel in the groove on either side of the trachea.

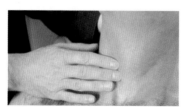

oxygen-rich blood around the body, and the force of the aorta recoil travels along the large arteries – it can be felt wherever an artery lies close to the surface of the skin. Use two fingers to feel for an adult's or child's pulse at the thumb side of the wrist, at the neck or on the front of the arm at the elbow joint. A baby's pulse is best felt on the inside of the upper arm.

It can be much trickier than most people imagine to determine whether someone has a pulse, so this check is often best left to those with medical experience. Remember that vital signs such as coughing, gasping, twitching or blinking also indicate a circulation, and anyone can check for those.

▽ Practice feeling for a pulse. Try on an adult and also on a child.

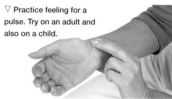

Dealing with shock

SEE ALSO

➤ What is first aid?, p12

➤ Full resuscitation sequence, p34

➤ Managing anaphylactic shock, p70

Shock is a serious condition caused by a sudden and dramatic drop in blood pressure. Without swift medical attention, shock can be life-threatening. It can be caused by any illness or injury that causes too little blood to circulate around the body, such as a heart attack or serious bleeding. This deprives the body of oxygen, leading to the pale, cold, collapsed state that typifies shock. This so-called physiological or circulatory shock must not be confused with the psychological or emotional shock that often occurs after a traumatic event.

Normally, the circulation provides a perfect balance between delivering oxygen and other nutrients to all cells in the body and removing toxic waste products. If this system fails and the amount of blood circulating around the body drops, the combined effect of a lack of oxygen reaching vital organs and a build-up of toxins leads to circulatory shock. If untreated or not attended to quickly enough, shock can be fatal.

WHAT CAUSES SHOCK?

Any trauma or illness that reduces blood circulation is capable of causing shock. Blood circulation can fail for many different reasons. If the heart is unable to pump effectively, after a heart attack for example, shock will follow. Abnormal heart rhythm can lead to shock. Electrocution can cause the heart to stop pumping blood.

Another common cause of shock is excessive loss of body fluids, which may be due to blood loss after a serious accident or fluid loss caused by extensive burns or prolonged diarrhea or vomiting. An adult is capable of losing up to 1 pint of blood without any effect; after a loss of 3.5 pints, symptoms of shock become apparent; and when the loss reaches 5 pints of blood, which is half the adult body's normal capacity, the end stages of shock, including loss of consciousness and heart failure, appear.

A severe head or spinal injury might affect control of the body's blood flow. The blood vessels may widen abnormally in severe infections and some types of poisoning. A severe allergic reaction in susceptible people may lead to the same symptoms – a very specific and rapidly life-threatening condition known as anaphylactic shock.

SIGNS AND SYMPTOMS OF CIRCULATORY SHOCK

➤ Pale or gray skin that feels cold and clammy.

➤ Fast, weak pulse.

➤ Profuse sweating.

➤ Fast, shallow breathing.

➤ Dizziness and faintness.

➤ Nausea and vomiting.

➤ Blurred vision.

➤ Thirst.

➤ Yawning, sighing, and gasping for air.

➤ Restlessness.

➤ Anxiety and/or confusion.

➤ Loss of consciousness.

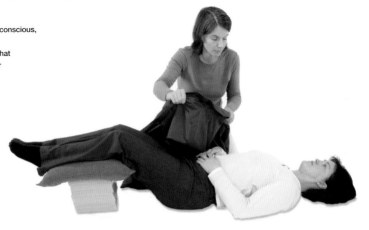

▷ If a person suffering from shock is conscious, they should lie down with their legs supported comfortably on an object that raises the legs above the level of their heart. (Do not raise legs that may be fractured, however.) The knees should be bent, as shown, to prevent straining the hamstring tendon at the back of the knee. You might want to pad the support with a folded blanket, garment, or cushion. Do not raise the head up on cushions, as this restricts the airway – place a blanket or similar under the head if needed. Once in position, cover the victim to keep them warm.

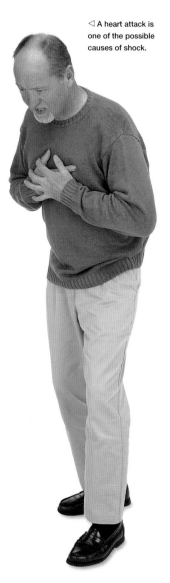

◁ A heart attack is one of the possible causes of shock.

FIRST AID FOR CIRCULATORY SHOCK

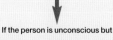

↓

If the person is unconscious, check DRSABC. Start resuscitating, if necessary. Get someone to control heavy bleeding, if possible.

↓

If the person is unconscious but breathing, put them in the recovery position. Stop any heavy bleeding.

↓

If the person is conscious, lay them down and calm them. Staunch any heavy bleeding.

↓

Call the emergency service, if you have not already done so.

↓

Check the body for fractures, wounds, and burns. Deal with these as necessary; make sure any heavy bleeding is controlled.

↓

Unless you think their legs may be fractured, place them on a low, padded support (so that the legs are higher than the heart).

↓

Cover the person with a blanket and try to keep them calm and reassured.

↓

Do not give them anything to eat or drink. Moisten an uncomfortably dry mouth with a wet flannel or towel.

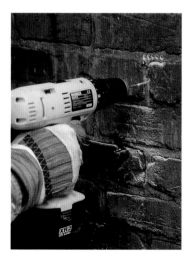

△ Electrocution is one of the traumas that can lead to circulatory shock. A common cause of electrocution around the home is using power tools or electrical gardening equipment.

SYMPTOMS OF SHOCK

In reaction to the reduced circulation of blood, the body directs blood to vital areas such as the heart and lungs, and away from the skin. This makes the skin cold and pale. The body releases epinephrine as an emergency response and this causes a rapid pulse and sweating. As the blood flow weakens further, the brain begins to suffer from lack of oxygen, leading to nausea, dizziness, blurred vision, and confusion. If blood circulation is not restored rapidly, the person will start gasping for breath and will soon lose consciousness.

WHAT YOU CAN DO TO HELP

If you think you have come across someone who is in shock, it is crucial to call the emergency services because medical help is always necessary. First-aid measures can help maintain the limited blood circulation to the brain, heart and lungs while waiting for expert help. Should the person slip into unconsciousness, you must assess them (ABC) and then administer life-saving techniques as necessary, for as long as you are able or until expert help arrives at the scene.

WARNING

Do not try to warm a shock victim by any means other than by covering with a blanket. Avoid hot water bottles, electric blankets, heaters, or any other form of direct heat, as overheating the body will increase the danger.

Managing anaphylactic shock

SEE ALSO
➤ What is first aid?, p12
➤ Full resuscitation sequence, p34
➤ Dealing with bites and stings, p104

Anaphylactic shock is a massive allergic reaction that can develop a short time after contact with a trigger substance. This is a potentially fatal condition caused by the body's inappropriate response to a substance that usually has no serious effect: a food, a drug, or an insect sting, for example. It is a form of circulatory shock, but the effects are so sudden and so dramatic that a susceptible person needs to carry an injection of epinephrine in case of accidental exposure. Once the condition has developed, the risk of anaphylaxis lasts for life.

What causes anaphylactic shock? The body's immune system overreacts to what it sees as a foreign body, even though, in most cases it would not cause any reaction. People become sensitized to a substance, often at an early age, and may not initially have any reaction to the substance – it will be the second and subsequent exposures that lead to anaphylaxis. From that time on, such people will remain at risk for the rest of their lives.

Even a tiny amount of the substance can set off a reaction – a trace of peanut oil in a sandwich might be enough for a person sensitive to nuts. Their body releases a massive amount of histamine; this makes their blood vessels dilate and leak fluid, and the lungs go into spasm, causing the symptoms of asthma. The most common causes of anaphylaxis are peanuts, sesame oil, fish, shellfish, dairy products, eggs, wasp or bee stings, latex, penicillin, other drugs or injections.

People known to be allergic to peanuts, for example, must be very vigilant when buying processed foods, ensuring that they check the ingredients label to check for nut traces. They must also take great care when ordering food in restaurants and even more so if buying food from street markets and stalls.

RECOGNIZING ANAPHYLAXIS

Anyone who has reacted to any substance – even to a mild extent – should be referred to an allergy specialist, because subsequent reactions can be sudden and severe. The specialist cannot always identify exactly

SIGNS AND SYMPTOMS OF ANAPHYLACTIC SHOCK

➤ Intensely itchy rash, often with white raised areas.

➤ A sudden drop in blood pressure (difficult to determine and not visible).

➤ Extreme anxiety, including a sense of imminent death.

➤ Swollen face, lips, tongue, and throat.

➤ Rapid pulse.

➤ Puffy eyes.

➤ Difficulty speaking or swallowing.

➤ Wheezing, tight chest, and breathing difficulty.

➤ Abdominal pain, feelings of nausea, and vomiting.

➤ Faintness.

➤ Loss of consciousness.

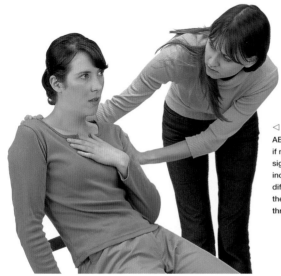

◁ Check through the ABC of resuscitation if necessary. Look for signs of shock, including breathing difficulty, swelling of the mouth, tongue or throat, and pale skin.

what has caused the reaction, but skin prick and blood tests may be useful In some cases of food allergy, a challenge test will be carried out in which minute quantities of the suspect allergen are ingested. This is the only certain way to confirm the allergen. Such a test is done only in a hospital setting under very strict guidelines and only if the patient and their family are happy to undergo it.

In some countries, desensitizing injections are given to reduce a person's sensitivity to a substance. However, this can induce anaphylaxis, and many people feel the risk is too great.

FIRST AID FOR ANAPHYLAXIS

Dial the emergency services. Help the victim sit up and keep them comfortable until medical help arrives.

If they lose consciousness, check breathing and circulation and place them in the recovery position. Monitor and record their vital signs every few minutes and be prepared to resuscitate .

People with a history of anaphylaxis should carry epinephrine injections with them. Check for a syringe and get them to inject themselves. Only administer an injection yourself if you are trained to do so – incorrect practice can cause very serious damage. If they continue to suffer severe symptoms, they should have a second injection.

If the victim is carrying a rescue inhaler for the relief of asthma this may help to relieve their breathing difficulty.

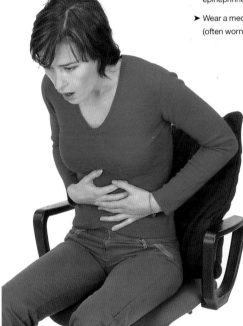

Insist that the sufferer go to the hospital, even if their reaction was mild and they feel better. Anaphylaxis can recur several hours after contact with the agent and it may be more serious next time around.

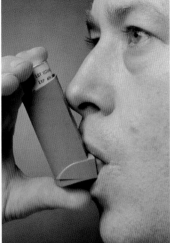
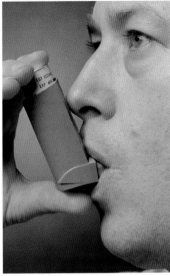

△ If the person is having difficulty breathing and they carry a rescue inhaler for the quick relief of asthma, this may ease their breathing. Always try to get them to take it themselves – only assist if absolutely necessary.

TIPS FOR ANAPHYLAXIS SUFFERERS

➤ If you are allergic to a food, be extra careful when eating out. Ask for detailed ingredients of any dishes you might order, and avoid anything that could contain the allergen.

➤ Read food ingredients labels – look out for lists hidden under sticky price tags. You may miss something vital otherwise. If in doubt, avoid it.

➤ Practice using epinephrine jabs – on an orange, not on other people. Be comfortable with the technique before an emergency occurs.

➤ Tell family, friends, and work colleagues what happens when you have an allergic reaction, and ensure that key people around you are properly trained in giving epinephrine. If your child is a sufferer, make sure their teachers and friends' parents know about the allergy and understand the importance of getting epinephrine administered.

➤ Wear a medical ID tag of some kind (often worn as a bracelet).

◁ Abdominal pain, nausea, and vomiting are among the common symptoms of anaphylactic shock.

Coping with a heart attack

SEE ALSO

➤ What is first aid?, p12

➤ Full resuscitation sequence, p34

➤ Cardiac compressions, p32

Heart attack is one of the leading causes of death in developed countries. For the best chance of survival, immediate hospital admission is necessary. To ensure that this happens you need to recognize when a person is possibly having a heart attack and call the emergency medical service without delay. The cause of a heart attack is nearly always a blockage in one of the major arteries supplying the heart muscle. There may be warning signs, such as angina, or a heart attack may occur suddenly, particularly in people at high risk.

A heart attack is also called a myocardial infarction or coronary thrombosis. This literally means the death of an area of tissue due to an interrupted blood supply. The coronary arteries, which supply the heart muscle, can become furred up with a fatty substance, a condition known as atherosclerosis. Eventually, one or more of these arteries becomes entirely blocked and part of the heart muscle dies as a result. This is a heart attack.

WHO HAS HEART ATTACKS?

Heart attacks become more common as we get older. However, some people are at greater risk of having a heart attack at an early age. These include:

• People with a family history of heart attacks – a close relative who has had a heart attack under the age of 60.

• Anyone with a high blood level of cholesterol. High levels of this fatty substance are linked to an increased risk of atherosclerosis, leading to heart attack.

• Smokers.

• People who are overweight.

• Anyone with high blood pressure.

• People with diabetes.

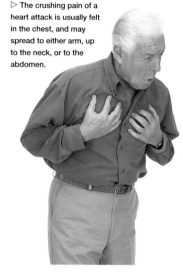

▷ The crushing pain of a heart attack is usually felt in the chest, and may spread to either arm, up to the neck, or to the abdomen.

• Female hormones give pre-menopausal women some protection against heart attacks, but after the menopause they are just as much at risk as men.

HOW TO AVOID HEART ATTACKS

If you are in a high-risk group, your doctor will monitor your condition on a regular basis and prescribe drugs. You may also be put on a special diet aimed at reducing the chances of your having a heart attack. For the majority of other people, the risk of heart attack can be reduced by the following guidelines:

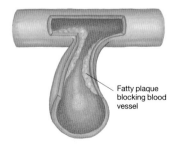

◁ This shows a cross-section of the junction between two arterial blood vessels. A fatty plaque has gathered and is constricting blood flow – atherosclerosis. If this occurs in arteries that supply the heart, a heart attack can occur.

Fatty plaque blocking blood vessel

SIGNS AND SYMPTOMS OF A HEART ATTACK

➤ Chest pain: "crushing" or "tight" pain, usually felt behind the breastbone. It may spread to an arm, up to the jaw, neck and teeth, or to the upper or middle part of the abdomen. (Note: some heart attacks are painless.)

➤ Pale/gray color or blue lips.

➤ Nausea.

➤ Sweating and clammy skin.

➤ Feeling restless.

➤ Rapid, weak pulse.

➤ Breathlessness.

➤ Loss of consciousness.

• Keep within the healthy weight range for your height and build.

• Take regular exercise (it is often best to check with a doctor before starting any exercise regime).

• Give up smoking.

• Eat a balanced diet that is low in animal fat, salt and processed food.

• Learn to manage stress.

WARNING

Beware a persistent pain that is like indigestion, which is not relieved by remedies for indigestion. Many people have died from a heart attack, having put up with what they thought was a bad bout of indigestion for a few days. If in any doubt, go to see a doctor.

FIRST AID FOR SUSPECTED HEART ATTACK

↓

Call the emergency services.

↓

Help the person into a sitting position, with the head and back supported, to minimize strain on the heart. Loosen any tight clothing and keep them warm.

↓

Keep them calm and monitor and record their breathing and circulation. Do not allow them to eat or drink.

↓

If they have any angina pills or a spray with them, they should take the pills or use the spray – usually under the tongue. If this does not alleviate the pain and they are fully conscious, give them one aspirin tablet to chew or swallow, unless they are allergic to aspirin or suffer from asthma.

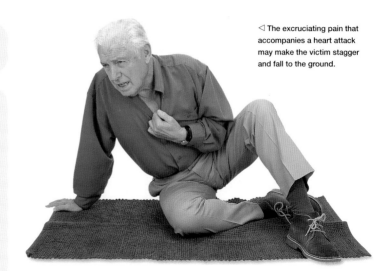

◁ The excruciating pain that accompanies a heart attack may make the victim stagger and fall to the ground.

ANGINA PECTORIS

Usually shortened to angina, the term angina pectoris literally means pain in the chest. Angina is caused by temporary blockage of one or more of the coronary arteries. The blockage causes pain that is usually relieved by resting, or special medication that dilates the arteries, or it may settle spontaneously. Angina may lead on to a full-blown heart attack. People at risk of angina are the same group as those at risk of heart attack. Those at risk should avoid the triggers that can bring on angina, which include excessive exercise, cold weather, heavy meals, and anxiety.

DEALING WITH ANGINA

➤ Ensure that the person is sitting down and resting.

➤ If they have had angina before and have an angina spray, let them administer it themself, or if necessary, help them to use it.

➤ If the pain is worse than normal or lasts for more than 20 minutes, or if the sufferer's condition starts to deteriorate, suspect a heart attack and call the emergency services.

▷ Make the person comfortable in a sitting position and get them to rest until the emergency services arrive.

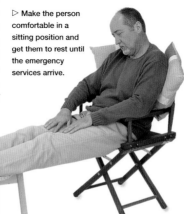

HEART FAILURE

A condition that often develops slowly over several weeks or months, heart failure occurs because the heart fails to pump efficiently enough to keep up with the body's demands. This results in gradually increasing shortness of breath on exertion, and fluid building up in the feet, ankles, legs, and abdomen.

However, an acute type of heart failure can develop when fluid suddenly builds up in the lungs, causing a sharp shortness of breath. This may occur alongside a heart attack or on its own, and requires emergency treatment. Sit the person upright, preferably with their legs over the side of a bed. Keep them calm, and do not let them move out of the bed. Call the emergency services immediately and be prepared to resuscitate.

SIGNS AND SYMPTOMS OF HEART FAILURE

➤ Breathing is fast, shallow and labored.

➤ Skin is cold, clammy and sweaty.

➤ Blue lips, skin, and nails.

➤ Sense of confusion and acute anxiety.

Dealing with an abnormal heart rate

SEE ALSO

➤ Full resuscitation
   sequence, p34
➤ Cardiac
   compressions, p32
➤ Coping with a heart
   attack, p72

Abnormal heart rate or rhythm, also known as arrhythmia, can cause palpitations and breathlessness. Occasional awareness of one's heartbeat is a normal reaction to fear or excitement, or it may be a sign of too much coffee or alcohol. Frequent palpitations may indicate disease, so this should always be investigated by a doctor. Arrhythmias are common after a heart attack, when the heart muscle is in a state of irritability; this is what often causes the heart to stop working altogether, otherwise known as cardiac arrest.

Everyone occasionally feels their heart "leap" – hopefully from love rather than fear, and sometimes for no apparent reason at all. That sudden thump, or feeling that the heart has missed a beat, is called a palpitation. This is only worrying when it becomes more than an occasional symptom. Frequent palpitations may be an indication of an illness, such as an overactive thyroid or heart disease. However, panic attacks and anxiety may also be the cause of palpitations, as may over-indulgence in coffee, cigarettes, alcohol, or illegal drugs.

WHAT CONTROLS HEART RATE?

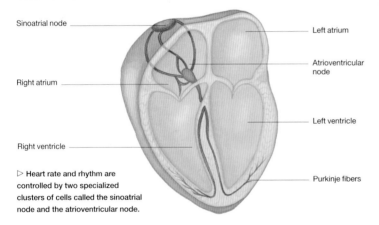

Sinoatrial node

Right atrium

Right ventricle

Left atrium

Atrioventricular node

Left ventricle

Purkinje fibers

▷ Heart rate and rhythm are controlled by two specialized clusters of cells called the sinoatrial node and the atrioventricular node.

HOW THE HEART RATE IS REGULATED

The heart is a muscle that contracts and relaxes continuously and rhythmically between 60 and 80 times a minute, on average, throughout our lives. Heart muscle is unique because it has its own conduction system, so it contracts without any outside control. Chemicals such as epinephrine or caffeine can alter the heart rate, as can anxiety, or a drop in blood pressure.

Each contraction of the heart muscle is controlled from within, by the conduction system. This system comprises groups of cells that charge up and fire spontaneously. One group of cells, called the sinoatrial (S/A) node, sets the rhythm for the rest of the heart – it acts as the heart's internal pacemaker. An electrical wave spreads from the S/A node through the atria, until it reaches a second node called the atrioventricular node. It then continues through a right and left branch, until it reaches the outermost parts of the heart. This contains specialized Purkinje fibers – a wiring system that transmits the impulses.

TYPES OF ARRHYTHMIA

Heart rate and rhythm may be either too high or too low. The most serious type of arrhythmia is ventricular fibrillation, which is caused by too high a heart rate in the ventricles (the lower heart chambers). This is the most common cause of death after a heart attack. In ventricular fibrillation, the heart "quivers", rather than beating in a coordinated fashion. The heart cannot pump blood efficiently in this state, and the person rapidly loses consciousness and will die as a result of cardiac arrest (when the heart stops) unless the heart can get back into a normal rhythm.

CARDIAC ARREST

A life-threatening emergency situation, cardiac arrest occurs when the heart stops beating. The most common cause is a heart attack, but there are many other causes. After a street accident, cardiac arrest may occur because of massive blood loss, or a collapsed lung. Cardiac arrest may occur in a pulmonary embolism, a condition in which blood clots form in the lungs. Electrocution or a lightning strike injury may cause a cardiac arrest. Asthmatics may have a cardiac arrest during a severe asthma attack.

Cardiopulmonary resuscitation is not a definitive lifesaving treatment for cardiac arrest, and can only keep the blood pumping around the body until specialized help is available. The only effective treatment is "defibrillation", in which a high-energy electric shock is applied to the chest wall. The sooner this is done after cardiac arrest, the more likely it is that the

FIRST AID FOR PALPITATIONS

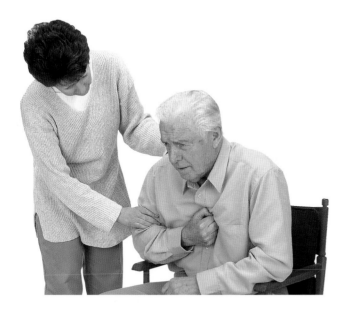

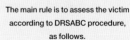

FIRST AID FOR CARDIAC ARREST

The main rule is to assess the victim according to DRSABC procedure, as follows.

Make sure the airway is clear and open. Check whether the person is breathing. If not, call the emergency services and start giving rescue breaths.

Assess for signs of circulation. If signs are absent, begin resuscitation, alternating 2 rescue breaths with 15 chest compressions.

Repeat this 2:15 ratio of breaths and compressions until emergency medical help arrives.

1 Sit the person down and reassure them if they are anxious. This may be all that is needed to settle the palpitations. Talk to them to find out whether they have experienced an abnormal heart rate before and whether they have a diagnosed heart condition.

2 If the palpitations do not settle after a few minutes but there are no other symptoms, call a doctor. If the person feels breathless, faint, or has chest pains, call the emergency services.

AUTOMATED EXTERNAL DEFIBRILLATOR (AED)

If someone suffers cardiac arrest in a public place, a defibrillator may be available on site. It should be used only by a trained operator.

➤ If you are already carrying out CPR, stop when the defibrillator and its operator are ready.

➤ Make sure you and any other helpers are not touching the victim while the machine is analyzing the heart or administering shocks.

➤ The prompts from the defibrillator should be followed until the paramedics arrive.

heart will return to a normal rhythm and resume pumping blood around the body.

Until recently defibrillators could only be used by trained paramedics and doctors. However, a new development has been launched in some areas. This is the automated external defibrillator, which requires some training but is much more user-friendly than the hospital types, and prompts the correct sequence of actions for its use. The rescuer needs to recognize that cardiac arrest may have occurred, and then to attach two sticky pads to the chest wall and switch on the machine. Such equipment is already kept at some busy public places, such as sports arenas, office buildings, and airports. This technology means that the average citizen, with minimal training, will be able to save a life.

SIGNS OF CARDIAC ARREST

➤ Loss of consciousness.

➤ Pale, blue skin.

➤ No sign of breathing.

➤ No pulse or heart sounds (for those with medical experience only).

➤ Dilated pupils that do not constrict when a light is directed at the eye (for highly trained first-aiders only).

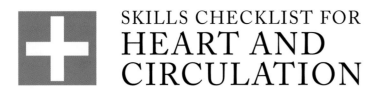

SKILLS CHECKLIST FOR
HEART AND CIRCULATION

KEY POINTS

- Effective blood circulation is essential for an individual to survive ☐

- Always call the emergency services out promptly to shock cases ☐

- Always call the emergency services out promptly if you suspect heart problems – they can quickly become life-threatening ☐

- Frequent heart palpitations must be investigated by a doctor – they are a symptom of various health problems ☐

SKILLS LEARNED

- An understanding of how the circulatory system works ☐

- Recognizing and dealing with circulatory shock ☐

- Recognizing, treating and avoiding anaphylactic shock ☐

- Recognizing and dealing with a heart attack ☐

- Recognizing and dealing with heart failure and angina ☐

- Dealing with palpitations and cardiac arrest ☐

BRAIN AND NERVOUS SYSTEM

The brain is the control center of the central nervous system, an extraordinarily complex set of mechanisms that is behind every function in the body and mind. Electrical and chemical signals rush around the body causing millions of actions every minute. However, the system is very delicate and easily damaged by injury or disease. Knowing what to do in the event of an accident affecting any part of the nervous system is of prime importance to the outlook for the injured person, and may even save their life. Even something as apparently minor as a headache may warn of a serious condition that must be investigated by a doctor.

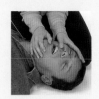

CONTENTS

Understanding the nervous system 78–79
Dealing with head injury 80–81
Coping with epilepsy 82–83
Recognizing a stroke 84–85
Coping with headache 86–87
Managing dizziness and fainting 88–89
Skills checklist 90

Understanding the nervous system

SEE ALSO

➤ What is first aid?, p12
➤ Dealing with head injury, p80
➤ Coping with headache, p86

The importance of the brain and the central nervous system to the rest of the body cannot be overstated. Every part of the body, and every bodily function, is under its control. For this reason, head and spinal injuries may prove particularly serious and have effects on many parts of the body at some distance from the injury. First aid is of the ultimate importance, particularly in maintaining the vital functions of breathing and circulation. Alert the emergency services without delay if you are in any doubt about the injured person's condition.

Human beings have a highly developed and sophisticated nervous system. The brain and nervous system are organized into many parts that serve specific and important functions – together they make up the body's main control center. All body sensations, muscle contractions, gland secretions, and a host of other complex interactions vital to life are relayed through the central nervous system.

HOW THE NERVOUS SYSTEM IS ORGANIZED

The nervous system is divided into two main sections – the central nervous system (CNS), which comprises the brain and the spinal cord, and the peripheral nervous system (PNS), which is made up of all the nerves that branch off the CNS. Nerves from the brain are called cranial nerves and those from the spinal cord are spinal nerves. The PNS is further broken down into nerves under voluntary control, such as those that control the muscles used for conscious movements, and nerves under involuntary control, such as those governing our internal systems – our heart rate and the changing size of the pupils in response to light, for example. The part of the system that regulates actions over which we have no voluntary control is known as the autonomic nervous system (ANS).

We take in information through our five senses – sight, smell, hearing, touch, and taste – and the brain acts on this information through the motor system. For example, when a small child's hand touches a hot oven, the brain receives a message via the senses and acts through the motor system to make the muscles move. The child immediately pulls the hand away from the painful stimulus.

THE CENTRAL NERVOUS SYSTEM

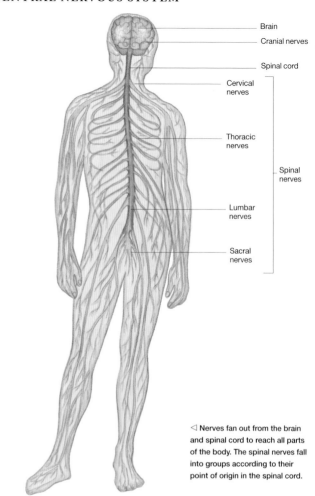

Brain
Cranial nerves
Spinal cord
Cervical nerves
Thoracic nerves
Spinal nerves
Lumbar nerves
Sacral nerves

◁ Nerves fan out from the brain and spinal cord to reach all parts of the body. The spinal nerves fall into groups according to their point of origin in the spinal cord.

Although this is a reflex action, the brain remembers the pain and the child will be wary of touching the oven in future.

CROSS-SECTION THROUGH THE BRAIN

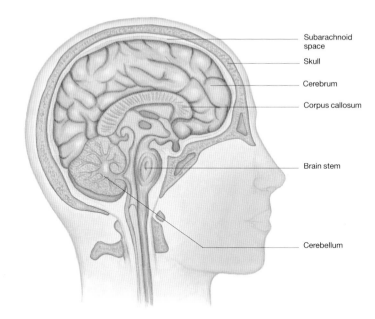

Subarachnoid space

Skull

Cerebrum

Corpus callosum

Brain stem

Cerebellum

MULTIPOLAR NEURONE

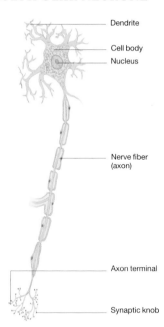

Dendrite

Cell body

Nucleus

Nerve fiber (axon)

Axon terminal

Synaptic knob

THE BRAIN

Our brain controls our thoughts, memories, speech, movements, and all the functions of the organs. Divided into three parts, the brain comprises the cerebrum, the cerebellum, and the brain stem.

The cerebrum forms the bulk of the brain: it controls sensation, movement, emotion, and intellect. The cerebrum is divided into two hemispheres, the left and the right. One of these hemispheres controls speech, and this is called the dominant hemisphere. In right-handed people, it is the left hemisphere, but left-handed people have their dominant hemisphere on the right. The effects of a stroke can, therefore, be very different depending on which hemisphere is affected. Damage to the left hemisphere will cause speech problems in a right-handed person, while a left-hander's speech will be unaffected.

The cerebellum controls coordination of movement, balance, and posture. People with damage to their cerebellum sometimes appear drunk and they may stagger, slur their words, and suffer from severe dizziness.

The brain stem regulates the heart rate and breathing, as well as coordinating activities such as coughing, sneezing, and swallowing. Life is impossible to sustain if the brain stem is damaged.

NERVES AND NEURONES

The nuts and bolts of the nervous system are cells called neurones and neuroglia. The neurones conduct electrical activity from one part of the body to another, while the neuroglia support and protect the neurones. Billions of these highly specialized cells are joined together to form nerves, which stretch from the brain or spinal cord to every part of the body.

Neurones in the brain are very densely packed and number around 1000 billion. Neurones in the spinal cord and around the body are very long and form an extensive communication system. The cell bodies of neurones are linked together by nerve fibers (axons), and the many projections coming off the cell bodies are called dendrites.

Nerve impulses in the form of electrical signals travel along the neurones at rapid speeds of up to 125 mph. With chemicals called neurotransmitters, signals from the brain are translated into effects at the target cell, for example in a muscle.

PROBLEMS WITH THE NERVOUS SYSTEM

Although peripheral nerves will regenerate if they are sewn back together fast enough, the central nervous system has no such ability. If the spinal cord is severed, it cannot heal or grow back. If nervous tissue is damaged, whether due to a stroke or multiple sclerosis, it is gone forever.

Problems with the nervous system can manifest themselves in a multitude of ways, but they are largely determined by the parts of the brain that are affected. Abnormal electrical activity causes epilepsy, degeneration of nervous tissue may cause dementia or Parkinson's disease, and processes that affect neurochemicals can trigger psychiatric conditions such as depression and schizophrenia.

Dealing with head injury

SEE ALSO

➤ What is first aid?, p12

➤ Full resuscitation sequence, p34

➤ Tackling skull and facial fractures, p152

Serious head injury is a medical emergency, particularly if the injured person loses consciousness. The first-aider should protect their airway, start resuscitation if necessary, and alert the emergency services without delay. A cut or bump on the scalp will lead to a suspicion of head injury, but serious internal injury is often not evident from external signs. It is worth remembering also that the very young and the elderly are especially likely to develop delayed reactions to relatively minor head injuries – so such cases need checking out.

Head injuries are potentially serious because they can damage the brain and surrounding blood vessels. Although the bony skull protects the brain, it also provides an enclosed space in which the brain can be easily shaken and damaged, and where there is little room for any swelling or bleeding following injury.

The main causes of head injuries are motor vehicle accidents, falls, and assaults.

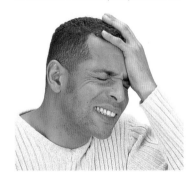

△ A sudden, crushing headache should always be investigated, particularly if it comes on at some point after a blow to the head.

TYPES OF HEAD INJURY

There are five main types of head injury, and people may have several simultaneously:

Cuts

Large cuts to the scalp look alarming, but are likely to be serious only if caused by a major blow. A large blow may cause brain damage.

Concussion

Symptoms such as loss of consciousness, short-term memory loss or headache after a head injury are termed concussion. The loss of consciousness may last up to six hours, and the loss of memory 24 hours, with little or no internal damage being suffered.

Contusion

Bruising, or contusion, may occur to the brain after an injury, and this causes swelling of the brain tissue. This may lead to much longer periods of unconsciousness

SIGNS AND SYMPTOMS OF SERIOUS HEAD INJURY

➤ Deep cuts or tears to the scalp, or goose egg swelling over the scalp.

➤ Nausea and/or vomiting.

➤ Severe headache.

➤ Drowsiness or difficulty being roused.

➤ Unequal sized pupils, or pupils that do not respond to light.

➤ Visual disturbance.

➤ Fluid flowing from eyes and/or mouth.

➤ Paralysis, numbness or loss of function over one half of the body.

➤ Problems with balance.

➤ Behaving as though drunk.

➤ Fits, confusion or unconsciousness.

CONTRECOUP INJURY

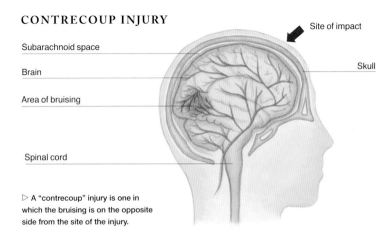

Subarachnoid space

Brain

Area of bruising

Spinal cord

Site of impact

Skull

▷ A "contrecoup" injury is one in which the bruising is on the opposite side from the site of the injury.

POSSIBLE SITE OF BRAIN INJURY FOLLOWING BLOW TO BACK OF HEAD

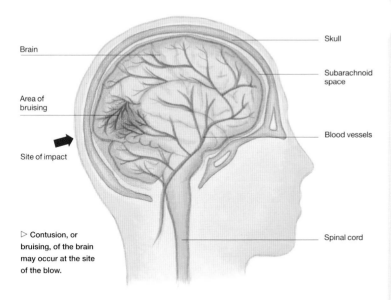

Brain

Area of bruising

Site of impact

Skull

Subarachnoid space

Blood vessels

Spinal cord

▷ Contusion, or bruising, of the brain may occur at the site of the blow.

Breathing in vomit while unconscious is the most common cause of death after a head injury. The first priority is to protect the victim's airway by tilting back the jaw. Always assume that they may have spinal injuries and protect their neck while trying to keep their airway open: if trained to do so, use the jaw thrust to open the airway. If they are not breathing, start resuscitation.

Carefully apply direct pressure to any scalp wounds that are bleeding, using a sterile dressing.

Watch for vomiting.

If the victim is conscious, lay them on the floor with head and shoulders slightly raised; if unconscious, place in the recovery position while protecting the neck.

Call the emergency services.

Monitor and record their level of response using AVPU. Reassure them if alert.

Continue to watch their breathing, circulation and level of consciousness until help arrives, and be prepared to resuscitate if necessary. Even if they regain consciousness, insist that they go to the hospital to be checked out.

---

following an accident, and possibly much longer periods of amnesia after regaining consciousness. In addition there may be signs of brain injury in other parts of the body, such as paralysis, numbness, or changes in breathing.

The bruising may be directly at the site of the injury, or it may be on the opposite side of the skull as the brain bounces away – this is called a contrecoup brain injury.

Hemorrhage

Bleeding within the skull, or hemorrhage, is a common consequence of head injury. The tough sheath (dura mater) attached to the inside of the skull is well supplied with blood vessels. These may be damaged and cause bleeding; sometimes the effects are delayed for several weeks after the injury.

Compression

The skull is an enclosed space, and if there is any swelling or bleeding within it, a point is reached when there is no more room for expansion. Compression of the

SIGNS AND SYMPTOMS OF RISING PRESSURE WITHIN THE SKULL

➤ Intense headache, worse when lying flat and/or with physical exertion.

➤ Vomiting.

➤ Unequal or dilated pupils.

➤ Weakness on one side of the body.

➤ Noisy, irregular breathing.

➤ Irritable or aggressive behavior.

brain can lead to quite severe damage and a wide range of symptoms. In extreme cases, it can cause brain tissue to squeeze out of the base of the skull – a condition known as coning. This is fatal so it is absolutely vital that any rise in pressure within the skull is recognized before this happens.

Even after seemingly minor head injuries, always be very vigilant for signs of increased cerebral pressure and get help promptly if you spot any.

Coping with epilepsy

SEE ALSO
➤ Responsiveness and the airway, p28
➤ The recovery position, p36
➤ Recognizing a stroke, p84

Epileptic fits, or "seizures", are caused by an instability of electrical activity in the brain. Such fits can be alarming, but there is usually no physical damage to the brain itself. There are over 40 types of seizure, which may be partial (affecting part of the brain) or generalized (affecting the whole brain). These many types range from an "absence" seizure (once called *petit mal*), where the sufferer simply seems to be daydreaming briefly, to a full-blown "tonic-clonic" fit (once called *grand mal*), where the sufferer writhes uncontrollably.

The nature of epileptic seizures depends on which part of the brain is affected. At one end of the scale, there is a brief "absence" of attention; at the other, the major jerking and total unconsciousness (tonic-clonic fit) traditionally associated with epilepsy. Partial seizures may develop into generalized ones. So, for example, someone might start off with one hand affected and progress to a complete tonic-clonic fit. It is reassuring to know that many people only ever have one fit during their lifetime.

WHAT CAUSES SEIZURES?
All kinds of things can cause a seizure:
• Brain damage caused by:
  – Head injury;
  – Difficulties at birth;
  – Reduced brain oxygen (for example, suffocation);
  – Brain problems (tumors, bleeding, swelling).
• Certain diseases (diabetes, liver failure).
• Certain poisons (such as pesticides).
• An inherited low "seizure threshold".
• A large intake of alcohol. Also, alcoholics commonly have seizures if they suddenly stop drinking alcohol.

• A high temperature (in children). Children up to the age of five years often have convulsions, typically as part of a feverish illness. They usually grow out of these in middle childhood. Feverish convulsions do not indicate that a child may develop epilepsy later on.
• The cause often remains unknown.

CHARACTERISTICS OF SEIZURES
In an absence seizure, the person typically stops what they are doing and stares into space for 10–15 seconds. They have actually lost consciousness briefly and are unaware of their surroundings. They will then continue as if nothing had happened, and will have no memory of the event.

In a tonic-clonic seizure, the person is fully unconscious for up to 10 minutes and may be very sleepy for an hour or two after the seizure. The main features include:
• A change in mood/behavior several hours or days before a fit – known as a prodrome.
• Immediately before the fit an imaginary smell or vision may be apparent, or a sense of déjà vu – called an aura.
• Sudden unconsciousness, followed by stiffening of the arms and legs – the tonic

phase. Then jerky movements of the limbs and face – the clonic phase.
• There may be loss of bladder control and the sufferer may bite their tongue.

HOW TO RECOGNIZE EPILEPSY
Someone who has fainted may jerk slightly – this is not epilepsy. There are many other non-epileptic causes of "funny turns".

A person who has had an epileptic seizure may come to in a confused state. It will help them to hear from a witness what has happened, particularly on the first occasion, as this can then be reported to the emergency medical service or the hospital.

Epilepsy is diagnosed by neurological tests. These include electroencephalography (EEG), in which brain activity is measured by attaching electrodes to the scalp, and a computerized tomography (CT) scan to exclude brain tumor and stroke. A person recently diagnosed with epilepsy needs reassurance and support to build up their confidence for leading a normal life.

COMMON TRIGGERS
➤ Excess alcohol.
➤ Tiredness.
➤ Emotion (stress/excitement).
➤ Failure to take medication regularly.
➤ Certain foods/not eating properly.
➤ Illness.
➤ Hormonal changes.
➤ Flashing lights.

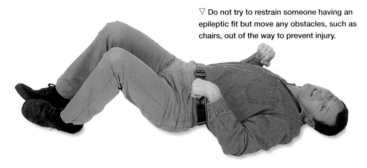

▽ Do not try to restrain someone having an epileptic fit but move any obstacles, such as chairs, out of the way to prevent injury.

FIRST AID FOR AN EPILEPTIC FIT

You may want to look quickly to see if the victim is wearing a medical ID tag, or is carrying a card that says they suffer from epilepsy and tells you what to do.

During the seizure: prevent any avoidable injury. Move any obstacles and loosen the clothing, especially around the neck. Never restrain the victim or put anything in their mouth.

After the seizure: put the sufferer into the recovery position and make sure that they have a clear airway – remove any obstacles if you can do so easily.

CALLING THE EMERGENCY SERVICES

If this is someone's first fit, call the emergency services, as a hospital assessment is necessary. There is usually no need to call for help for a routine seizure suffered by a diagnosed epileptic. However, you should call if:
- They do not stop fitting after 5 minutes.
- The fit is worse than usual: more prolonged or violent.
- They suffer a series of fits with short gaps.
- Serious injury has occurred.
- The person remains unconscious for more than 10 minutes.

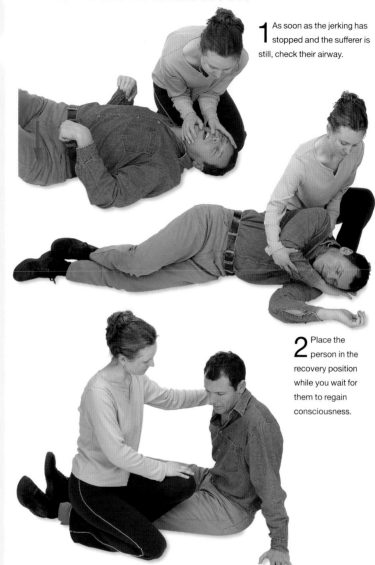

1 As soon as the jerking has stopped and the sufferer is still, check their airway.

2 Place the person in the recovery position while you wait for them to regain consciousness.

3 Explain to them what happened. Find out whether this has occurred before, and if it has not, send them to the hospital. Ask whether they would like you to contact anyone.

HOW IS EPILEPSY TREATED?

Epilepsy is usually controlled with anticonvulsant drugs, taken until the sufferer has been seizure-free for 2–3 years. Women with epilepsy considering pregnancy should speak to their doctor first as they may have to be put on a different anticonvulsant drug.

WARNING

People with epilepsy should not swim alone or cycle in traffic-dense areas. Driving is not allowed for up to a year, or even longer, after diagnosis, depending on state law and the individual case. Cases are reviewed regularly, and driving may be permitted again if the epilepsy is well controlled.

Recognizing a stroke

SEE ALSO

➤ Dealing with an abnormal heart rate, p74
➤ Coping with headache, p86
➤ Managing dizziness and fainting, p88

Strokes are caused by a sudden stoppage of the blood supply to part of the brain. They are usually the result of a blood clot or a ruptured artery, and vary in severity: some leave no lasting effects, others cause paralysis on one side of the body, and some prove instantly fatal. Although more common in elderly people, people who smoke, have high blood pressure, or take the combined oral contraceptive pill are at increased risk of having a stroke. First-aid treatment aims to maintain breathing and circulation until the emergency services arrive.

A stroke occurs when the blood supply to a part of the brain is cut off. This may be caused by a blood clot in a vessel in the brain or by bleeding into the brain. A stroke's short- and long-term effects depend on which part of the brain is affected.

A stroke tends to occur very suddenly with very little warning. If you find yourself having to administer first aid to a probable stroke victim, it is important to act swiftly and ensure the emergency services are called without delay.

WHAT CAUSES A STROKE?

Generally, strokes tend to affect older people, and people with high blood pressure or a circulatory problem.

There are also a number of other factors that can increase a person's risk of having a stroke. These include taking the combined oral contraceptive pill, having a high blood cholesterol level, being diabetic, smoking, and being overweight.

Atherosclerosis

Atheroma is a thick, fatty substance that builds up in the arteries over the years, gradually narrowing them and eventually blocking them altogether. This condition, known as atherosclerosis, slows the flow of blood around the body and encourages the formation of blood clots. If a blood clot occurs in one of the cerebral arteries, it will cause a stroke.

Embolism

A fragment of material traveling through the bloodstream, often a piece of blood clot, is called an embolus. An embolus may arise in the heart, travel to the brain and cause a stroke. Anyone with a heart valve abnormality or an abnormal heart rhythm is more likely to develop an embolus.

Aneurysm

Some people are born with a weakness in one of the arteries at the base of the brain; this is called an aneurysm. It may leak, causing warning headaches, but often it will suddenly burst, causing a severe and often fatal stroke.

HOW TO RECOGNIZE A STROKE

Sometimes there may be prior warning signs of an imminent stroke, with the person feeling very unwell and suffering a severe headache and copious vomiting. The initial symptoms usually happen quickly over minutes or hours, and the situation may deteriorate progressively over several days.

Usually, the part of the body affected is on the opposite side to the side of the brain affected. If the person is right-handed then a left-sided stroke will usually affect their speech. If left-handed, the opposite is true. Occasionally a person may be totally unaware that they have a right or left side at all. For example, they might eat food only from the side of the plate that they are aware of.

CROSS-SECTION OF BRAIN AFTER A STROKE

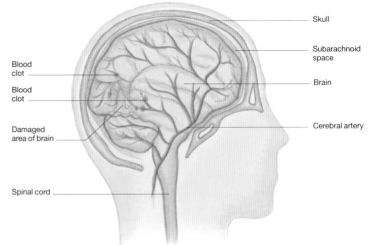

- Skull
- Subarachnoid space
- Brain
- Cerebral artery
- Blood clot
- Blood clot
- Damaged area of brain
- Spinal cord

△ A common cause of stroke is a blood clot in a cerebral artery, which supplies blood to the brain. This will starve nearby tissue of oxygen and other nutrients, which will cause temporary or permanent loss of function.

CAN STROKE BE PREVENTED?

Although none of us can escape the increased risk of having a stroke that comes with growing older, there are a number of measures we can take to reduce the risk.

Smoking increases the risk of a stroke occurring by several hundredfold, and high blood pressure is also closely linked to a higher chance of having a stroke. People with high levels of cholesterol and other fats in their blood will develop atherosclerosis; this causes a build-up of a fatty substance that blocks the arteries and may cause a stroke, among other diseases. All these factors can be controlled by diet, exercise, abstension from smoking and, if necessary, with drugs.

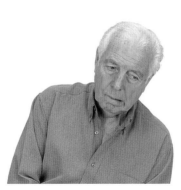

▷ In many stroke victims, the side of the face droops and they may be unable to speak, smile, or swallow without dribbling. There may be loss of sensation in one arm. These symptoms often don't appear until a little while after the initial stroke.

SIGNS AND SYMPTOMS OF A STROKE

➤ Sudden, severe headache.

➤ Dizziness.

➤ Loss of consciousness.

➤ Confusion and slurred speech that could be mistaken for drunkenness.

➤ Dribbling when trying to smile, speak, or swallow.

➤ Inability to speak or understand words.

➤ Weakness or complete loss of the ability to use one side of the body.

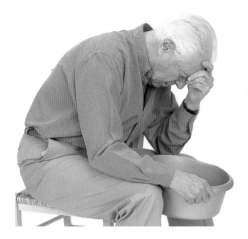

◁ Stroke victims may vomit copiously. Make sure they are not in a position where they might inhale their vomit, as this can prove fatal.

FIRST AID FOR STROKE

Assess according to DRSABC, and be prepared to resuscitate if necessary.

If you know it is a stroke, call the emergency services – prompt aid is vital.

If the victim is unconscious, open the airway and check breathing and circulation. Be prepared to resuscitate if necessary. Put them in the recovery position in case they vomit (stroke victims often lose their gag reflex).

If conscious, lay them on their back with head and shoulders comfortably raised.

Look quickly for a medical ID tag. They may be suffering from another condition, such as diabetic hypoglycaemia.

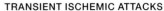

Call the emergency services if not called already. Do not give any food or water.

TRANSIENT ISCHEMIC ATTACKS

A transient ischemic attack (TIA) is like a mini-stroke. Symptoms are short-lived and totally disappear within 24 hours. TIAs are often a warning sign of a full-blown stroke, with about a 10 percent risk that a stroke will happen within a year. The sufferer should be investigated urgently for the cause of the TIA in order to prevent either a recurrence or a full stroke. They will probably be put on aspirin by their doctor, to thin the blood and make clotting less likely.

Coping with headache

SEE ALSO
➤ Dealing with head injury, p80
➤ Recognizing a stroke, p84
➤ Tackling skull and facial fractures, p152

Headaches are such a common complaint that very few people will go through life without experiencing them. Usually a headache is associated with stress, tension, overwork, or too much alcohol; it quickly passes with self-help remedies and there is no need for concern.

However, it is important to be aware that severe, persistent, or recurrent headaches may have a more serious underlying cause and should be investigated by a doctor. A person experiencing a migraine attack for the first time should also seek the advice of a doctor.

Everybody suffers from headaches at some time in their life and their cause is usually obvious. Persistent headaches that do not ease with simple painkillers, or severe ones that start suddenly, may mean you should see a doctor. Headaches have many different causes, including alcohol, caffeine-withdrawal, lack of fresh air, dehydration (a very common cause, often arising from excess alcohol), stress, menstruation and sinusitis, but very few causes are in any way life-threatening.

Headache following head injury is common and may last for months and even years after the accident. Seek medical attention if there are other symptoms, such as fever, fainting, fits or any discharge from the ears or nose.

WHEN TO SEE A DOCTOR
A person with any of the following types of headache should be seen by a doctor:

➤ Sudden onset.

➤ Persistent headaches.

➤ Associated with a fever and neck stiffness.

➤ Accompanied by a rash.

➤ Following head injury.

➤ Feels like "the worst headache ever".

➤ Accompanied by persistent or severe vomiting.

➤ Worse when lying flat or straining.

➤ Accompanied by confusion, drowsiness, or loss of consciousness.

➤ Accompanied by numbness, tingling of the limbs, or any other neurological problem.

➤ Regular headaches starting after the age of 50.

TYPES OF HEADACHE

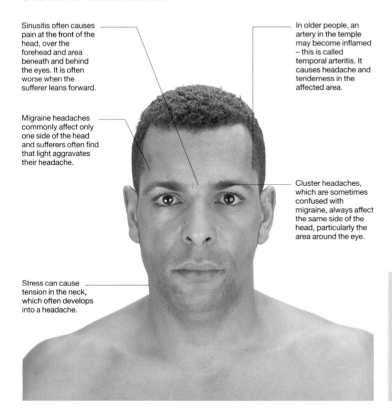

Sinusitis often causes pain at the front of the head, over the forehead and area beneath and behind the eyes. It is often worse when the sufferer leans forward.

Migraine headaches commonly affect only one side of the head and sufferers often find that light aggravates their headache.

Stress can cause tension in the neck, which often develops into a headache.

In older people, an artery in the temple may become inflamed – this is called temporal arteritis. It causes headache and tenderness in the affected area.

Cluster headaches, which are sometimes confused with migraine, always affect the same side of the head, particularly the area around the eye.

WARNING
Any severe headache that persists for several days should be investigated promptly by a doctor. There may be a serious underlying cause, although in most dangerous conditions, such as a brain tumor or stroke, additional symptoms usually accompany the headache.

MIGRAINE

Migraines are a problem often passed down through generations of a family. Migraine is believed to be caused by blood flow changes in the brain, which lead to chemicals being released that act on the blood vessels in the brain. This causes severe pain, vomiting, and visual problems. The root of these changes is as yet unknown, although the neurotransmitter serotonin may play a big role, as does the food enzyme, tyramine (see "Triggers" box).

Recognizing migraine

Migraines are usually felt on one side of the head, and they might last up to three days. In some people, a migraine attack is preceded by a warning called an aura. This is primarily visual, such as seeing zigzag lines or spots in the field of vision. There may be other symptoms present such as dizziness, tingling, temporary speech difficulties, and

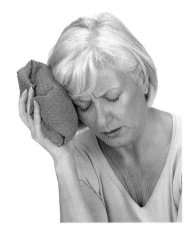

△ Wrapping a bag of frozen vegetables in a cloth and placing it against the headache site may ease the pain a little. Heat applied in the same way may also work.

blurred vision. Since visual problems often accompany migraine it is not advisable to attempt to drive during an attack.

Treating migraine

A large selection of drugs is available to prevent and treat migraine. Both over-the-counter and prescription drugs are available, and it is best to discuss the options with your physician. You need to consider the frequency of attacks, how long each attack lasts, and the extent to which the debility affects everyday life.

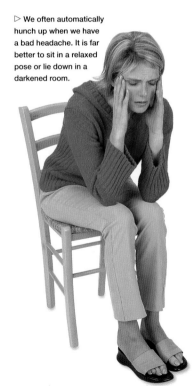

▷ We often automatically hunch up when we have a bad headache. It is far better to sit in a relaxed pose or lie down in a darkened room.

MIGRAINE TRIGGERS

➤ Stress, or relaxing after stress.

➤ Strong smells, loud noises, flickering screens.

➤ Premenstrual hormonal surge.

➤ Contraceptive pill.

➤ Missing meals.

➤ Foods such as: chocolate, aged cheese, cured/pickled foods, citrus fruit, monosodium glutamate (MSG), cola drinks, red/fortified wine, caffeine. (The enzyme tyramine plays a part here.)

HOME REMEDIES FOR ROUTINE HEADACHES

➤ Over-the-counter painkillers.

➤ An ice pack or heating pad over the site of the headache.

➤ Bed rest, preferably in the dark.

➤ Relaxation techniques.

➤ Complementary remedies, including herbal remedies such as feverfew, valerian, lavender and betony. Never take feverfew with any blood-thinning drugs and always check the safety of a herbal preparation in case you have a condition that makes its use unsafe.

➤ Massage and acupressure.

There are over-the-counter drugs that combine acetaminophen with an anti-sickness treatment, and some people find that ibuprofen helps.

Some people find complementary treatments, such as lavender or betony and homeopathic remedies, very effective.

▽ Nausea and vomiting are very common symptoms of a migraine attack.

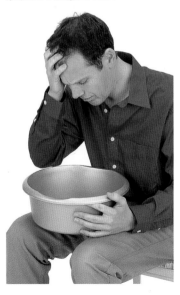

Managing dizziness and fainting

SEE ALSO
➤ What is first aid?, p12
➤ Dealing with head injury, p80
➤ Coping with headache, p86

Dizziness, or a feeling of unsteadiness, is a common complaint and is usually a momentary sensation of no consequence. Dizziness may lead to fainting, which is a short-lived loss of consciousness that usually resolves the giddiness. A brief dizzy spell, with or without fainting, can be caused by a hot, stuffy atmosphere, fatigue, anxiety, emotional shock, lack of food, blood loss, or standing still for too long. Vertigo, or the sensation that your surroundings are spinning for no apparent reason, may have a more serious cause.

The main issue with dizziness is whether or not it is caused by a balance disorder.

CAUSES OF DIZZINESS

Non-vertigo dizziness might be felt as wooziness or light-headedness and may be due to anything from low blood sugar (not eating regularly) to high blood pressure, anemia, or wax in the ears. If this type of dizziness occurs regularly, you should see your doctor, who will determine whether an underlying condition is to blame. The dizziness will have to be controlled, so that activities such as driving can be continued.

One common trigger for dizziness is standing up suddenly. This is often caused by your blood vessels not adjusting fast enough to accommodate a changed body position. It can also happen if you bend down or turn around very quickly. If this persists, see a doctor.

CAUSES OF VERTIGO

Balance is controlled by a part of the inner ear called the labyrinth, and also centrally in the brain. A problem with any part of this system might cause dizziness. The dizzy sensation in this case is more dramatic and is known as vertigo – the person feels their surroundings spinning around them alarmingly (like the result of drinking too much alcohol or going on a fairground ride).

Vertigo is often due to a viral infection of the labyrinth, known medically as labyrinthitis, which may last a few weeks but from which complete recovery is usual. It responds well to medication that controls the dizziness and nausea that often accompany true vertigo.

Another reasonably common, but unfortunately life-long, illness that causes dizziness is Ménière's disease. In this instance, typical symptoms that accompany the vertigo include intermittent deafness and tinnitus (noises heard in the ear that are similar to an aircraft taking off). This condition usually develops in middle age and is treated with drugs.

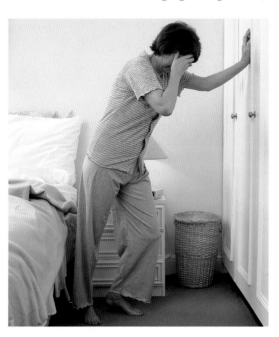

▷ If you get dizzy on standing up suddenly, for example when you first get up in the morning, lean against the wall in case you faint and then kneel or sit down till the dizziness clears. When you get up again, do so more slowly than you did the first time.

WHEN TO SEE A DOCTOR

Most types of dizziness are short-lived but you should see your doctor if any of the following apply:

➤ Dizziness happens regularly.

➤ You have vertigo rather than light-headedness.

➤ Other symptoms, such as deafness, earache, ear popping, tinnitus, nausea or vomiting accompany the dizziness.

➤ There is a family history of Ménière's disease.

➤ You are taking any medication that could be causing the dizziness.

Your main concern should be to stop the sufferer from hurting themself or others, for example if they are driving a car when dizziness strikes.

Sit the sufferer down. If the dizziness continues, lay them flat so that if they faint they won't hurt themself.

Unless they have sustained a head injury, raise their legs higher than their head.

Ask whether this has happened before, and whether they have any anti-dizziness medication that you could get for them. Call a doctor if they are very distressed or request medical help.

FAINTING

This occurs when there is a temporary lack of oxygen to the brain. It may happen for many reasons, including hunger, a sudden change of atmosphere from cold to warm, or standing still for a long time. If a person stands still without regularly clenching their calf muscles, the blood pools in their legs and they may faint as the brain does not receive enough oxygen. By fainting, the body is able to get blood and oxygen back up to the brain again – and so the person "comes to" as the brain recovers its function.

Fainting can often cause worry about more serious complaints such as brain tumors or epilepsy. The following features distinguish simple fainting from other causes of brief unconsciousness:

• There may be certain brief sensations that warn of a fainting episode: a sense of narrowed vision or of voices becoming distant, for example.
• The victim's skin looks very pale and feels clammy to the touch.
• The victim's pulse becomes slow.
• When they recover, there is no prolonged drowsiness (as there is with epilepsy).
• They may jerk slightly after they pass out, but there is no epileptic-type fit.

Check that the person is breathing. If so, lay them flat on their back and raise their legs higher than their head (unless they have a head injury/pains).

Loosen their clothing – especially around the neck – and if the atmosphere is hot and stuffy, open doors and windows.

If they don't wake up after a few minutes, recheck their ABC, place in the recovery position, and call the emergency services. Monitor their breathing and circulation until help arrives.

Tell them exactly what happened when they fainted; this witness information may be vital in distinguishing a simple faint from something more alarming. The victim should see their doctor if there were any unusual signs, such as loss of bladder control or drowsiness, after the faint.

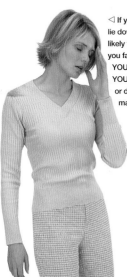

◁ If you feel dizzy, try to sit or lie down – you will be less likely to hurt yourself in a fall if you faint. NEVER SIT WITH YOUR HEAD BETWEEN YOUR LEGS if you feel faint or dizzy – this could make things worse.

◁ In fainting cases, support the person's legs above the level of their head so that blood returns quickly to the brain and resolves the dizziness. If possible, keep their knees slightly bent. Do not raise their legs if they have sustained a head injury or have sudden/persistent head pains, or if you suspect bad leg injuries.

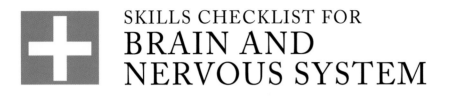

SKILLS CHECKLIST FOR
BRAIN AND NERVOUS SYSTEM

KEY POINTS

- After someone has sustained any blow to the head, be very vigilant for further problems ☐

- Never try to restrain someone who is having an epileptic fit ☐

- Get emergency aid to a stroke victim as fast as possible ☐

- Persistent or unusual headaches or dizziness should be investigated by a doctor ☐

SKILLS LEARNED

- Recognizing the signs of a serious head injury ☐

- Dealing with a head injury ☐

- What to do if someone has an epileptic fit ☐

- Recognizing and dealing with a stroke ☐

- Knowing when to consult a doctor about headaches ☐

- Giving first aid for dizziness and fainting ☐

- Knowing when to consult a doctor about dizziness and fainting ☐

7

OTHER MEDICAL EMERGENCIES

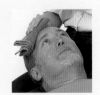

This chapter describes what to do in the event of a range of potentially critical situations. In some of them, including antenatal emergencies, emergency childbirth, and diabetic crisis, the emergency medical service is needed, but there is action you can take to minimize risk before the paramedics arrive. Others are conditions that can usually be dealt with by home first-aid action but that might develop into more serious conditions requiring expert help; these include allergies, bites and stings, and heat and cold disorders. More common symptoms, such as abdominal pain, nausea and vomiting, and fever, are also covered.

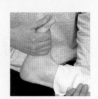

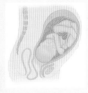

CONTENTS Coping with antenatal emergencies 92–93

Helping with emergency childbirth 94–95

Managing diabetic conditions 96–97

Dealing with nausea and vomiting 98

Tackling diarrhea, fever and cramp 99

Dealing with abdominal pain 100–101

Coping with allergy 102–103

Dealing with bites and stings 104–105

Managing heat and cold disorders 106–107

Skills checklist 108

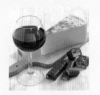

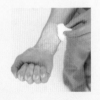

Coping with antenatal emergencies

SEE ALSO

➤ CHILDREN'S LIFE
SUPPORT, p43

➤ Helping with
emergency
childbirth, p94

➤ Bleeding from
orifices, p142

Situations sometimes arise in pregnancy that call for immediate action. These include bleeding, severe abdominal pain, headache, continuous vomiting, breaking of the waters, and lack of fetal movements. The first priority is to call the emergency services and explain what has happened so they can warn the hospital. While waiting for specialist help, keep the mother calm and reassure her that help is on the way and that the baby will be fine. You should be prepared to monitor her condition and take appropriate action if it changes.

Problems in pregnancy may occur that require getting to the hospital quickly, and occasionally rapid action is needed prior to reaching the hospital, but you should always seek medical advice if you are in any doubt at all about a pregnant woman's symptoms.

If you are a male first-aider treating a woman who is not known to you, she may be reluctant to confide in you, and you should seek help from another woman.

COLLAPSE IN PREGNANCY

Any woman of fertile age who suddenly collapses should be considered possibly to be pregnant. The main concern is that the collapse may be due to an ectopic pregnancy, a life-threatening condition.

A woman who is heavily pregnant should not be laid on her back if she collapses. The pregnant uterus lies on the vessels that feed blood back to the heart, so resuscitation and cardiac compressions will be effective only if she is turned slightly onto her left side, so that these vessels are not constricted in any way.

BLEEDING IN EARLY PREGNANCY

Any bleeding during the first eight weeks of pregnancy could be due to an ectopic pregnancy, in which the baby develops in one of the fallopian tubes. There is often, but not always, low pelvic pain before the bleeding starts. In this case, the pregnant woman should see her doctor urgently, even if the bleeding is very light.

If there is any abdominal pain with the bleeding, or if the woman feels unwell, particularly if she is pale, dizzy, or prone to fainting, it is important to seek a doctor's advice urgently.

Miscarriage

Another possible cause of bleeding in early pregnancy (up to 23 weeks) is miscarriage, and the woman should see her doctor

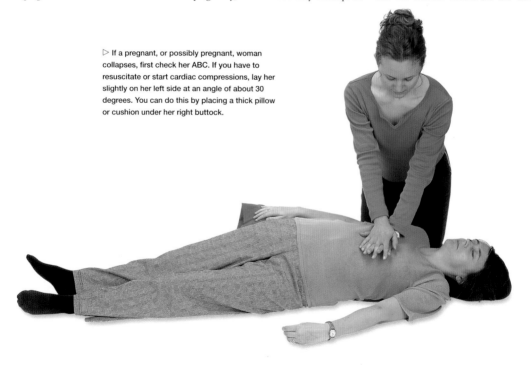

▷ If a pregnant, or possibly pregnant, woman collapses, first check her ABC. If you have to resuscitate or start cardiac compressions, lay her slightly on her left side at an angle of about 30 degrees. You can do this by placing a thick pillow or cushion under her right buttock.

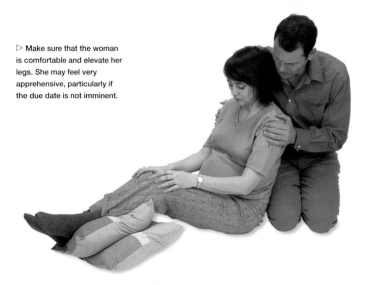

▷ Make sure that the woman is comfortable and elevate her legs. She may feel very apprehensive, particularly if the due date is not imminent.

urgently or go to hospital, depending on the severity of symptoms. Sometimes there is only a very small amount of blood and very little abdominal pain. This is usually called a threatened miscarriage, and bed rest and avoidance of sex may be the only advice from the doctor.

In other cases, the bleeding from a miscarriage may be extremely heavy and accompanied by cramp-like pains in the lower abdomen. There may even be symptoms of shock when the miscarriage has become inevitable, and there may also be visible parts of the placenta and fetus in the blood. (These should be kept and given to the paramedics.) Such severe symptoms require admission to hospital, where it is likely that an operation will be performed under anaesthetic to ensure that the entire contents of the uterus are removed.

▽ In case a pregnant woman passes out, put her in the recovery position, as lying on the left side is best while waiting for the emergency services to arrive.

BLEEDING IN LATE PREGNANCY

Any bleeding after 23 weeks should be taken very seriously, and the woman should be taken to a doctor immediately. It may only be a harmless "bloody show", the discharge of the mucus plug that sits in the cervix until near the end of pregnancy. However, it may be a sign that the placenta is bleeding, or has started to rupture from the uterus. These placental conditions are known as placenta previa (in which there is painless bleeding) and placental abruption (in which there is severe pain). Both conditions can threaten the baby's life.

THE AMNIOTIC SAC

The membranes surrounding the baby in the uterus normally rupture at the onset of labor. This may release a gush of amniotic fluid or a more gentle leakage. Sometimes, however, the waters can break before the baby is ready to be born and the woman will have to be admitted to hospital to protect the baby from infection.

ACTION FOR BLEEDING IN PREGNANCY

In early pregnancy with painless bleeding:
➤ Make the woman as comfortable as possible.
➤ Make sure that she is wearing a sanitary napkin.
➤ Get her to see a doctor the same day.

In early pregnancy with heavy bleeding and the passing of clots:
➤ Lay her flat and elevate her legs.
➤ Monitor her breathing and circulation every few minutes in case she collapses.
➤ Seek medical advice urgently.

In pregnancy after the 23rd week:
➤ Lay her on her left side.
➤ Keep a close eye on her breathing and circulation.
➤ Call the emergency services.

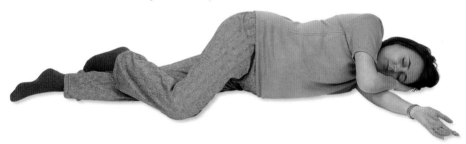

Helping with emergency childbirth

SEE ALSO

➤ Full resuscitation sequence, p34

➤ CHILDREN'S LIFE SUPPORT, p43

➤ Coping with antenatal emergencies, p92

It is not usually first-time mothers who deliver on the kitchen floor but the more experienced second- and third-timers, whose labors are less predictable and occur at a faster pace. Knowing what to do if a woman goes into labor is essential first-aid knowledge. Although the mother herself does most of the work during labor and birth, there are a number of things you can do to help. Newborn babies sometimes struggle to breathe, and you might have to provide crucial help. Bringing a new life into the world is an unforgettable experience.

Although there may be few signs that labor is imminent, sometimes the baby's movements are less frequent a day or two before labor begins. As a general rule, a mother should feel her baby move at least ten times a day even just before labor starts. However, there is much variation, and she need only be concerned if she feels a significant drop in fetal activity: she should seek medical advice if this happens.

LABOR

There are three stages of labor. The first stage starts with contractions and ends when the cervix is fully dilated. The second stage begins as the baby descends through the birth canal and ends when the baby is born. The third stage is when the placenta or afterbirth is delivered.

First stage

During the first stage the cervix dilates to allow the baby's head through at the second stage. The first signs of labor come on at this stage – the contractions. These are regular pains that start like a much more intense version of period pain, felt across the lower abdomen. They come and go every 5-20 minutes, lasting up to 30 seconds. The mother may also feel the "bag of waters" breaking, as the amniotic fluid around the baby gushes out. If the fluid is brownish, rather than clear yellow, the baby may be in distress, and hospital delivery is essential.

Second stage

During this stage the baby will be delivered. Prepare a clean, comfortable area for the birth and make sure the emergency services are on their way. Let the mother get into whatever position feels comfortable for her. She now has an overwhelming urge to push with each contraction. She may involuntarily open her bowels: try to clear away the feces without contaminating the vulval area and risking infecting the baby.

The baby is ready to be born when you can see the head sitting behind the vulva at the vaginal entrance. The mother should now pant through the urge to push, to prevent the baby shooting out too fast.

As the baby's head arrives, it will normally be facing the floor. Support the head with your hand beneath it – the head naturally turns 90 degrees at this stage. Let it come naturally and do not pull. As soon as the baby's head is out, check to see if the

FIRST AND SECOND STAGES OF LABOR

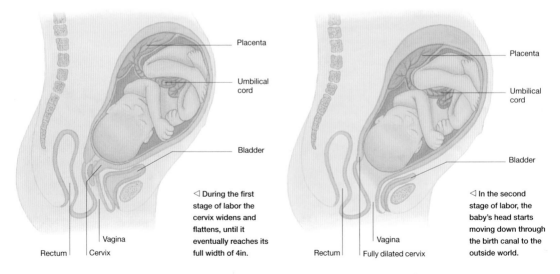

Placenta

Umbilical cord

Bladder

Vagina

Rectum   Cervix

◁ During the first stage of labor the cervix widens and flattens, until it eventually reaches its full width of 4in.

Placenta

Umbilical cord

Bladder

Vagina

Rectum   Fully dilated cervix

◁ In the second stage of labor, the baby's head starts moving down through the birth canal to the outside world.

umbilical cord is around the neck. If it is, check that it is loose and then slip it carefully over the baby's head. Continue to support the baby throughout the rest of the delivery. The shoulders should appear next, usually after a short delay.

The rest of the body arrives quickly after this. The emerging baby will be slippery, so be careful not to drop it. Keep the baby level with the mother's vagina until the cord stops pulsating (about 20 seconds) then gently lift the baby onto the mother's abdomen. Do not cut the umbilical cord, but leave it attached for professional treatment.

The baby should start to cry at this point and can be wrapped in a warm towel or blanket. If there are no signs of breathing, remove obvious obstructions from the mouth and immediately give 2 rescue breaths with your mouth over the baby's mouth and nose. Continue following the standard basic life support routine for a baby.

Third stage

The placenta may not be delivered until up to an hour after the baby's arrival. It should arrive naturally without any action by you. Place the placenta in a plastic bag, to be examined in the hospital. With the mother's consent, gently massage the uterus to reduce the chance of hemorrhage. The uterus can easily be felt just above the pubic bone.

DELIVERY OF THE BABY

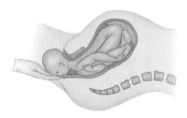

1 Most babies come out with the back of their heads facing upward and their faces pointing downward.

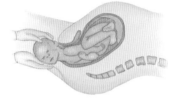

2 Support the head rather than pulling on it, to avoid causing any damage to the nerves supplying the neck and shoulder area.

3 When most of the body has emerged, keep it at the same level as the mother. Make sure you hold the baby carefully as it will be covered in blood and amniotic fluid and will be very slippery.

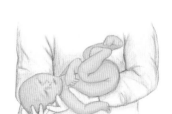

4 Hold the baby in a tilted position, with the head slightly lower than the rest of the body, in case of vomiting.

HOW TO PREPARE FOR AN EMERGENCY DELIVERY

If a pregnant woman is having continuous contractions, or is trying to push, there will be no time to get her to hospital and you must prepare for an emergency delivery. First, call the emergency services. The dispatcher can give you step-by-step instructions while the paramedics are on their way. Listen carefully. What they say may well contain the following advice, but always stick to their instructions.

Use a large plastic sheet to cover the lowest and firmest bed available, or clear a space on the floor. Find two or three clean sheets.

Find a blanket to keep the baby warm, clean towels, warm water for washing, sanitary napkins for the mother, disposable gloves and plastic bags.

Mother and baby are vulnerable to infection, so take all possible precautions to prevent its spread. Keep away anyone with a cough or cold. Wash your hands.

Check that the mother has removed any clothing that might obstruct the birth.

Wear gloves, and ideally change them whenever you have been in contact with potentially contaminated material, such as blood or feces.

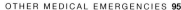

Managing diabetic conditions

SEE ALSO

➤ Responsiveness and the airway, p28

➤ The recovery position, p36

Diabetes is a condition in which the body cannot control sugar levels in the blood. This can create all kinds of symptoms, from excessive thirst to loss of consciousness. There are over 120 million people with diabetes worldwide. However, most of them are able to live normal lives because their diabetes is carefully controlled with insulin, drugs, and in some cases with diet alone. Since a diabetic crisis can be life-threatening it is important to recognize the signs of an impending episode and to take appropriate first-aid action.

People with diabetes mellitus have a problem with control of blood glucose. The body obtains glucose from sweet and starchy foods such as cakes, bread, and potatoes. The glucose is absorbed into the blood through the gut and provides fuel for all our body cells.

In people without diabetes, blood glucose levels are regulated by insulin, a hormone produced by the pancreas. Diabetes means the pancreas produces too little or no insulin. A diabetes sufferer's blood sugar levels are not controlled properly, which may cause symptoms that can develop into a crisis.

WHAT ARE THE TYPES?

There are two main types of diabetes mellitus – insulin-dependent (Type I, which accounts for 10–25 percent of cases) and non-insulin dependent (Type II, the remainder of cases). Type I usually develops before people reach the age of 40; Type II tends to begin after 40, often in people who are overweight.

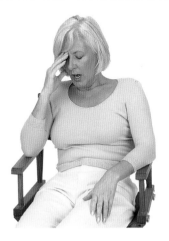

▷ Feeling very tired most of the time is a common sign of untreated diabetes.

SIGNS AND SYMPTOMS OF DIABETES

Type I diabetics become ill very quickly over several weeks. Type II diabetics may be symptom-free for many months or years before the condition is discovered. Symptoms include:

➤ Passing urine often, in large amounts.

➤ Exceptional thirst.

➤ Tiredness.

➤ Blurred vision.

➤ Weight loss, despite healthy appetite.

➤ Recurrent boils.

➤ Abscesses.

➤ Genital thrush.

▷ The pancreas is an elongated gland that secretes insulin. It actually lies just behind the stomach, but has been shown in front here so that it can be seen clearly.

LOCATION OF THE PANCREAS

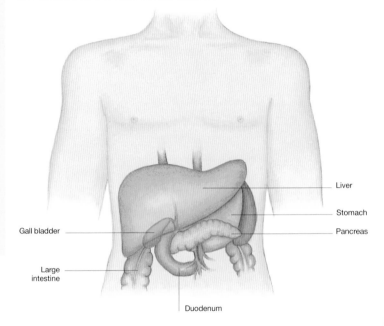

Liver

Stomach

Pancreas

Gall bladder

Large intestine

Duodenum

FIRST AID FOR HYPOGLYCEMIA AND HYPERGLYCEMIA

IF UNCONSCIOUS:
Follow DRSABC and call the emergency services. Do not try to give the person anything to eat or drink. If breathing, place in the recovery position and monitor breathing while waiting for help to arrive.

IF CONSCIOUS:
Help the person sit or lie down and loosen tight clothing. For hyperglycemia, call the emergency services. For hypoglycemia, give a sweet drink such as cola or fruit juice, or some squares of chocolate. Do not give "diet" or diabetic drinks of any kind. If the person responds, give more food or drink until they recover, then let them rest. If they do not respond, call the emergency services.

Do not administer insulin, if you find it on the person. If they are properly alert, they will take it themself. If not, look for clues about their condition so you can inform the emergency services: a medical ID tag/card, an insulin "pen", glucose tablets, medication, or a blood-testing kit.

CAUSES OF DIABETES

Both types of diabetes can sometimes run in families. Conditions that may lead to diabetes include obesity and disorders of glands such as the pancreas (pancreatitis, for example), the adrenals and the thyroid. However, very little is really known about the causes.

HOW IS DIABETES TREATED?

In both types of diabetes diet is crucial: high in complex carbohydrates (e.g. brown rice, wholemeal bread) and low in sugar and fat. It may help to lose weight, exercise regularly, and stop smoking, but always consult your doctor about diet and exercise first. Type I diabetes requires daily injections of insulin; Type II can often be controlled by diet alone, but sometimes tablets and occasionally insulin are needed.

WHAT CAN GO WRONG?

There are some long-term health risks associated with diabetes, but the only likely emergencies are hypoglycemia or, less commonly, hyperglycemia.

Hypoglycemia

This crisis, often called a "hypo" or "low", results from too little blood sugar. It can be caused by lack of food, too much exercise, shock, or stress, and can be so sudden that the person is unable to take the necessary action, (generally, eating some form of sugar). See Signs and Symptoms box.

Hyperglycemia

This results from too high a level of blood sugar, sometimes caused by too much food, forgetting to take tablets, or by a virus. It develops more slowly than hypoglycemia, except in children or with viruses, but is more difficult to treat and is likely to need medical attention. A viral illness unsettles the blood sugar balance, making a person with diabetes dehydrated, with abnormal levels of sodium and potassium and acid in the blood. This makes them very ill and may even lead to a coma. See Signs and Symptoms box.

SIGNS AND SYMPTOMS OF BLOOD SUGAR PROBLEMS

Hypoglycemia

➤ Rapid onset of symptoms.

➤ Hunger.

➤ Weakness/hand tremors/staggering.

➤ Feeling faint or dizzy.

➤ Sweating.

➤ Pale color.

➤ Strong. rapid pulse.

➤ Confused/aggressive/uncooperative/ uncharacteristic behavior that may be mistaken for being intoxicated.

➤ Slurred speech.

➤ Drowsiness; may become unconscious.

➤ Dry skin.

➤ Convulsions/fits are possible.

Hyperglycemia

➤ Extreme thirst.

➤ Dry skin.

➤ Rapid pulse.

➤ A smell of acetone (like nail-varnish remover) on the breath.

▽ Cola or fruit juice, a few squares of chocolate or a milky sweetened drink are good first-aid choices for hypoglycemia.

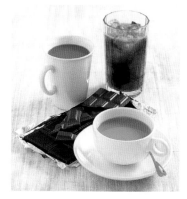

Dealing with nausea and vomiting

SEE ALSO
➤ Dealing with head injury, p80
➤ Coping with headache, p86
➤ ACTION ON POISONING, p185

Nausea and vomiting are common conditions that are usually short lived and have no serious consequences. They can arise from all kinds of causes, most commonly food poisoning, travel sickness, migraine, viral infection, allergic reaction, a drug side-effect, or pregnancy.

However, persistent nausea and vomiting may also be symptoms of a more serious condition, such as appendicitis, which will need to be investigated by a doctor. Prolonged vomiting can lead to dehydration, which can quickly become a medical emergency.

There are many causes of nausea and vomiting. Most of them are "self-limiting", which means they will settle without the need for further treatment or investigation. However, nausea and vomiting may be the beginning of a serious illness, and if they persist, or if dehydration sets in, the sufferer should be seen by a doctor.

CAUSES OF NAUSEA
Common reasons for nausea and vomiting include:
• Motion sickness.
• Migraine.
• Food poisoning.
• Viral gastroenteritis.
• Pregnancy.
• Drug side-effect.

More serious causes of nausea and vomiting, such as head injury, appendicitis, hepatitis, urinary tract infection, and bowel obstruction, will usually be accompanied by other symptoms such as headache, abdominal pain, yellow conjunctiva (whites of eyes), fever, frequent and burning urine, or abnormal bowel movements, which may range from loose and frequent to entirely absent for a few days.

TREATMENT FOR VOMITING
Urge the person to drink small sips of iced fluid, every 30 minutes or so, and to refrain from eating for 12 hours. When vomiting stops and the appetite returns, eat bland foods such as rice. If there are signs of dehydration, they need to see a doctor.

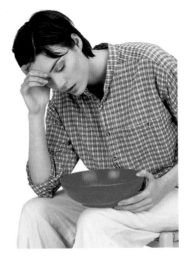

△ Seek immediate medical assistance if vomiting is accompanied by a headache that might be due to head injury.

▷ Encourage someone who is vomiting to drink a little plain water every half an hour in order to prevent any danger of dehydration.

SIGNS AND SYMPTOMS OF DEHYDRATION

Mild
➤ Headaches.
➤ Thirst.
➤ Dark urine.
➤ Dry, scaly-looking lips and tongue.

Moderate
➤ A fast pulse.
➤ No urine passed in over 24 hours.
➤ Breath smells of nail-varnish remover.
➤ Sunken eyes.

Severe
➤ The skin remains in folds even after letting go of a pinch.
➤ Drowsiness.

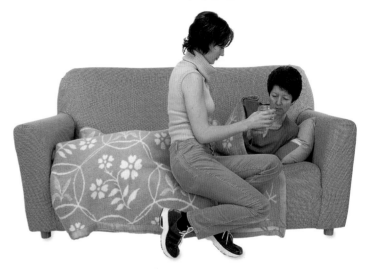

Tackling diarrhea, fever and cramp

SEE ALSO
➤ Dealing with nausea and vomiting, p98
➤ Dealing with abdominal pain, p100

Diarrhea is a common complaint that usually clears up on its own, although persistent cases should be investigated. Fever is usually a symptom of infectious illness. If the temperature is very high or persists, see a doctor. With fever and diarrhea, replacing fluid is all-important.

Cramp is another common problem, and one that may be exacerbated by fever (or any other factor that raises body temperature). Cramp spasms occur when muscle fibers over-contract. This often happens after exercise, due mostly to a build-up of lactic acid in the muscles.

DIARRHEA

Characterized by loose, frequent bowel movements, diarrhea usually gets better without treatment. It may be accompanied by vomiting, and is commonly caused by gastroenteritis, which may be viral or caused by contaminated foods – especially shellfish, meat, milk, or egg products – that have not been cooked properly or kept cool enough in storage. Diarrhea may occur in many other illnesses, from harmless conditions such as earache to bowel cancer. Even constipation can lead to diarrhea, as loose stools start to overflow the blocked-up bowel. Medical help should be sought if:

• Diarrhea persists beyond 7–10 days.
• The stools are blood-stained.
• Dehydration is developing.
• There is fever.
• There is persistent abdominal pain.
• It occurs in babies or young children.

FEVER

A raised temperature is a sign that the body is fighting infection or illness. It makes people feel tired and shivery, and they may have cold-like symptoms, feel nauseous, or even vomit. Other symptoms that often accompany fever include diarrhea and a burning sensation when passing urine.

It is useful to have a thermometer in your medicine cabinet, particularly if you have children. The most common methods for taking a temperature are: oral or under the arm, using a mercury or a digital thermometer; and with a digital strip that is placed on the forehead.

Acetaminophen brings down a temperature. Keep the person cool by sponging with lukewarm water or fanning. Increase fluid intake to make up that lost in sweating and protect against dehydration.

TAKING TEMPERATURE

Normal body temperature varies slightly depending on where, and at what time of day, it is taken:

Method	°F
Under arm	97.7
Oral	98.6

CRAMP

Cramp is usually felt at night when we are most immobile, and it happens most commonly in the calf muscles. Getting out of bed and walking around is the best way to relieve cramp, or try massaging the affected muscle or pulling the toes toward you as far as they will go.

Cramp occurs more often during pregnancy, and may also be a sign of serious circulation problems, particularly in older smokers. Anyone experiencing regular cramp when exercising, which is relieved by rest, should see a doctor.

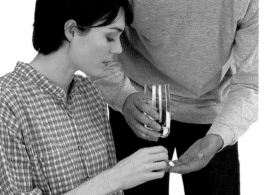

◁ Adults can be offered acetaminophen tablets or capsules, taken with water, to bring down a raised temperature.

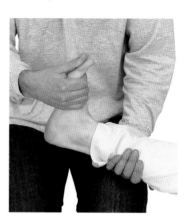

▷ In order to relieve calf muscle cramp, extend the leg through the pain and the cramp will disappear.

Dealing with abdominal pain

SEE ALSO

➤ Coping with antenatal emergencies, p92
➤ Dealing with nausea and vomiting, p98

Abdominal pain is one of the most common symptoms, with causes ranging from menstruation to appendicitis or even pneumonia. When helping someone with abdominal pain, you need first to ascertain the likely cause. Try to find out when the pain started, where it is sited and how severe it is. Accompanying symptoms, such as vomiting or vaginal bleeding, will help your assessment. Call a doctor if the pain is severe and prolonged, and if there is unexpected vaginal blood, or blood in the motions, vomit, or urine.

Of all the areas in the body, apart from the chest, the painful abdomen probably causes the most worry. Abdominal pain is very common in all age groups, and even recurrent pain may be due to completely benign and treatable causes.

In attending a person with abdominal pain, it is important to be able to make a distinction between a minor episode that will pass without any problems and a serious, possibly life-threatening, condition such as an ectopic pregnancy.

WHERE AND WHY ABDOMINAL PAIN ARISES

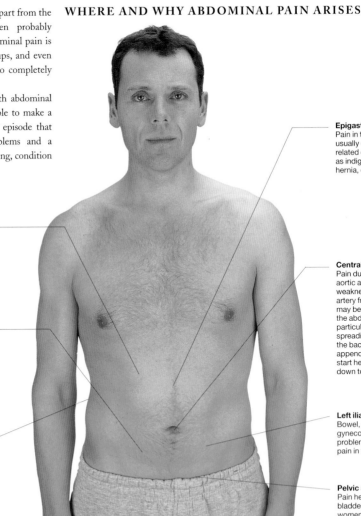

Epigastrium
Pain in this area is usually due to stomach-related conditions, such as indigestion, hiatus hernia, or peptic ulcer.

Right upper quadrant
The gallbladder, liver and pancreas lie in this area. Pain here is often due to gallstones or pancreatitis.

Central abdomen
Pain due to a rupturing aortic aneurysm (a weakness in the main artery from the heart) may be felt all over the abdomen, but particularly in this area, spreading through to the back. Pain from appendicitis may often start here and then move down to the right.

Right iliac fossa
This is typically where the pain of appendicitis is felt, although bowel, kidney and gynecological problems can cause pain here.

Left iliac fossa
Bowel, kidney or gynecological problems can cause pain in this region.

Right and left loin
This is where the kidneys lie, and pain from them is often felt here, spreading down to the lower pelvic areas.

Pelvic area
Pain here is often due to bladder problems or, in women, may have gynecological causes (including ordinary period pain).

ASSESSING ABDOMINAL PAIN

Before you start to consider what might be causing the abdominal pain, you should bear in mind the following considerations:

- Remember that the pain may not just be over a specific organ as it can be "referred" to other areas. This is especially true in appendicitis.
- Any woman of childbearing age with abdominal pain might be pregnant.
- Very ill or old people do not necessarily have a high temperature with serious causes of abdominal pain.
- People taking regular anti-inflammatory medication for arthritis or muscular pain can suffer perforation of their stomach with no pain at all. The first sign may be shock as they start bleeding internally.

CAUSES OF ABDOMINAL PAIN

It is not only the site of the pain that gives clues to its origins. Hollow organs such as the intestine and renal tract tend to cause pain that comes and goes in waves, rather like labor pains, and this is often called "colic". Pain due to peritonitis, where the membrane that lines the abdominal cavity becomes inflamed, is a constant, uninterrupted ache. Pains that occur around the time that the bowels open are usually due to a bowel-related problem.

SIGNS OF POTENTIALLY SERIOUS ABDOMINAL PAIN

- ➤ Nausea and vomiting.
- ➤ Diarrhea or constipation.
- ➤ Back pain.
- ➤ Shallow, fast breathing.
- ➤ Fever.
- ➤ Signs of developing shock – rapid pulse and sweaty, cold skin.
- ➤ A bulging or rigid abdominal wall.
- ➤ Tenderness on pressing the abdomen.
- ➤ A lump or mass in the abdomen.
- ➤ Any bleeding from the rectum, in the urine, or non-menstrual vaginal bleeding.

There may be other clues to the origin of the pain, such as symptoms relating to the kidneys (including a burning when passing urine and passing urine often or not at all).

The duration of the pain is important. Regular bouts of pain that settle after a few days may be due to irritable bowel syndrome or diverticulitis. Severe pain of sudden onset is more likely to be due to a serious condition such as appendicitis.

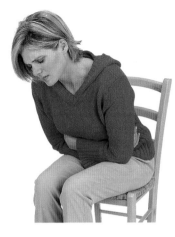

△ Always consider pregnancy as a possible cause of abdominal pain in any woman of childbearing age.

FIRST AID FOR ABDOMINAL PAIN

Have a receptacle within reach of the sufferer in case of vomiting.

GENERAL, NON-ACUTE STOMACH/ABDOMINAL ACHES:
Keep the sufferer comfortable and give them fluids little and often, rather than a glassful that may be vomited straight back. A hot-water bottle or heating pad placed on the painful area may ease the pain. If the pain does not settle, call a doctor.

ACUTE STOMACH/ABDOMINAL PAIN:
If there is severe or sudden acute pain, or pain accompanied by fever, call the emergency services. Give nothing to eat or drink with acute abdominal pain, and never apply heat if there is fever or acute pain (for example, applying heat to an inflamed appendix would be very dangerous).

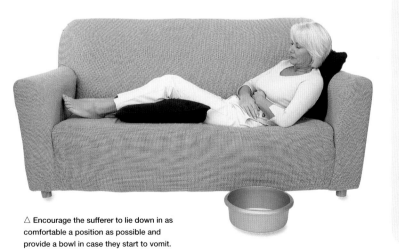

△ Encourage the sufferer to lie down in as comfortable a position as possible and provide a bowl in case they start to vomit.

Coping with allergy

SEE ALSO

➤ LUNGS AND
  BREATHING, p53
➤ Managing
  anaphylactic shock,
  p70
➤ Dealing with bites and
  stings, p104

Allergic responses may be minor or they may be severe. At worst, an allergen can cause anaphylactic shock, which demands immediate medical help to prevent serious illness and even death. People with allergic illnesses, such as asthma and eczema, are likely to develop allergic responses to other allergens. A relatively minor response on the first exposure may be followed by a much more dramatic response the next time. You should be familiar with the first aid necessary to assist the person and know how to prevent exposure in future.

The immune system is designed to protect us, but in allergy it works against us. Normally harmless substances, such as pollen or cat fur, are called allergens, because they can cause an allergic reaction if they come into contact with the immune system of a susceptible person. The immune cells act as if the allergens are dangerous invaders and the cells release damaging chemicals, such as histamine, in order to eradicate the invader. This causes allergic symptoms in the sufferer.

Once sensitized to a particular allergen, the immune system will react to it in every future contact. This may cause inflammation of the eyes, nose, throat, lungs, skin, or digestive system, causing a wide variety of symptoms from wheezing and running eyes to vomiting. The respiratory allergens such as pollen, dust and animal hairs tend to lead to fairly mild

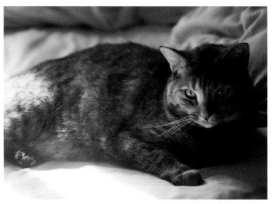

◁ Cats are well-recognized causes of allergic reaction, causing the sufferer to wheeze and sneeze within minutes of entering the same room.

reactions, while allergens such as penicillin or bee stings may be much more severe.

At worst, an allergic reaction can cause anaphylactic shock, with the risk of serious illness and death.

HOW TO SPOT AN ALLERGY

Allergic reactions vary depending on which part of the body is reacting to the allergen. Respiratory allergies tend to cause hay fever or asthma. Intestinal allergies can cause diarrhea and vomiting as well as stomach pain. Skin allergies may cause a rash called hives or urticaria, or result in dermatitis.

You may start to recognize a seasonal pattern to certain symptoms, or notice that they only happen when there is a cat in the house or when mowing the lawn. Certain blood tests can help identify if a reaction is allergic or not, but they cannot tell you

reliably what the allergen is. Skin prick tests are not very reliable, especially for food allergies.

FOOD ALLERGY OR INTOLERANCE?

Many people believe they have allergies to foods when, in fact, they have a food intolerance. A food intolerance is due to a lack of one or more of the digestive enzymes

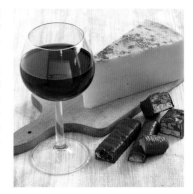

▷ These foods can produce a food intolerance reaction rather than an allergic reaction.

COMMON ALLERGENS

Almost any substance can be an allergen but these are the most common culprits:

➤ Foods – fish, shellfish, milk, nuts, eggs, chocolate, wheat, and soya.

➤ Antibiotics – penicillin, tetracycline.

➤ Other drugs, such as insulin.

➤ Venoms – wasp, bee, snake.

➤ Dust, pollens, and molds.

➤ Chemicals in plants.

➤ Iodine-containing dyes used in certain X-ray investigations.

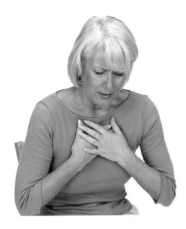

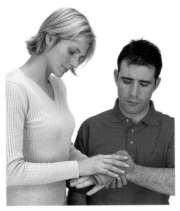

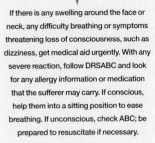

FIRST AID FOR ALLERGIC REACTION

If there is any swelling around the face or neck, any difficulty breathing or symptoms threatening loss of consciousness, such as dizziness, get medical aid urgently. With any severe reaction, follow DRSABC and look for any allergy information or medication that the sufferer may carry. If conscious, help them into a sitting position to ease breathing. If unconscious, check ABC; be prepared to resuscitate if necessary.

△ Coughing, a tight chest, and breathing difficulty may be potentially worrying signs of an allergy that is affecting the respiratory system.

△ Try using a wrapped ice pack, or a bag of frozen vegetables, to reduce the pain and inflammation of an insect sting or bite.

Try ice on swellings due to insect bites; scrape off the stinger and elevate the affected part in a high sling if possible.

that break down food, such as those that digest lactose or monosodium glutamate.

A true food allergy should be suspected if the person has repeated symptoms, such as abdominal pain, diarrhea, nausea, vomiting, and cramps, after eating a particular food. The only way to test for a food allergy is to follow an exclusion diet and reintroduce the excluded food to see if there is a recurrence of the symptoms.

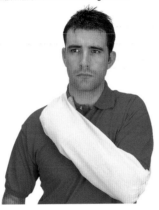

△ If you are dealing with an insect sting, elevate the affected part of the body in a sling if this is possible.

Antihistamines can be bought over the counter and may help with a nettle-type rash common in skin allergies. Use only on advice from a pharmacist.

Calamine lotion and ice are useful for itchy rashes or insect bite reactions.

KEEPING HOUSE-DUST MITES UNDER CONTROL

➤ Try not to have too many carpets in the house – floorboards, tiles, vinyl flooring or linoleum are healthier.

➤ Keep the house well ventilated and dust-free.

➤ Buy dust-resistant pillows and mattresses or mattress covers, or vacuum the mattress daily.

➤ Put soft toys into the freezer every six months to kill the house-dust mites.

➤ Avoid sheepskin underlays, as they attract house-dust mites.

➤ Use damp cloths rather than dusters for cleaning around the house.

Anti-allergy nose drops can be bought over the counter and can be useful for hayfever-type reactions.

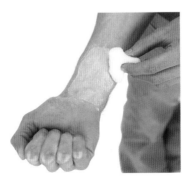

△ Calamine lotion is a cooling first-aid remedy for itchy rashes and insect bites.

In the long term, avoiding the allergen is the best option, as in not having pets or mowing the lawn early in the morning or in the evening when pollen is less troublesome.

Dealing with bites and stings

SEE ALSO

➤ What is first aid?, p12

➤ Dealing with breathing difficulties, p56

➤ Coping with allergy, p102

Domestic animals, insects, snakes, and sea creatures may all present a hazard either at home or when traveling. Any bite or sting is potentially dangerous, and however careful you are to avoid them, accidents happen. Dogs can inflict very nasty wounds, and in certain countries they may carry rabies; jellyfish and other sea creatures may inject poison; parrots and cats can produce wounds; and some people are allergic to bee and wasp stings. Knowing the correct first aid to administer in the event of an accident gives peace of mind.

Some basic knowledge of how to treat any problems arising from contact with poisonous snakes and insects can be particularly useful when you are traveling. Even bites and stings that are not venomous may cause infection or an allergic reaction.

HUMAN AND ANIMAL BITES

The most common way of sustaining a human bite is "in reverse", when one person punches another in the mouth, and teeth break the skin of their knuckle. The joint underlying this knuckle area usually becomes infected, and surgery may be needed to open it up and clean out the infection. Cat bites and scratches also often lead to infection, especially on the hand and face.

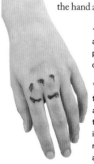

◁ Human bites need antibiotics, and possibly surgery, to clear any infection.

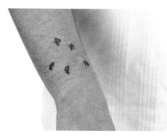

▽ A dog bite must be thoroughly cleaned and the question of tetanus (and rabies in certain countries) resolved with the attending doctor.

FIRST AID FOR A BITE

Clean the wound thoroughly with soap and water and dress with sterile gauze and bandage.

Seek medical assistance if there is any doubt about tetanus cover or if the bite is severe. A human bite on the hand or face will need antibiotic treatment.

Watch for swelling, redness and pain up to 48 hours after the bite, and go to the doctor for antibiotics if these symptoms develop.

SYMPTOMS AND SIGNS OF A VENOMOUS BITE

➤ Puncture marks in the skin.

➤ Feeling generally unwell.

➤ Lack of appetite.

➤ Abdominal pains.

➤ Rash, headache or fever.

➤ Muscle spasms.

➤ Joint pains.

WASP AND BEE STINGS

In a susceptible person, wasp and bee stings can cause an allergic reaction. Infections also commonly occur after stings. Suspect an allergy if there is heavy swelling, dizziness, fainting, difficulty breathing, nausea or vomiting, hives, or a tight throat or chest: take the sufferer to a doctor. If there are signs of anaphylactic shock, call the emergency services.

A bee may leave behind a sting attached to a poison sac. Do not squeeze the sac, but scrape it off carefully with a fingernail or blunt knife, and wash the area with soap and water. Place ice over the sting to reduce swelling and pain. Taking an oral antihistamine may be advised, in case an allergic reaction develops.

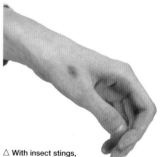

△ With insect stings, watch out for swelling, redness or pain, as this may indicate bacterial infection. Never squeeze a sting left in the skin as this will release more venom. Use a clean fingernail, blunt knife or credit card to scrape it off – carefully but decisively.

SNAKE BITES

Poisonous snakes release venom when they bite, which can cause pain and swelling, abdominal pain, vomiting and diarrhea. Dizziness due to blood pressure dropping may also occur, and the skin may become pale, cool, and increasingly sweaty, indicating that shock has occurred.

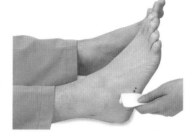

△ Stem bleeding from a bite using firm pressure with an absorbent dressing, ideally a gauze swab.

◁ Elevate the head and shoulders and splint the bitten part of the body. If the leg is bitten you can use the other leg as a makeshift splint.

FIRST AID FOR SNAKE BITE

Follow DRSABC. Do not bite, cut, squeeze, suck or apply ice or a tourniquet to the bite.

Calm the victim and keep them as still as possible, so the poison does not spread.

Call the emergency service or get the victim to medical help quickly. Identify the snake to the dispatcher so that the correct anti-venom can be prepared.

If you cannot get medical help or advice within 30 minutes, bandage the bitten part firmly, but not so tightly that it stops blood reaching or leaving the affected part. Splint the bitten part to rest it.

SEA CREATURES

Some marine animals can inflict damage, either by puncturing the skin with spines, or by injecting venom. Many of them are invisible as they blend with the sand and rocks, such as stingrays and stonefish. If you step on a spiny creature such as a sea urchin, the spines break off in the foot, causing pain. The embedded spines must be removed and wounds disinfected.

Lethal jellyfish are found in some parts of the world, notably in Australia. They inject a neurotoxin that stops muscles working, which leads swiftly to respiratory arrest and suffocation.

FIRST AID FOR A MARINE STING

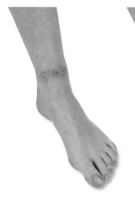

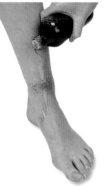

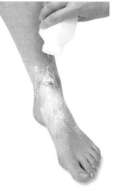

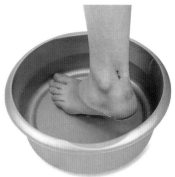

1 Get the victim out of the water as quickly as possible. Watch for problems with breathing, and start resuscitating if necessary.

2 Pour liberal amounts of vinegar or seawater onto a jellyfish sting to stop any further venom from being released.

3 Apply talcum powder to make any stinging cells stick together. Brush the powder off gently.

4 For a marine puncture wound, place the injured part in hot water for at least 30 minutes. Call the emergency services in case anti-venom is needed.

Managing heat and cold disorders

SEE ALSO

➤ Dealing with breathing difficulties, p56

➤ Dealing with shock, p68

➤ Dealing with nausea and vomiting, p98

It takes time for our bodies to get used to a different temperature. The brain controls our response to hot and cold conditions mainly by altering sweat production and the amount of blood circulating in the body. If it is not given sufficient time to adapt to excessive temperature change, we may become ill – sometimes dangerously so. Temperature disorders in which the sufferer overheats include heatstroke, heat exhaustion (which may lead to heatstroke) and heat cramps; extremes of cold can cause frostbite and hypothermia.

HYPOTHERMIA

Caused by cold conditions, hypothermia occurs when the body's core temperature drops below 95°F. It is most common:

• In a poorly heated home, particularly in infants, the elderly, and people who are frail, chronically ill or undernourished.

• In cold, exposed outdoor conditions, such as in mountainous regions, or at the scene of traffic accidents. Temperatures do not have to be freezing. It is more likely to occur in wet and windy conditions.

• During or after immersion in cold water.

The elderly are particularly vulnerable to hypothermia in the winter months: they may sit still for long periods, they may not be able to eat properly or heat their home sufficiently, and their metabolism is slower than that of a younger person.

Diagnosis can be difficult, and unconscious hypothermia sufferers may be mistaken for dead. However, due to the body's reduced need for oxygen when very cold, even prolonged resuscitation efforts have been successful.

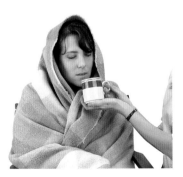

△ Give a shivering person a warm drink, such as sweetened tea. Do not give alcohol.

FIRST AID FOR HYPOTHERMIA

BASIC PRINCIPLES:
• Prevent further heat loss • Get urgent help • Rewarm the person gradually • Follow DRSABC

Keep the movement of the sufferer to a minimum, and very gentle. Sudden movement can cause heart problems.

IF OUTDOORS
Keep the victim in shelter. Replace wet clothing with dry, ideally warmed (e.g. from dry, warm bystanders). Cover the person's head and insulate them against cold from the ground. Wrap them in something warm such as a sleeping bag or plastic bags (leave the face uncovered), or ideally a survival bag.

IF INDOORS
Replace any cold, damp clothing. Rewarm gradually in a generally warm room by covering with layers of blankets.

If alert enough to eat/drink, give hot, sweet fluids (no alcohol) and a little high-calorie food. Do not apply direct heat (hot-water bottles or heaters), massage or rub the skin, or get the victim to exercise.

SIGNS AND SYMPTOMS OF HYPOTHERMIA

Mild – body temperature 95°F or less

➤ Sufferer feels very cold.

➤ Uncontrollable shivering.

➤ Stumbling, poor coordination, slurred speech, mild confusion, odd behavior.

Deep – body temperature 91.4°F or less

➤ No sensation of cold.

➤ Shivering stops.

➤ Drowsy, becoming unconscious.

➤ Breathing slows.

➤ There may be no detectable pulse.

HEAT EXHAUSTION

Due to excessive loss of water and salt from profuse sweating, heat exhaustion often occurs after heavy exercise and on hot days. If not treated promptly, heat exhaustion can prove fatal or develop into heatstroke.

SIGNS AND SYMPTOMS OF HEAT EXHAUSTION

➤ Occurs gradually over several hours.

➤ Body temperature may be normal, but may rise to 100.4–104°F.

➤ Headache, dizziness, tiredness, nausea.

➤ Cold, pale, clammy skin and sweating.

➤ A rapid, weak pulse.

➤ Feeling faint or actually fainting.

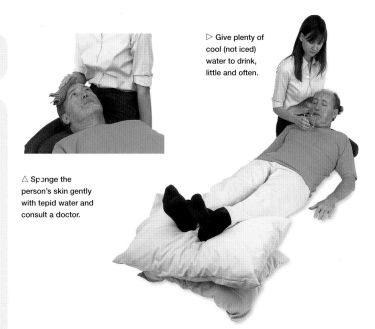

▷ Give plenty of cool (not iced) water to drink, little and often.

△ Sponge the person's skin gently with tepid water and consult a doctor.

FIRST AID FOR HEAT EXHAUSTION

Follow DRSABC and call the emergency services if necessary or if the condition seems worrying or severe.

Move the victim into a cool room with air-conditioning or a fan. Lay them down with their feet raised to improve blood flow to the brain. Sponge with tepid water until their temperature drops to 100.4°F.

Give plenty of cool water to drink. Follow this with an oral rehydration solution or make a salted drink by adding 1 teaspoon salt to 1 quart water and give half a cup every 15 minutes. Monitor their condition.

If the sufferer cannot drink because of nausea or vomiting, or there is no improvement after 1 hour, call the emergency services. A doctor should, in any case, be consulted after recovery.

HEATSTROKE

A very serious condition, heatstroke is often fatal. It may start as heat exhaustion, but if the body does not cool down, its heat-regulating mechanism fails, and body tissues start to heat up. Muscles and major organs begin to break down. Heatstroke tends to happen mainly in a very hot environment or with a fever.

Certain people are more vulnerable to heatstroke, such as the elderly, the disabled and infirm, those with diabetes, the obese, and alcoholics. Some drugs, especially antidepressants, diuretics, and sedatives, can increase susceptibility.

Dealing with heatstroke

A person suffering from heatstroke needs urgent medical attention. Call the emergency services without delay and, while waiting for them, follow these steps:
- Having followed DRSABC, move the person out of the sun to a cool place. Remove excessive clothes.
- Lay them flat unless they have heart problems. In this case, sit them up.
- Watch for breathing problems.
- Cool the person down but do not immerse them in water – this makes blood vessels in the skin shrink and so delays cooling. The best way to cool down

SIGNS AND SYMPTOMS OF HEATSTROKE

➤ Similar to heat exhaustion but with no sweating.

➤ Pulse is strong and rapid.

➤ Temperature is over 105.8°F.

➤ Sudden delirium, with confusion and agitation.

➤ Convulsions, coma and death.

a hot person is to spray their skin with water and then put them near a fan.

HEAT CRAMPS

These may happen after excessive exercise, or exercising in very hot weather. The muscle cramps occur as a result of loss of salt and water from sweating. People may also feel sick and dizzy. First-aid treatment involves moving the sufferer to a cool place and giving them fluids with added sugar.

PREVENTING HEAT PROBLEMS

Follow these important tips whenever you are in hot conditions:
- Stay in the shade and use air conditioning when it is available.
- Drink 9–10$\frac{1}{2}$ pints of fluid per day if sweating a lot in a hot climate or because of exercise or fever, and avoid excessive alcohol. (Normal daily fluid intake is 3$\frac{1}{2}$–5 pints; dark urine is an indication that you must drink more.)
- Avoid over-exertion and take frequent cool showers.
- Ensure adequate ventilation indoors.
- Wear a hat at all times when outside.
- Avoid going out when the sun is at its hottest – between 11 a.m. and 3 p.m.

SKILLS CHECKLIST FOR
OTHER MEDICAL EMERGENCIES

KEY POINTS

- Unusual symptoms in pregnancy should always be dealt with urgently ☐

- Always consider blood-sugar problems when the cause of collapse is unknown ☐

- Although usually self-limiting, nausea and vomiting can point to serious conditions ☐

- Consult a doctor for persistent or severe abdominal pain ☐

- Always seek rapid medical help in the event of a serious allergic reaction or snake bite ☐

SKILLS LEARNED

- What to do for collapse and bleeding in pregnancy ☐

- Assisting at the birth of a baby ☐

- Coping with a diabetic crisis ☐

- Dealing with sickness, diarrhea, fever, cramp and dehydration ☐

- Recognizing severe abdominal pain ☐

- Coping with allergic reactions and bites and stings ☐

- Dealing with temperature-related conditions: hypothermia and heatstroke ☐

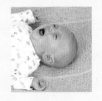

CHILDHOOD PROBLEMS

8

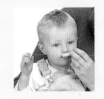

Babies and young children can deteriorate alarmingly quickly when they are ill. It is therefore wise to take seriously any symptoms they may have. Symptoms such as fever, vomiting, diarrhea, breathing difficulties, coughs, abdominal pain, and headache may be signs of routine, non-threatening childhood complaints, but they could signal something more serious. As a preventive measure, you should leave your child only with trusted and experienced family child care providers or at licensed preschools where you can be sure that your child will receive good care in the event of developing an illness.

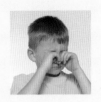

CONTENTS
Recognizing childhood illness 110–111
Dealing with problems in babies 112–113
Coping with fever 114
Dealing with vomiting and diarrhea 115
Managing abdominal pain 116–117
Coughs and breathing difficulty 118–119
Tackling headaches 120–121
Managing other problems 122–123
Skills checklist 124

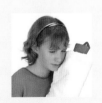

Recognizing childhood illness

SEE ALSO

➤ CHILDREN'S LIFE SUPPORT, p43
➤ Dealing with problems in babies, p112

Babies and young children can become seriously ill within a very short space of time. It is vital that the parents and any other carers are familiar with what is normal for that particular child and, therefore, know when something is wrong. Very often children are unable to articulate exactly what the problem is and so you have to be prepared to make an informed guess about the cause. Whenever you are in any doubt about the health of a child you should consult a doctor or go to the hospital immediately, no matter what time of day, or night, it is.

Children are not simply miniature adults – their bodies are different and respond differently to illness and trauma. The responses of a baby will differ to that of a toddler, and the responses of a 7-year-old or a teenager will differ too. Children may not be physically or emotionally able to articulate how or why they feel ill, or where it hurts. This is why it is always important to listen to their parents. Parents may not be certain of what the problem is either, but they know that "something is not right" with their child.

Doctors always find time to see children, as they know how difficult it can be to judge childhood illness, and that problems may develop rapidly. At the same time, being able to deal with the common, short-lived childhood illnesses and with emergency situations yourself may allow you to avoid seeking unnecessary medical help or to improve matters until further medical help is available.

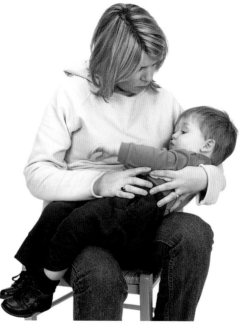

◁ The young sick child will probably be clingy and tearful. Look closely for any signs of illness.

▽ The sick child is usually unhappy and subdued, although they may be unable to explain exactly what is wrong.

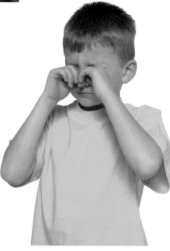

ASSESSING AN ILL CHILD

Children react differently to illness at different ages. So, a baby's small nasal passages and inability to mouth-breathe make a cold a very distressing experience that affects sleep and feeding, whereas an older child tolerates the symptoms more easily. There are, however, a few pointers to illness that apply more generally:

➤ How alert is the child? If they show interest in their toys and in people around them, this is a good sign. If they are slumped, silent, and inert in an adult's lap, you should be concerned.

➤ Look for rashes or abnormal skin color, for example a grayish pallor may indicate a very sick child.

➤ Identify any areas of pain. You can ask an older child where the pain is, but in babies and younger children you may have to use your intuition.

➤ Is there any restricted movement in the arms or legs? The child may be protecting an injured limb.

➤ Babies' cries can offer clues – a high-pitched cry is often a sign of illness.

RECOGNIZING A SERIOUSLY ILL CHILD

Children get seriously ill very quickly, and tend to recover as suddenly. Potentially worrying signs include:

➤ Altered consciousness: not engaging with people, unusually agitated or apathetic, drowsy, or unrousable.

➤ Breathing quickly, noisily or not at all.

➤ Gray/white/blue skin color.

➤ Sunken eyes, caked and dry lips and tongue that suggest dehydration.

➤ Weak pulse.

➤ Hot trunk and head but cold limbs.

➤ Pupils are unequal/do not react to light.

➤ Aversion to light.

➤ Stiff neck.

➤ Weak, high-pitched cry.

➤ No spontaneous movement.

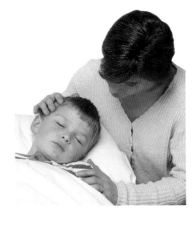

△ If the child is extremely apathetic and drowsy, consult a doctor immediately.

▷ If the child exhibits no sign of illness other than not being her usual self, then she may be unhappy. Childhood depression often goes unrecognized.

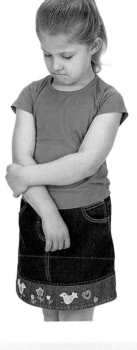

A REASSURING MANNER

Always try to calm a sick child – children soak up, and respond to, mood and atmosphere very readily. Being reassuring and friendly lessens their fear, which may, in turn, lessen their pain and distress. If you come across a situation where you are dealing with distraught parents as well as an ill child, the key thing is to put both the parents and the child at ease before attempting to examine the child. Chat calmly to the parents before addressing their child at all, and try to gather as much information about the situation as possible. Then keep the child occupied by playing and chatting quietly with them.

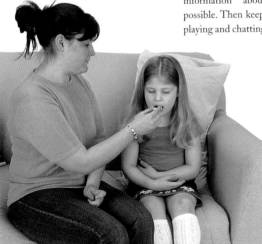

◁ Giving your child acetaminophen syrup is a good first line of treatment for any type of pain or feverish illness.

FIRST AID FOR A SERIOUSLY ILL CHILD

Follow DRSABC, and start to resuscitate if necessary. If unconscious but breathing, put in recovery position (hold those under 1 year in the babies' recovery position). The emergency services must be called.

If the ABC is adequate but the child is struggling to breathe, you must still call the emergency services. Sit the child up and keep them as calm as possible while waiting for help to arrive.

If breathing is adequate but your child is feverish, give them acetaminophen syrup and call your doctor for further advice.

Dealing with problems in babies

SEE ALSO

➤ CHILDREN'S LIFE
   SUPPORT, p43
➤ Recognizing
   childhood illness,
   p110
➤ Coping with fever,
   p114

Young babies commonly suffer from a number of problems, most of which are perfectly normal. Crying is a baby's main method of communication so a change in the pattern or type of crying may indicate that something is wrong. Parents soon become attuned to their infant's crying. Problems that commonly affect babies include feeding and sleeping difficulties, colic, diaper rash, and teething. Symptoms such as fever or diarrhea should never be attributed to minor baby problems: seek your doctor's advice if such symptoms develop.

New babies arrive after a long and sometimes seemingly endless nine months. It seems that there is ample time to prepare for their arrival, and yet so often these tiny, innocent beings arrive in their expectant households like miniature missiles. This is especially true for first-time parents, who before the birth can rarely see past the labor to the daily care routine beyond.

New babies don't know that they are meant to sleep at night and be more awake during the day. They have no routine – but their parents are often used to rigid schedules that they have stuck to for many years before their child's arrival. In the first few weeks, babies seem to do nothing but sleep, feed, and cry, in an entirely random way. It helps to know what to expect.

CRYING

A baby's cry has a remarkably unsettling effect on its parents, especially the mother. Other people may hardly notice the noise but the mother will find it very hard to ignore. There is a good reason for this, rooted in evolution. When a mother is breastfeeding, she is the only person who can feed the baby, and if their cries did not make her run to them, they would starve. Crying is a baby's only means of communication.

Most parents quickly recognize that their baby has different cries. Sometimes it will be the weak, "don't leave me" cry of the tired baby left to fall asleep in their crib; at others, the alarmed and heart-rending cry of the hungry baby. A very sick baby may have a high-pitched cry that sounds odd

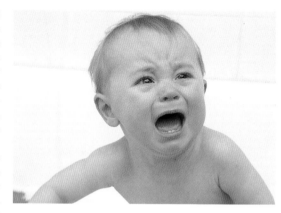

◁ The cry of a sick child is noticeably different to their normal cry. Parents can usually recognize a cry that is simply asking for cuddles or food.

and frightening, or may be too weak to cry at all. Some babies hardly seem to cry while others never seem to stop.

Babies cry for many reasons including hunger, tiredness, pain, colic, and dirty diapers. Babies differ in their tolerance of discomfort: some can have a filthy diaper and not fret at all, while others cannot bear even to be just a little wet.

▷ A colicky baby may cry inconsolably for many hours, but is not ill and feeds well.

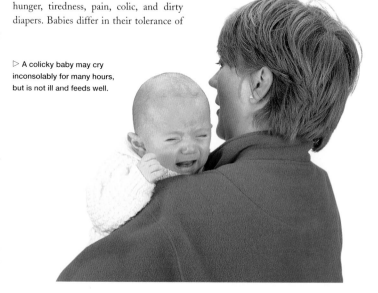

➤ Rock your baby gently or walk around with your baby either in your arms or in a baby sling.

➤ Put your baby into the baby carriage and wheel it around inside, or, if convenient, go out for a walk with the baby.

➤ Rub or massage your baby's abdomen and feet, following the path of the digestive system.

➤ Try giving your baby dimethicone drops 20 minutes before a feed.

➤ Dill, fennel and chamomile are age-old traditional herbal remedies for colic – look out for the special herbal preparations for babies that are now available.

➤ If you are breast-feeding, then you should try to rest during the day if at all possible – this will help to replenish your supply of milk, ready for the evening feeds.

➤ Making sure that you always drink plenty of fluids, and eat good, nutritionally balanced meals, will help to keep your milk supply going well.

▽ Diaper rash can be alleviated by regularly leaving the baby on a towel with no diaper, allowing the circulation of air.

COLIC

Characterized by very sudden attacks of stomach pain, colic causes infants to draw up their legs and cry inconsolably for several hours, day after day. No one knows what causes colic, which makes it rather difficult to treat. Colic often follows a definite pattern: it occurs at specific times of the day, usually in the evening, and it peaks at two to three months of age, improving or disappearing altogether by around six months.

Parents of colicky babies need to be reassured that there is nothing at all wrong with their child; and they will often need emotional support, or someone else to look after the baby for awhile.

RASHES

Babies often have blotchy skin when they arrive, and a few weeks out of the womb, their skin often becomes dry and spotty.

Milia

These little white "milk spots" appear round the nose of a newborn's face. They usually disappear after a few weeks.

Diaper rash

Babies have very sensitive skin, and so it is not surprising that it sometimes becomes sore from contact with urine and feces.

To reduce the likelihood of diaper rash occurring, always change your baby if the diaper is dirtied or wet. Using a liberal application of a barrier cream at each change helps protect the skin. Also, give your baby some time, after a bath or during the day, when they are without a diaper.

When a baby is teething or ill, especially with diarrhea or fever, they are much more susceptible to diaper rash. Be aware of this and make sure you do not delay changing their diaper.

If there are little red and white spots either within or outside the general rash area (yeast diaper rash), the baby may have thrush. Over-the-counter creams are available for this condition.

PREVENTING DIAPER RASH

➤ Use a barrier cream on the diaper area all the time – such as petroleum jelly or zinc oxide cream.

➤ Try to use only water for cleansing in the early weeks, as the skin may react to wipes or lotions.

➤ Change diapers regularly, rather than waiting for them to start leaking through clothes.

➤ If a baby's skin is beginning to look a little red, try leaving them on a towel without a diaper for a while. This will allow some air to circulate around the area.

TEETHING

Some babies cut their teeth with very little fuss, while others seem to have a lot of trouble. The incisors at the front of the mouth usually arrive fairly painlessly around 6 months, but the bigger teeth at the back (molars), which arrive later, can cause a lot of upset.

Rubbing the gums with special teething gel and giving liquid acetaminophen may help. For some babies, biting on a hard object, such as a special teething ring, can help to relieve the pain.

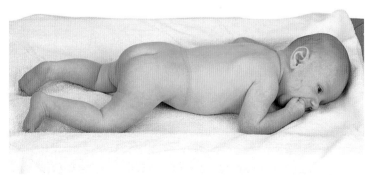

Coping with fever

SEE ALSO

➤ Recognizing childhood illness, p110

➤ Dealing with problems in babies, p112

Fever is usually a sign of infection – although it can be caused by immunization or being overdressed or in an overheated room – and there is a risk that it can lead to seizures in young children. Try simple ways of bringing the temperature down first – such as removing clothing and bedding and reducing the room temperature. Sponge the child's skin with tepid water and perhaps give acetaminophen. Keep a look-out for other symptoms that might give a clue as to the cause of a fever, and always call a doctor if you are concerned.

For many of us, the fear of fever in a child stems from the worry that the child will have a seizure if we cannot bring the fever down. There is also the worry about what might be causing the fever.

A child's temperature often rises for up to 24 hours or even longer with no other obvious signs of infection, such as an earache, a sore throat, or an ordinary cold. In many ways, it is reassuring when the first signs of a runny nose and cough appear, as the cause of the temperature then becomes obvious.

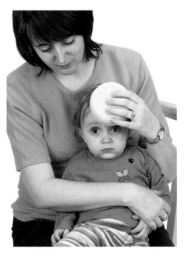

△ A feverish child will benefit from gentle sponging with tepid water.

NORMAL TEMPERATURE

Under arm/forehead	97.7°F
Oral	98.6°F

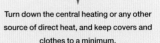

FIRST AID FOR A CHILD WITH A FEVER

Turn down the central heating or any other source of direct heat, and keep covers and clothes to a minimum.

Give your child acetaminophen syrup (never aspirin) to bring down their temperature. Babies under 3 months should not have acetaminophen unless your doctor advises it.

Sponge the child's body and forehead with tepid water. Avoid using a fan – it may make them shiver, which will generate even more heat.

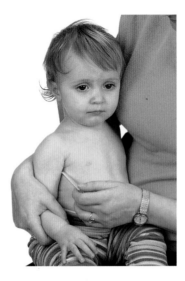

△ A digital strip thermometer on the forehead is the easiest way to take a baby's temperature.

▷ You can take a child's temperature using a conventional thermometer under the arm.

DANGER SIGNS AND SYMPTOMS

➤ Infant under 3 months old.

➤ Fever over 104°F.

➤ Infant refusing feeds.

➤ A rash that does not disappear when a glass is pressed on it.

➤ Fever persists over 48 hours without any obvious source of infection.

Dealing with vomiting and diarrhea

SEE ALSO
➤ Recognizing
  childhood illness
  p110
➤ Dealing with
  problems in babies
  p112

Extremely common symptoms in babies and children, diarrhea and vomiting usually clear up quickly without any special treatment. Viral gastroenteritis and food intolerance are common causes. If diarrhea and/or vomiting is profuse and persistent there is a danger of dehydration, particularly in babies and very young children. It is important to make sure the child drinks plenty of clear fluids for the duration of the illness. If other symptoms develop or there is no improvement after 48 hours, you should seek a doctor's advice.

DEHYDRATION DANGER

What cannot be stressed enough with these childhood complaints is that babies and children are more prone to dehydration than adults because they are less able to replace fluid losses.

BABIES

Vomiting and diarrhea without a serious cause occur quite often in babies because their digestive systems are still immature.

A small amount of vomiting after feeding is perfectly normal. Some babies are prone to bringing up a lot of their feeds each time, which is worrying only if the baby is not gaining weight. Babies may vomit as a sign of a general infection.

You should ask for medical advice about:
• Sudden onset of vomiting.
• Unwell baby with a fever.
• Green-stained vomit.
• Projectile vomiting.
• Signs of dehydration.
Breast-fed babies have runny, bright yellow stools that smell like soft cheese; babies on formula often have dark green, liquid bowel motions. Diarrhea is different – watery, frequent, and often foul-smelling stools.

OLDER CHILDREN

There are many causes of vomiting and diarrhea in children, but the most common is viral gastroenteritis. Although this will get better without treatment, dehydration may develop if the child does not drink enough. Encourage your child to drink clear, diluted fluids and avoid fizzy and milk-based drinks. An alternative is to use oral rehydration sachets, which can be bought from the pharmacist.

▽ A child who is vomiting may be drowsy and listless. Take the child's temperature and consult your doctor if you are worried.

FIRST AID FOR A BABY WITH VOMITING AND/OR DIARRHEA

Stop formula feeds for 12 hours. Give rehydration fluids from the pharmacist, then try half-strength formula feeds.

↓

If breast-feeding, do not stop, but include bottles of water between feeds.

↓

Continue to give regular feeds, and seek medical help if the problem persists for more than 48 hours or if you are worried.

FIRST AID FOR A VOMITING CHILD

Give sips of fluid to the child in small amounts, and at frequent intervals. This way, the fluid is more likely to stay in the stomach.

↓

If they feel feverish, try giving them some acetaminophen.

↓

Keep them off food while they are vomiting. Once it settles, try bland foods such as rice, soup, and bread.

SIGNS AND SYMPTOMS OF DEHYDRATION

➤ The soft spot on top of a baby's head becomes sunken.

➤ The eyes become sunken and hollow-looking.

➤ The lips are parched and the tongue is dry.

➤ Urine production falls. A baby's diaper may remain dry all day.

➤ They may be drowsy and listless.

➤ The pulse is raised.

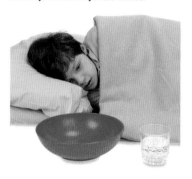

Managing abdominal pain

SEE ALSO

➤ Coping with fever, p114

➤ Dealing with vomiting and diarrhea, p115

Abdominal pain is a very common symptom in young children, and it is usually short-lived. It can occur for a wide range of reasons, which may or may not affect the digestive tract. Children tend not to suffer from indigestion, but anxiety and even migraine can cause stomachache. However, there are a few serious conditions that require immediate medical attention, and you should be alert for other symptoms that might signal such a situation. If you have any doubts, you should always consult a doctor immediately.

Children often complain of stomachache, but the pain will usually disappear spontaneously. Even children admitted to hospital with stomach pain are often sent home with no definite diagnosis. Children often experience physical symptoms as a result of unhappiness or anxiety. For example, a child who complains of recurring stomach pain may have problems at school or at home.

CAUSES OF ABDOMINAL PAIN

In children, abdominal pain is often not connected with the digestive system and may have causes such as a twisted testis or migraine, which in young children tends to affect the stomach rather than the head.

Urinary tract infections, which are particularly common in girls, can cause abdominal pain. Even a general infection, such as a cold or flu, might give a child a stomachache – this is due to the glands swelling in their abdominal cavity as well as the head and neck area.

The type of pain and its location often give valuable clues to what might be causing it, but it is often difficult for a child to describe the pain accurately or to tell you exactly where it is situated. Accompanying symptoms, such as fever, diarrhea or vomiting, can help to narrow down the possible causes but you should never hesitate to contact your doctor if you are at all concerned.

FIRST AID FOR A CHILD WITH ABDOMINAL PAIN

Try to find out exactly where the pain is and when it occurs. Is the pain there all of the time or does it relate to opening the bowels or urinating?

Do not give the child any medicines or anything to eat or drink.

A wrapped hot-water bottle placed on their stomach can be extremely comforting.

If the child is vomiting or is suffering from diarrhea, then they should avoid solid foods for 12–24 hours. Give them small amounts of fluid at frequent intervals.

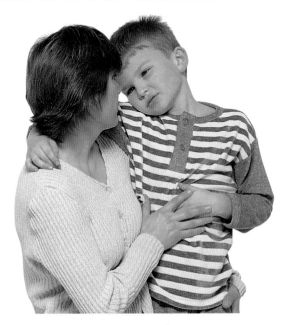

◁ Talk to your child to try to assess whether the abdominal pain has an emotional rather than a physical cause.

PAINFUL CONSTIPATION

If you have never seen the distress that constipation – passing infrequent hard stools – causes in a baby, this may seem an odd condition to discuss in a first-aid book. However, it is one of the commonest causes of abdominal pain in children, and it is very useful to be aware of this fact.

A baby who screams and strains at the same time, while drawing up their knees, may be constipated. They may pass very hard, pellet-like stools or not have any bowel movements for a few days. It often happens briefly when babies who are bottle-fed change to a formula designed for older infants. A baby who has had bowel difficulties from birth may have a problem with the nerves that supply the gut – this is known as Hirschsprung's disease. It is a serious condition that always requires surgical treatment.

Constipation may begin to be a problem during potty training. Parents should be aware that this can impede the learning process, as it is obviously unpleasant for the child – a situation to look out for and handle carefully. A child might also pass one large, hard motion that tears their anus. If they then start holding onto their stools to avoid pain, this could set up a vicious cycle which may eventually lead to the child being unable to control their bowel motions and soiling themselves. Plenty of fluids and gentle laxatives are needed to stop this scenario from developing – the earlier the better.

WHEN TO CALL THE DOCTOR

Call the doctor if a child's abdominal pain is accompanied by any of these symptoms:

➤ Sudden, severe pain that does not settle, usually in the lower right abdomen.

➤ A swollen abdomen.

➤ Vomiting.

➤ Signs of dehydration such as dry lips and mouth, no urine passed for several hours, noticeably sunken eyes.

➤ A lump in the stomach.

➤ Pain that has lasted intermittently for 24 hours and is getting worse.

APPENDICITIS

The appendix is a tiny tube attached to the intestine that may become blocked and inflamed. Children of all ages can develop appendicitis. Pain often starts around the navel, and after a few hours shifts to the lower right-hand side of the abdomen, where the appendix is sited. The child may vomit, lack appetite, or have a fever and bad breath. There is a danger of perforation, so if you think appendicitis is a possibility you should seek a doctor's advice or go to the hospital without delay.

INTUSSUSCEPTION

Usually occurring between the ages of 3 months and 2 years, intussusception must be treated as an emergency. The cause is unknown, but the result is that a section of intestine folds into itself, like the sleeve of a sweater. The child will be in severe pain and highly distressed. Vomiting may occur and a red, jelly-like stool may also be passed. If any of these symptoms occur, you must call the emergency services right away.

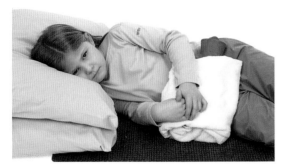

◁ A wrapped hot-water bottle placed on the child's stomach can be comforting and may also relieve the pain.

WARNING

Call the emergency service if your child has any of the following symptoms:

➤ Pain that has lasted continuously for over 6 hours.

➤ Pain in the groin or testes.

➤ Greenish-yellow vomit.

➤ Red material in the feces.

Coughs and breathing difficulty

SEE ALSO

➤ CHILDREN'S LIFE SUPPORT, p43

➤ Recognizing childhood illness, p110

➤ Dealing with breathing difficulties, p56

Colds and coughs are very common in young children but they are not usually a cause for concern, and home remedies can generally provide relief. Occasionally, however, a child may experience severe difficulty in breathing: this constitutes an emergency, and you should call the emergency service immediately. Causes of breathing difficulty range from asthma to choking, and some childhood infections, such as bronchiolitis. Breathing difficulty can be life-threatening and is alarming for both parent and child; never hesitate to call for help.

Children's air passages are smaller than adults', and so they are more likely to become blocked. A child can be unwell with a cough and a runny nose, but this is seldom likely to lead to any serious breathing problems. However, some conditions can lead to sudden breathing problems that may require first aid or emergency medical treatment.

COUGH

All too common in childhood, coughs and colds are rarely serious. Sometimes the type of cough may give clues to what is causing it. A barking cough and hoarse voice is characteristic of croup, a viral infection affecting the larynx and vocal chords. It usually occurs at night. The noise can be very alarming, sounding somewhat like a seal barking, but you should stay calm as alarming the child will make the attack worse. Humidifying the atmosphere with steam can help.

A cough that comes in paroxysms so that at the end of the coughing fit, the child has to take such a deep breath that they make a "whooping" noise, is characteristic of whooping cough. Vomiting with the coughing is common . This condition is less common since the advent of the whooping cough vaccine.

NOISY BREATHING

Children may make all sorts of noises when they breathe, but this does not always indicate difficulties with breathing. Some types of noise may help to pinpoint what the problem is likely to be.

Wheezing

Usually heard when a child breathes out, wheezing is a rather musical noise, often said to be similar to a seagull's cry. Most people associate wheezing with asthma, but wheezing can also be due to viral infections, principally a viral infection called bronchiolitis. This is mostly seen in infants under 1 year and may require hospital admission if they have feeding problems, but is usually self-limiting. They may go on to develop asthma, but many do not.

Noisy in-breaths

A harsh noise made as a child breathes in ("stridor") comes from the upper airways. It is caused by the airways being blocked or narrowed. Croup causes this type of noise, but it may also be due to inhaling a foreign body or very rarely due to a bacterial infection called epiglottitis.

TIPS FOR TACKLING CHILDREN'S COUGHS

➤ Use a humidifier or boil some pans of water to create a steamy atmosphere in the kitchen, or take the child into the bathroom and run the hot faucet or shower. Do this twice an hour if necessary.

➤ Place a wet towel on a warm radiator to humidify the air in a bedroom.

➤ Menthol and eucalyptus oil added to a bowl of warm water, or on the pillow or sheets, can help to ease a cough caused by an infection.

➤ Never smoke in the house.

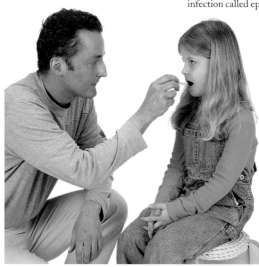

◁ Giving your child liquid acetaminophen can help reduce a fever and may make them feel much better.

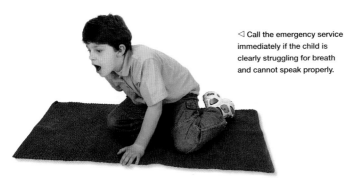

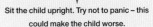

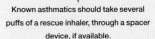

◁ Call the emergency service immediately if the child is clearly struggling for breath and cannot speak properly.

Grunting

This noise can indicate serious breathing difficulties in a baby, and often pneumonia in an older child.

Snuffling

Babies will often snuffle when they have a cold. They then find it difficult to sleep and feed, which disturbs both them and their parents. However, most babies manage to find a way over this temporary problem without too much difficulty.

▽ If your child is on asthma medication and they start to cough or wheeze, they should use a quick-relief "rescue" inhaler to dilate the airways, preferably using a spacer device to assist uptake of the drug.

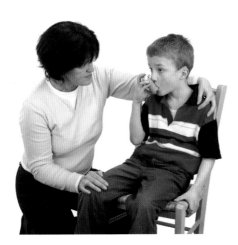

ASTHMA

Childhood asthma can be hard to recognize – for example, it often shows itself as sudden coughing fits or night-time coughing rather than wheezing. Children with asthma may cough, wheeze and, in severe attacks, have extreme breathing problems that require hospitalization. As asthma is potentially life-threatening it is essential to recognize the symptoms that need hospital treatment.

A child who has been diagnosed with asthma will have one or more inhalers, which normally keep the condition well controlled. Occasionally, maybe in the summer when the pollen count is high or if the child has a bad cold, the asthma does not respond to the normal treatment and breathing difficulties develop. This may mean that it is necessary to make a reassessment of the medication that the child is taking.

An asthmatic child with obvious breathing difficulties can become seriously ill very rapidly, so never hesitate to call the emergency services or take them to the hospital.

FIRST AID FOR SEVERE BREATHING DIFFICULTY

Sit the child upright. Try not to panic – this could make the child worse.

Known asthmatics should take several puffs of a rescue inhaler, through a spacer device, if available.

Call a doctor or the emergency services, depending on the severity of the problem.

WARNING

Call the emergency services immediately if:

➤ Breathlessness and noisy breathing start suddenly, especially after choking.

➤ Breathing is so labored that a baby or child is unable to feed/eat or drink.

➤ The child cannot speak in proper sentences or even utter sounds.

➤ The child is drowsy or confused.

➤ There is a visible "sucking in" of the rib cage as they breathe in and out.

➤ The child stops breathing altogether for more than a few seconds.

➤ The lips turn blue.

Specific asthma danger signs:

➤ Too breathless to speak or feed/eat.

➤ Breathing rate over 50 breaths/minute.

➤ Pulse over 140/minute.

➤ Blue lips.

➤ Very wheezy chest turning into no wheezing – no air is getting through.

➤ Fatigue/exhaustion.

➤ Drowsiness/agitation.

Tackling headaches

SEE ALSO

➤ Recognizing childhood illness, p110

➤ Coping with fever, p114

Headaches are a very common complaint in childhood. Usually, the headache passes quickly without the need to consult a doctor. Often a headache can signal the beginning of a childhood infectious illness, so look out for other symptoms. Occasionally, a headache can be a sign of a serious condition, such as meningitis, that requires urgent medical help. On the other hand, a headache may have its root in something as simple as a child having stayed out a little too long in the sun or not having drunk enough fluid.

Because most children often complain of having a headache, the difficulty is knowing when to worry about it and seek help, and when to assume it has a self-limiting cause and will settle down by itself. Younger children obviously may not be able to articulate that they have a headache, but their actions may suggest it, for example they may dislike having their head moved, or be very irritable when moved at all, or they may be very sensitive to bright light or noise.

COMMON TYPES AND CAUSES OF HEADACHES

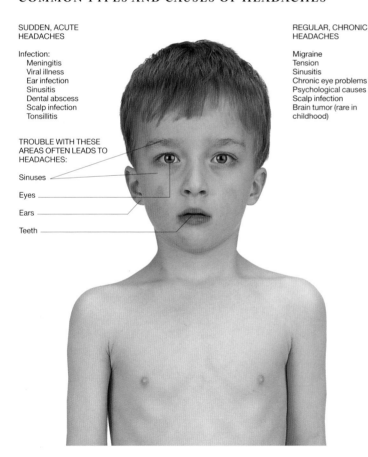

SUDDEN, ACUTE HEADACHES

Infection:
 Meningitis
 Viral illness
 Ear infection
 Sinusitis
 Dental abscess
 Scalp infection
 Tonsillitis

TROUBLE WITH THESE AREAS OFTEN LEADS TO HEADACHES:

Sinuses

Eyes

Ears

Teeth

REGULAR, CHRONIC HEADACHES

Migraine
Tension
Sinusitis
Chronic eye problems
Psychological causes
Scalp infection
Brain tumor (rare in childhood)

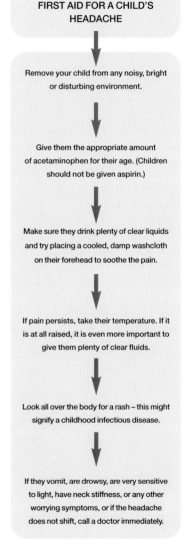

FIRST AID FOR A CHILD'S HEADACHE

⬇

Remove your child from any noisy, bright or disturbing environment.

⬇

Give them the appropriate amount of acetaminophen for their age. (Children should not be given aspirin.)

⬇

Make sure they drink plenty of clear liquids and try placing a cooled, damp washcloth on their forehead to soothe the pain.

⬇

If pain persists, take their temperature. If it is at all raised, it is even more important to give them plenty of clear fluids.

⬇

Look all over the body for a rash – this might signify a childhood infectious disease.

⬇

If they vomit, are drowsy, are very sensitive to light, have neck stiffness, or any other worrying symptoms, or if the headache does not shift, call a doctor immediately.

WHEN IS A HEADACHE SERIOUS?

Your child's behavior and distress level can indicate how serious the headache is, but you should always seek medical advice in the following circumstances:

➤ If the pain comes on suddenly.

➤ If it is accompanied by vomiting, irritability, fever, drowsiness, rash, and/or neck stiffness.

➤ If the headache lasts longer than 24 hours.

➤ If the headache is recurrent and starts early in the morning.

➤ If headaches are becoming increasingly severe and more frequent.

➤ If the pain is not relieved by simple, over-the-counter painkillers.

➤ If the headache immediately follows an accident.

➤ If the headache occurs some hours after the child has suffered a bump on the head.

▷ The meningitis rash caused by meningococcal bacteria has a dark red/blue, paint-speckled look. Test for it by pressing a clear glass against the rash to see if it fades. If you can still see the rash through the glass, call the emergency services.

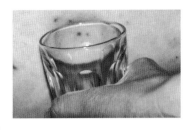

MENINGITIS

A headache can be a sign of meningitis – an infection of the linings covering the brain that is caused by either a bacterium or a virus. It is very worrying for all parents, and difficult to recognize, as it may resemble other, lesser infections.

While a headache is often a principal symptom of meningitis, other signs – such as high fever, drowsiness, neck stiffness, light sensitivity, and/or profuse vomiting – may be more obvious. A child who has been mildly unwell and then worsens should be examined by a doctor. In bacterial meningitis, there may be a characteristic rash, but this is one of the later symptoms. (Babies with any kind of meningitis may just be non-specifically unwell and do not generally suffer from neck stiffness.)

A WORD ON RASHES

Children often develop rashes when they are unwell. As well as meningitis, infections such as chicken pox, measles, and German measles have a specific rash that helps diagnose the condition. Many unspecific viral infections cause a child to have a rash, often as their temperature settles and they improve. Drug allergies may cause rashes that resemble nettle stings.

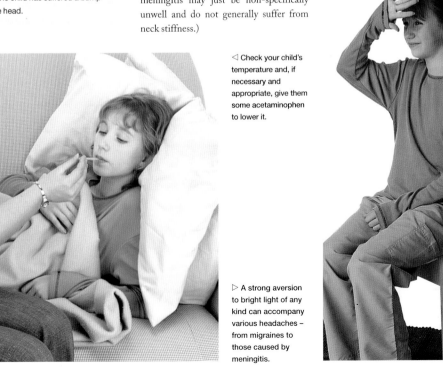

◁ Check your child's temperature and, if necessary and appropriate, give them some acetaminophen to lower it.

▷ A strong aversion to bright light of any kind can accompany various headaches – from migraines to those caused by meningitis.

Managing other problems

SEE ALSO

➤ Recognizing childhood illness, p110

➤ Coping with fever, p114

➤ Managing abdominal pain, p116

Children's immature immune systems make them very susceptible to a range of minor infections, such as earache and sore throat. It is not uncommon, particularly during the winter, for children to have endless colds and other infections, but these are rarely of an emergency nature and can be dealt with safely at home. Toothache tends to affect older children; it is important to look after teeth from babyhood to prevent tooth decay later. If your child is feeling feverish and generally unwell, do not overlook the possibility of a urinary tract infection.

Children are more prone than adults to mild infectious illnesses, probably because their immune systems are still developing and they have countless opportunities to pick up infections from other children. Sometimes these illnesses have serious consequences, such as short-term deafness or lots of time off school, but for the most part, they are minor, self-limiting problems that can be treated at home.

EARACHE

Practically every child has an earache at some stage during a normal year. It often starts after a cold, the pain from the earache being caused by a build-up of infection behind the eardrum – a condition called otitis media. Pus builds up behind the drum, causing an unbearable increase in pressure that may be relieved when the eardrum finally bursts and lets the pus out. Antibiotics are prescribed for such severe cases. Earache may also be caused by an infection in the outer ear canal, a toothache that is radiating out to the ear, or a foreign body in the ear. It can also accompany tonsillitis.

Sometimes a thick, gluey fluid remains in the ear after otitis media and makes the child temporarily deaf for up to six months. Your doctor may examine the ear six weeks after the otitis media, and refer the child to an ear, nose and throat specialist if further treatment is necessary.

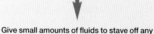

FIRST AID FOR A CHILD WITH EARACHE

Try giving your child acetaminophen syrup – it is very effective at relieving earache pain.

Give small amounts of fluids to stave off any mild dehydration that can worsen the pain.

Give the child a wrapped hot-water bottle to hold against the ear – it is comforting and pain-relieving.

Prop up the child with pillows or cushions – this may be more comfortable.

WHEN TO SEE A DOCTOR IF YOUR CHILD HAS EARACHE

These are the main pointers for when to seek expert advice:

➤ If the child has a high fever, especially if the fever lasts for longer than about 24 hours.

➤ If there is fluid or blood coming out of the ear.

➤ If the child is not drinking, or is generally unwell.

➤ If there is any deafness.

▽ Liquid acetaminophen is usually a highly effective way for a parent to relieve pain caused by earache or a sore throat.

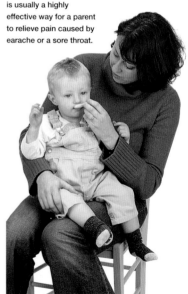

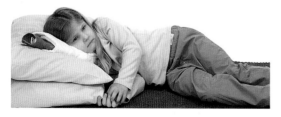

◁ Lying with the affected ear against a wrapped hot-water bottle may help to ease earache pain.

TOOTHACHE

Toothache may be due to an infected tooth, in which case the pain is often throbbing and there may be obvious swelling around the gum area. It may settle by itself, but if it lasts longer than 24 hours the child should see a dentist.

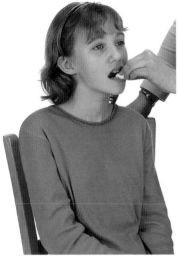

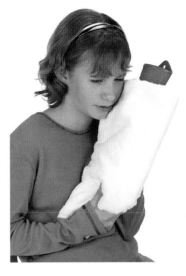

FIRST AID FOR TOOTHACHE

↓

Give your child acetaminophen syrup.

↓

Unless an abscess is suspected, try placing a wrapped hot-water bottle against the cheek where the tooth can be felt.

↓

Soak a small roll of gauze in oil of cloves and hold it against the painful tooth.

↓

Arrange for the child to see a dentist as soon as possible.

△ Try soaking a small roll of gauze in oil of cloves and placing this on the offending tooth – it is an effective pain-reliever and is anti-flammatory.

△ Another good way to relieve the pain of toothache is to hold a wrapped hot-water bottle against the cheek (but not if an abscess is suspected).

SORE THROAT

Most sore throats in children are caused by self-limiting viral infections and can be helped simply by giving your child acetaminophen syrup and plentiful fluids. Unless the child cannot swallow fluids or is very hot and unwell, they will usually get better after a few days without needing to see a doctor. However, do keep watch for a high temperature.

URINARY TRACT INFECTIONS

Children can also develop infections in their urinary tract. The problem with a urinary infection is that it could be a sign of an abnormal kidney system. If it is not detected and treated immediately with antibiotics, the infection may also cause scarring of the kidney system and, ultimately, over a long period of time, kidney failure.

Babies and young children may not seem to have any urine-related symptoms but just be unwell with a fever, vomiting, diarrhea, and feeding difficulties. If a child is hot and unwell for a few days with no other obvious cause for the fever (such as a cold, cough, or runny nose), they may have a urinary tract infection. The doctor will take a sample of urine for culture and analysis to tell if there is any infection.

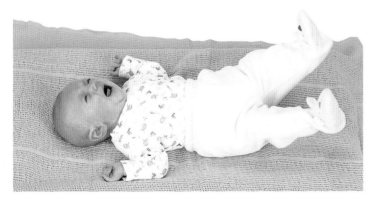

◁ Sore throats can be hard to diagnose in babies. A doctor may be able to tell by shining a light into the back of the throat while the baby is crying.

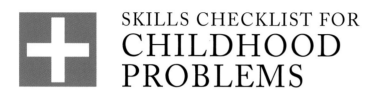

SKILLS CHECKLIST FOR
CHILDHOOD
PROBLEMS

KEY POINTS

- Babies' and children's bodies function differently from those of adults ☐

- A baby or child can become seriously ill very rapidly – within the space of a few hours ☐

- Always be on the look-out for dehydration ☐

- If in doubt about a baby's or child's health, consult a doctor immediately ☐

- If abdominal pain, headache, or breathing problems in a young child do not resolve quickly, get help; always seek help urgently if you suspect meningitis ☐

SKILLS LEARNED

- Recognizing a seriously ill child ☐

- Managing babies' crying, diaper rash, teething, and colic ☐

- Treating fever, vomiting and diarrhea ☐

- Dealing with abdominal pain and recognizing appendicitis ☐

- When to seek medical assistance for a child with breathing difficulties ☐

- When to seek medical assistance for headaches in a child ☐

- How to recognize meningitis ☐

- Action for earache, toothache, sore throats, and possible urinary tract infections ☐

9

WOUNDS AND BLEEDING

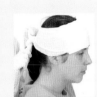

Minor wounds can be carefully cleaned and dressed at home. Any large wound, or a wound that is severely bleeding or contains foreign matter, must be professionally cleaned and treated in the hospital. If you are in any doubt about whether or not a wound needs stitching, take the injured person to the hospital – the more promptly this is done, the better the outcome is likely to be. Protecting the first-aider from infection is another important issue when discussing wounds – you will find dealing with blood and other body fluids covered elsewhere.

CONTENTS

Types of wound 126–127

Wounds and wound healing 128–129

Tackling embedded objects 130–131

Treating infected wounds 132–133

Dealing with major wounds 134–135

Coping with severed body parts 136

Managing crush injuries 137

Controlling severe bleeding 138–139

Recognizing internal bleeding 140–141

Bleeding from orifices 142–143

Miscellaneous foreign bodies 144–145

Skills checklist 146

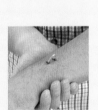

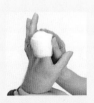

Types of wound

SEE ALSO

➤ Tackling embedded objects, p130

➤ Coping with severed body parts, p136

➤ Miscellaneous foreign bodies, p144

Even minor wounds can become infected and cause real problems with the injured person's health. However, most bites, grazes, and cuts heal without too much trouble and can easily be treated at home. It is important that you are aware of the type of wound sustained so that you can carry out the appropriate first aid, described in detail on the following pages. Some wounds, such as puncture wounds, are more likely to cause damage to the underlying tissues and organs, so they need professional assessment by emergency personnel.

There are two main types of wound: closed and open. Closed wounds are usually caused by a blunt object, and vary from a small bruise to serious internal organ damage. A bruise the size of the injured person's fist would cause substantial blood loss. Open wounds range from surface abrasions to deep puncture wounds. Identifying the wound type helps you decide whether damage to underlying structures is likely.

ABRASIONS

Abrasions tend to be caused by a blunt object applied at an angle, or by falling onto, or sliding along, a hard or rough surface. A knee, ankle, or elbow is a common place for an abrasion arising from a fall or slide.

SIMPLE LACERATIONS

These are clean-edged cuts, such as those caused by a knife or broken glass, and they may be deep. The wounds may look relatively harmless, but there can be considerable damage to underlying tendons, nerves, blood vessels, and even organs. Deep lacerations may be life-threatening, especially if the injury is around the chest or abdomen. Bleeding from them can take some time to stop. Superficial cuts often heal quickly and well, as the edges come together cleanly.

COMPLEX LACERATIONS

Rough tears or wounds with jagged edges are often seen in motor vehicle accidents. They may cause heavy bleeding (although some large lacerations show little bleeding). As the object that caused the wound may be dirty, the risk of infection is high.

PUNCTURE WOUNDS

Often caused by long, needle-like objects, these can be tricky to assess, as the size of the external wound gives no clue to how deep it goes (and the extent of tissue damage). Professional assessment may be needed.

BITES

All bites carry a high risk of infection, with human bites almost invariably becoming infected – a doctor should see any human bite at all, in case antibiotics are needed.

BRUISES

A bruise is discoloration of unbroken skin, caused by blood escaping from a vessel. This may be minor, as from a small area of broken capillaries after a bump, or may indicate internal bleeding. Most look more alarming than they are, and gradually disappear. A new bruise is usually red or purple; older ones are brown, yellow, or greenish.

SCARRING

The extent of scarring after an injury will vary depending on the individual.

➤ Children's skin is usually flawless and so any scarring will show up more clearly than in an adult. However, children also heal much more quickly and more effectively. A childhood scar will often fade completely over time.

➤ Some people are unlucky and their skin forms what are known as keloid scars. In these cases, cut or wounded skin heals over-enthusiastically, forming huge, often unsightly, scars.

GRITTY WOUNDS

Dirty or gritty wounds must be cleaned in hospital to remove foreign bodies from the wound and prevent infection.

GUNSHOT WOUNDS

Guns can inflict many types of wound, and bleeding can be external and internal. Handguns, low-caliber rifles, and shotguns fire fairly low-velocity projectiles, which usually stay in the body, while high-velocity bullets from military weapons often leave entry and exit wounds. High-velocity bullets create powerful shock waves that can break bones and cause widespread tissue damage.

AMPUTATIONS

The cutting or tearing off of body parts needs urgent treatment. Keep the severed part dry and cool and take it to hospital along with the injured person, as reattachment may be possible.

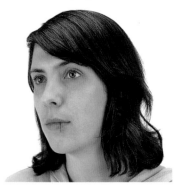

△ A cut that extends beyond the outer edge of the lip should be professionally treated. The cut edges need to be matched up exactly so they heal with minimal scarring.

TYPES OF WOUND

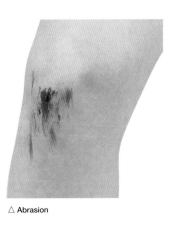

△ Abrasion

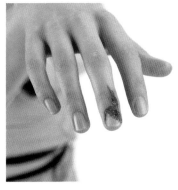

△ Complex laceration

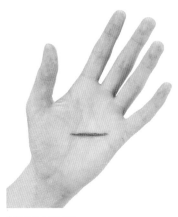

△ Simple laceration

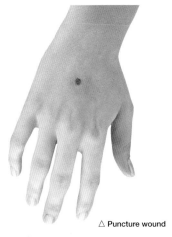

△ Puncture wound

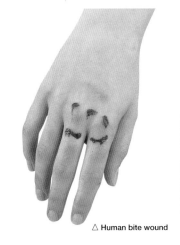

△ Human bite wound

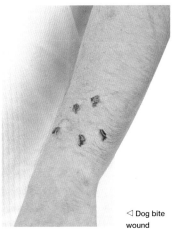

◁ Dog bite wound

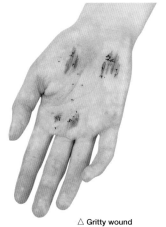

△ Gritty wound

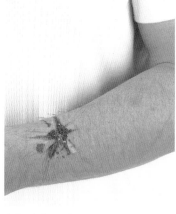

△ Gunshot wound

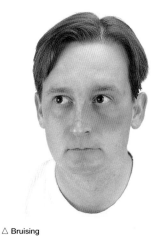

△ Bruising

Wounds and wound healing

SEE ALSO

➤ Dealing with major wounds, p134
➤ Controlling severe bleeding, p138
➤ Recognizing internal bleeding, p140

It is very useful for a first-aider to understand both how wounds affect the body as a whole, and how the body heals itself. Remember that any major loss to the body's constantly circulating blood supply is a potential emergency, as it can lead progressively from a drop in blood pressure through to fainting, unconsciousness, loss of breathing and heartbeat, and death. It is vital to grasp the basic issues of wound care – including stemming blood loss and preventing infection – and also to be able to tell a minor from a major wound.

Our skin has many important functions. Nerves in the skin let us feel temperature, pain, touch, and pressure. We get rid of water, salts, and toxins through our skin, and changes to the flow of blood to the skin also help us to control our body temperature. The skin produces vitamin D, which helps to keep our bones strong and healthy. Our skin protects the tissues lying beneath it from infection, trauma, dehydration, and the harmful rays of the sun. The skin is our first line of defense and is easily damaged.

THE HEALING PROCESS

A superficial wound, such as a surface burn, involves only the topmost layer of skin, called the epidermis. This can heal very quickly, in one to two days. A deeper wound takes longer to heal.

As blood rushes into the wound, it clots and effectively seals the wound. The wound then fills with white cells which kill any bugs and absorb foreign matter. However, in a large or dirty wound, the

INSIDE A BLOOD VESSEL

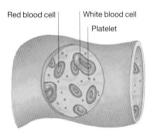

Red blood cell | White blood cell | Platelet

△ Important constituents of wound-healing: white and red blood cells and platelets.

HOW A WOUND HEALS

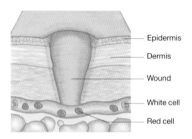

Epidermis
Dermis
Wound
White cell
Red cell

1 A large wound in the skin penetrates both the epidermis and the dermis.

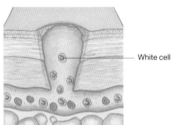

White cell

2 Blood rushing into the wound forms a clot as it exits. White cells fight infection.

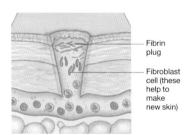

Fibrin plug
Fibroblast cell (these help to make new skin)

3 Strands of fibrin form a plug that slowly shrinks. New tissue forms underneath.

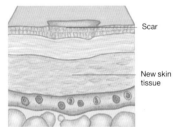

Scar
New skin tissue

4 The plug forms a scab, which eventually drops off. A scar remains.

white blood cells may be outnumbered and so infection begins. The wound may also be too big to allow clotting to stop the bleeding, resulting in continual blood loss (and, potentially, shock).

The body does all it can to reduce the bleeding from a wound. Damaged blood vessels within the wound go into spasm, and may stay in spasm for anything up to several hours. At the same time, platelet cells from the blood help to form a "plug" that may be enough to stop bleeding in a small wound. The body also uses a complex series of processes in the blood to produce strands of a substance called fibrin. These stick together to form a substantial protective plug, beneath which new skin tissue forms.

CLOTTING PROBLEMS

When someone's blood clots too easily, a clot may form in an unbroken blood vessel. This condition – "thrombosis" – is more

CLEANING AND DRESSING A WOUND

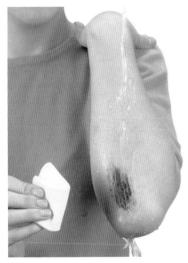

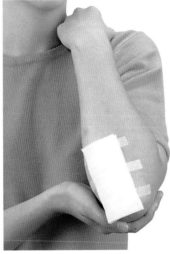

1 Expose the wound and clean it well (grit and dirt can cause infection and slow healing). Control any bleeding with direct pressure.

2 Cover small wounds with an adhesive dressing, larger wounds with a non-adhesive sterile dressing and bandage.

likely in those who have had major surgery, in smokers, and after long-distance travel. If the blood is slow to clot – as in people taking blood-thinning medication or those who have the inherited condition hemophilia – severe bleeding may occur after relatively minor injuries.

WARNING

➤ Any penetrating injury that could have pierced a body cavity, for example an injury in the chest or abdomen, should be treated very seriously, even if it looks small and insignificant.

➤ If broken glass was involved, the wound will need to be X-rayed.

➤ Wounds caused by sharp implements, such as knives and glass, may have caused damage to tendons or nerves under the skin.

➤ It may well be relevant for the person to have tetanus protection; they may need to get this from a doctor.

MINOR AND MAJOR WOUNDS

A minor wound is a small wound that stops bleeding easily and is neither too deep nor infected. A brief look at the wound, and finding out how it occurred, will help you to make your assessment and proceed accordingly. You should treat it as a major/serious wound, and seek qualified medical aid, if:

• The bleeding is not stopped by an adhesive dressing.
• The wound looks as if it could be deeper than $^1/_8$in, or appears to need stitching.
• You suspect that there might be damage to underlying structures such as nerves and tendons – for example, if there seems to be any loss of function or numbness in the affected part.
• There is potential for infection.
• The wound may leave ugly scarring, as in facial wounds.
• The wound covers a large area.

Stitching is needed on some wounds, to stop bleeding or prevent infection. Never use steri-strips (adhesive tape

closures designed for smaller wounds) unless you are medically qualified, as incorrect use can lead to abscesses.

KEEPING WOUNDS DRY

A wound must stay fairly dry in order to heal. Wounds kept enclosed and damp are more likely to become infected and can take longer to heal. If the pad of a dressing becomes wet, it should be carefully changed for a dry one. Some small, minor wounds, grazes, and open blisters respond well to exposure to the air – provided dirt or dust are unlikely to get into them.

FIRST AID FOR MINOR WOUNDS

Wash your hands thoroughly with soap and water. Cover any wounds or sores on your hands with waterproof dressings. Wear gloves if possible. Avoid coughing, sneezing or talking over the wound.

Take a brief look to find out how and where the wound was caused.

Clean the wound with an antiseptic wipe. If this is not available, wash the wound with gently running water.

Dry the wound with a gauze swab and cover with a sterile dressing and bandage.

Advise the injured person to keep the wound clean and dry for the next few days. They should show it to a doctor if there is a risk of infection.

Tackling embedded objects

SEE ALSO
➤ Dealing with major wounds, p134
➤ Miscellaneous foreign bodies, p144

A "foreign body" that has lodged within a wound can cause infection. The object may be relatively easy to remove, as is usually the case with a splinter. However, if you are in any doubt about your ability to remove it safely and cleanly, leave it until you can get professional help. This is essential if the object is large or deeply embedded. A foreign body will usually set up an infection around the site within hours so this problem should be promptly resolved. An embedded object left in the wound could cause an infection of the bloodstream.

Even tiny embedded objects can be very painful, and they may travel and cause further problems – such as pressure on a nerve or an annoying lump. Remove an embedded object (or any foreign body) only if the injury is minor and it is easy to do so; otherwise, get medical help. Sometimes doctors decide to leave an embedded object in place, because it is more risky to remove it than to leave it where it is.

SMALL SPLINTERS

A small splinter of wood, metal or glass may come out if you gently squeeze the skin on either side. If it is protruding from the skin, it may be easy to remove with a pair of sterile tweezers. Sterilize them in boiling water for a few seconds, or hold them in a gas flame, and allow to cool before using. Pull the splinter out at the angle it went in. (A soft wood splinter may need professional aid, as it falls apart easily.) If the splinter does come out, encourage bleeding by squeezing either side of the site. Wash the wound and apply an adhesive dressing.

WARNING
If you cannot see a splinter, be very wary of trying to remove it. Small objects under the skin often become surrounded by pus after a few days, and then pop out easily. Glass is very difficult to find and does not always show up on X-rays. Even a foreign body that does show up on an X-ray can be hard to locate, so removal is best left to experts. Whether or not a person has tetanus cover may affect your assessment.

FISH HOOKS

These can be very sharp and often get stuck in people's fingers. The barb means you can't pull them back out the way they went in.
• Your first priority is to get medical help.
• Ask if the person has tetanus cover; if not, medical aid is particularly important.
• Remove a hook only if no medical help is available, especially if you can't see the barb.

• If the barb is visible, use pliers to cut the barb off and then pull the hook out.
• If you know that there is a barb, but cannot see it, do not try to pull the hook out unless no medical help is available. The person may require an anaesthetic before this is done, so it is best to take them to a doctor. If you do have to remove it, a doctor should still examine the wound as soon as possible.

DEALING WITH FISH HOOKS

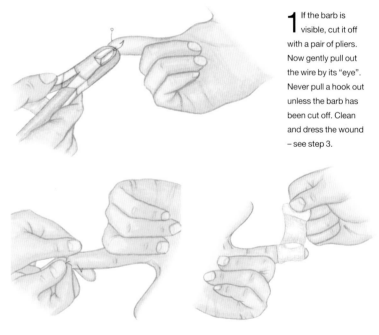

1 If the barb is visible, cut it off with a pair of pliers. Now gently pull out the wire by its "eye". Never pull a hook out unless the barb has been cut off. Clean and dress the wound – see step 3.

2 If the barb is not visible, and no medical help is available, push the hook firmly but carefully through the wound until the barb emerges. Cut the barb off and remove the wire.

3 When the wire is out, clean the wound with an antiseptic wipe or running water. Pad the wound with sterile gauze and bandage it. Seek medical help as soon as possible.

DRESSING ARM WOUNDS WITH EMBEDDED OBJECTS

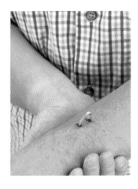

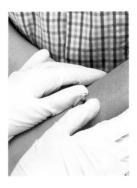

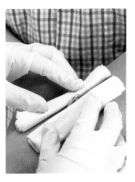

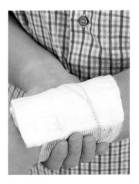

1 Do not try to remove this kind of embedded object as you may cause further damage. Your aim is to deal with bleeding and protect the area from infection, and to get aid promptly.

2 If the wound is bleeding, apply pressure to the surrounding area with your hands. Never apply pressure directly onto an embedded object. Elevating the wounded part will also help.

3 Place padding around the object. If possible, as it would be here, build this padding up until it is as high as the embedded object, ready to bandage over smoothly.

4 Bandage over the padding (or on either side of the object if it is a long one and still protrudes). Apply no direct pressure to the object. Keep the wound elevated and get the person to the hospital.

LARGE EMBEDDED OBJECTS

If a large object is embedded in the wound, you should not try to remove it but should seek urgent medical help. This is especially important if the injury is to the chest or abdomen. The object may have cut through large blood vessels or even be embedded in the heart, but while it remains in the wound, it may act as a plug and prevent further bleeding. You could do just as much damage pulling it out as occurred as the object went in.

If someone is impaled, on railings for example, never attempt to get them off as you may aggravate internal injuries and cause severe bleeding. Instead, help the person to stay still and try to support their weight in as comfortable a position as possible. Cover them with a coat or blanket to keep them warm, and call the emergency service immediately, or ask a helper to do so. Tell the dispatcher how the person is impaled, as the emergency service will need to bring specialized cutting equipment. Reassure the injured person that help is on its way, and keep talking to them to keep them calm.

▷ Small children playing with pencils is one of the many everyday situations that can turn into an embedded object incident – children frequently embed pencils in their face or staples in their fingers. Keep a careful eye on children.

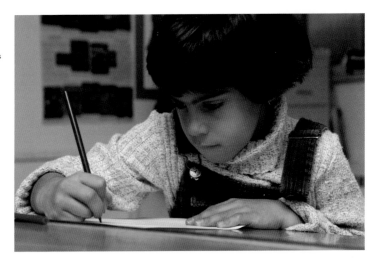

Treating infected wounds

SEE ALSO
➤ Types of wound, p126
➤ Tackling embedded objects, p130

When a wound becomes infected, it will need very careful monitoring and handling. If not treated correctly, the wound may become increasingly infected, spreading to a larger and larger area of the body. An infected wound can also lead to poisoning of the bloodstream, a serious condition known as septicemia. Bites, whether inflicted by a human or a dog, cat or other animal, are all likely to cause infection unless the site of the wound has been professionally cleaned and treated. The person will often need to take antibiotics.

Sometimes a wound becomes infected despite having been cleaned and dressed correctly, and kept clean and dry. Certain types of wound are prone to infection – bites, for example, and particularly human or cat bites. If there is a lot of blood under a wound and this is not cleared out and its reappearance prevented, or if a wound is deep and dirty, then infection is more likely. Some people are more vulnerable to infection. These include those with diabetes, those with a compromised immune system (due to drugs or illness), and alcoholics.

There are usually many warning signs that a wound has become infected, giving plenty of time for it to be treated with antibiotics and drainage if necessary.

SIGNS AND SYMPTOMS OF INFECTION

➤ An infection may start to show itself within a few hours of the injury, or may not appear for several days.

➤ Be aware of pain around the site of the wound – often an early sign of infection.

➤ Watch for any redness, tenderness, swelling under the wound or pus, or for the start of a fever.

➤ Swollen glands (armpit/groin).

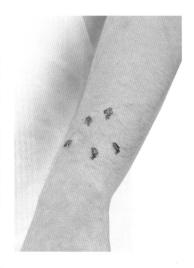

▷ This wound, caused by a dog, will need to be assessed by a doctor. Antibiotics may be given as a preventive measure.

FIRST AID FOR INFECTION

Cover the wound with a sterile dressing and bandage in place. Leave the surrounding area visible, so that you can monitor signs of infection – vital information for the doctor.

Elevate and support the infected area if possible. For example, if a forearm is infected, the elbow could be supported on a stack of books.

Get the injured person to a doctor as soon as possible.

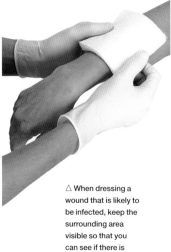

△ When dressing a wound that is likely to be infected, keep the surrounding area visible so that you can see if there is spreading infection.

WOUNDS THAT ARE PRONE TO INFECTION

Any wound can become infected, but certain kinds are more at risk:

➤ Bite wounds: animal or human.

➤ Wounds/scratches from human nails or the claws of animals.

➤ Stab (penetrating) wounds.

➤ Wounds sustained while working: in soil or manure; in or around waste or excrement; with animals.

➤ Wounds from dirty tools or objects, for example sustained while gardening or working on a construction site.

➤ Wounds with embedded objects, especially softwood splinters, grit, and plant thorns.

SIGNS OF INFECTION

You may notice the first signs of infection in and around a wound within hours, but it frequently takes longer to manifest itself. The infection may not surface until a day or two after the injury, when the person may have more or less forgotten it.

Pain, redness, tenderness, and swelling are all signs of infection. The injured person may also experience fever and notice pus oozing from the wound.

SPREADING INFECTION

Infection may spread under the skin (cellulitis) and/or into the bloodstream (septicemia). Cellulitis may appear even without an obvious wound, and is often from an unsuspected insect bite.

If the wound is near a joint, infection may spread into the joint. This is particularly true of human bites on the knuckles – these may be "self-inflicted", occurring when someone aims a punch at another's face and sustains a laceration to the knuckles from their victim's teeth. Some people, such as those with the disease osteoarthritis, may develop a joint infection with no actual wound.

You should suspect cellulitis if there is a spreading redness and swelling beyond the wound site. The glands in the armpits, neck or groin may be sore and tender, and there may be a red line going up the limb toward the glands.

Suspect septicemia if the injured person feels unwell with a fever, thirst, shivering, and lethargy. A joint infection may be present if the joint feels hot or swollen, or if it is exceedingly painful, especially with movement. All these conditions require medical treatment – as a first-aider, your priority is to recognize the likely symptoms and get the person professional medical assistance.

TETANUS

A bacterium commonly found in soil and animal feces, tetanus can contaminate the tiniest of wounds. In general, the dirtier the wound, the greater the chance of infection, but some 20 percent of people with tetanus infection have no obvious wound through which the infection could have entered. It may take 3 months for signs of the disease to develop, although it is usually obvious within 2 weeks.

Tetanus is a particularly vicious disease. The tetanus bacterium produces a neurotoxin that causes painful muscle spasms (lockjaw) as well as having a detrimental effect on the heart. People still develop this infection worldwide, and it is a huge killer. However, you can be vaccinated against the disease – both as a general preventive and if an injury is sustained that puts you at greater risk of developing it.

Tetanus immunization

The usual tetanus immunization program in Western countries starts at the age of 3 months, is boosted around 4 years old and in adolescence, and then every 10 years. If an injured person has not had a booster for 10 years, they will require another booster to ensure that they do not develop the infection. If they are elderly or from abroad, they may need the whole three-dose course, and if the wound is very dirty, they may be given an extra tetanus booster or even some anti-tetanus protein if they have never had any tetanus immunization.

If there is any doubt about tetanus cover, it is best to assume the person is not covered and take them to the hospital.

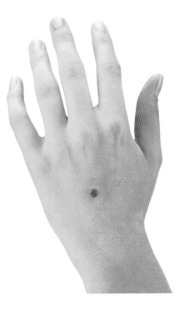

△ Penetrating wounds caused by needle-like objects or cats' teeth are prone to infection.

TETANUS-PRONE WOUNDS

The following wounds are particularly prone to infection with tetanus.

➤ Those contaminated with soil or feces.

➤ Old wounds (more than 6 hours).

➤ Puncture wounds.

➤ Wounds with a poor blood supply.

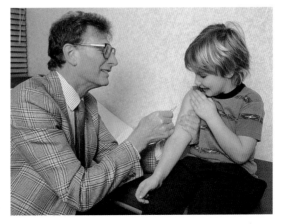

◁ A child is given the tetanus vaccine (combined with diphtheria and pertussis vaccines). When dealing with anyone with a wound, no matter how clean it looks, always try to check if their immunization against tetanus is up to date. Elderly people in particular may never have had any routine tetanus boosters.

Dealing with major wounds

SEE ALSO

➤ Controlling severe
  bleeding, p138
➤ Recognizing internal
  bleeding, p140
➤ Managing rib
  fractures, p160

The two main priorities when treating major wounds are to stop the bleeding and get help as fast as possible. You must call the emergency services as fast as possible because heavy blood loss is very serious, and because the wound may conceal further internal injury. Try to dress the wound effectively if you can, although large wounds will usually need professional cleaning and stitching in the hospital's emergency department. While you wait for the paramedics to arrive, keep the injured person warm and reassure them that help is on the way.

Large wounds may bleed profusely and signify greater problems internally. When wounds are over the abdomen or chest, particular care must be taken to avoid exacerbating the situation. You should not attempt to remove an object embedded in a wound (see page 130), nor should you try to stop the bleeding by applying a tourniquet (see page 136).

If possible, wear protective gloves to treat the bleeding; otherwise wash your hands well both before and afterward. Once you have stopped the bleeding, brushed any debris off the wound (do not wash it), and dressed it, call the emergency services if this has not already been done by a helper.

The injured perrson may lose consciousness and may develop symptoms of shock. Do not leave them alone except to call for help. Keep them warm while you wait for the emergency services to arrive.

BASIC FIRST AID FOR MAJOR WOUNDS

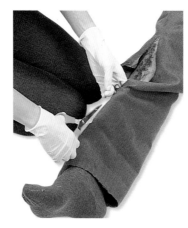

1 Wear protective gloves. Expose the wound. Do not drag clothing over the wound, but cut or lift aside the clothing.

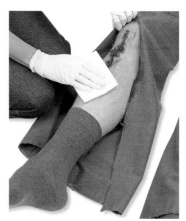

2 Using a gauze pad, clear the wound surface of any obvious debris such as large shards of glass, lumps of grit, or mud.

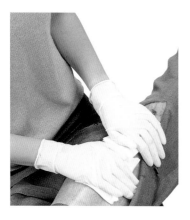

3 Control bleeding with direct pressure and then by elevating the limb.

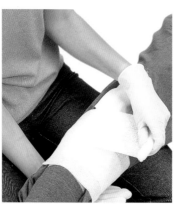

4 Once bleeding is controlled, apply a bandage to the wound.

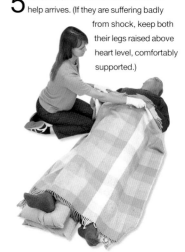

5 Keep the person warm and rested until help arrives. (If they are suffering badly from shock, keep both their legs raised above heart level, comfortably supported.)

ABDOMINAL WOUNDS

There are many organs within the abdominal cavity, all of which may become injured and bleed profusely with little sign of external damage. Any penetrating injury to the abdomen could damage the internal organs, and might also introduce infection into the abdominal cavity, leading to peritonitis. If a penetrating object – such as a knife or a piece of metal – remains in the wound, it should be left where it is, or even more damage may be inflicted.

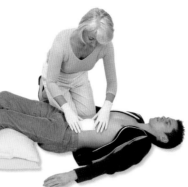

△ When dealing with abdominal wounds, raise and support the injured person's knees to relax the abdominal muscles and reduce pain.

CHEST WOUNDS

Take great care when dealing with any injury in the chest area. Look out for breathing difficulty, a penetrating wound, or a "flail chest" (multiple rib fractures causing unusual movement). These conditions can indicate life-threatening damage that needs emergency attention.

In many cases, especially after a high-speed automobile accident or a fall, the person may have fluid or bruising in the lungs, which will make them very short of breath. You can do little in this case except keep the person sitting up and supported, and reassure them, until help arrives.

First-aid efforts are potentially life-saving when someone has an injury that penetrates the chest wall. This may occur as a result of a rib fracture (even a person with a simple rib fracture may perforate a lung if they bend at an awkward angle), a stabbing or a gunshot injury, for example. The victim may end up with air entering the lung cavity as they breathe in, and this will eventually lead to lung collapse. If the lung is perforated, air escapes out of the lung into the space between the lung and the chest wall, and will again cause the lung to collapse. These cases need urgent help.

FIRST AID FOR AN ABDOMINAL WOUND

Lay the person on a firm surface and raise their knees. Loosen any tight clothing and call the emergency services.

If there are organs visible, do not touch or try to replace them. Cover them with a plastic bag or food wrap to stop them drying out or sticking to dressings.

Dress other wounds with large sterile dressings. If blood seeps through these, apply further dressings on top.

Leave any penetrating objects in place and stabilize them with bulky dressings.

If the person starts to vomit or cough, support the wound. If they lose consciousness, check the airway and be prepared to resuscitate. Place them in the recovery position.

FIRST AID FOR A CHEST WOUND

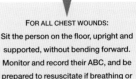

FOR ALL CHEST WOUNDS:
Sit the person on the floor, upright and supported, without bending forward. Monitor and record their ABC, and be prepared to resuscitate if breathing or circulation stops.

Summon emergency help urgently, using a bystander if possible.

FOR PENETRATING CHEST WOUNDS:
Leave any penetrating object in place and keep it still with your hand(s).

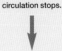

Seal the wound immediately using the injured person's hand placed flat on the hole. If this is impossible, use your own gloved hand.

Place a large sterile dressing over the wound and cover completely with a plastic bag or several layers of film. Secure with firm bandages, or with adhesive tape on three sides of the dressing, so that air trapped in the chest can escape when the person breathes out.

IMPORTANT NOTES:
• Do not let further air enter the wound while applying bandages.
• Adhesive tape may not adhere well to sweaty skin: you may need to keep a hand on the dressing to maintain the seal.
• The priority is to seal the hole completely and get help rapidly.

Coping with severed body parts

SEE ALSO

➤ What is first aid?, p12
➤ Full resuscitation sequence, p34
➤ Dealing with shock, p68
➤ Controlling severe bleeding, p138

When a person loses a finger, hand, toe, ear, or limb as the result of an accident, there may be considerable bleeding and the person is likely to suffer shock. Your priorities are to stop the bleeding and to get the person to the hospital or summon the emergency services immediately. It is vital that you take the body part with you as it may be possible for it to be reattached. Keeping it cool improves the chances of this, but you should not freeze or place ice directly next to the body part. It is also important that you do your best to keep the injured person calm.

A severing of a body part by whatever means, whether accidental or surgical, is known as an amputation. Accidental amputations are most commonly the result of occupational injuries inflicted by power tools or industrial machinery; they also can often occur during a motor vehicle accident. The body part may be torn, crushed, or sliced off. The smaller parts of the body such as fingers and toes are most likely to be involved.

The main priority in the case of an amputation is to stop the bleeding, but also to remember to take the amputated body part to the hospital with the injured person. If a body part is kept at 39.2°F, there is a chance that it can be sewn back or "re-implanted" within 12–24 hours.

If you have to take a severed body part to hospital, keep it dry and cool – wrapped in plastic, then protected with padding and placed in ice. **Do not**:

• Let ice or water come into direct contact with the part – this causes tissue damage.
• Use dry ice or chemical additives.
• Freeze the part.
• Use fabric or fluffy dressings, as the fibers may stick to the part.
• Wash the part, especially with soap or disinfectant.

WARNING

Tourniquets are emergency devices for stemming bleeding – the simplest form is a very tight bandage. Tourniquets risk making the tissue damage even worse by cutting off its blood supply, and thus necessitating even more of the limb being amputated. They also lessen the chances of successful re-implantation. This is why they should never be used in first aid, except by highly trained professionals under specific circumstances.

FIRST AID AFTER AN AMPUTATION

Follow DRSABC and if necessary, administer basic life support.

Control bleeding by applying direct pressure using gauze dressings, and elevation. Cover the wound with a sterile dressing and secure with a bandage.

Call the emergency services. Tell the dispatcher that the case involves amputation.

If pressure does not stop the bleeding, press harder and elevate higher. Do not use a tourniquet (see Warning box).

To protect the amputated part, wrap it in plastic, then in gauze, then in another plastic bag, then in ice. Mark the package with the person's name and time of injury.

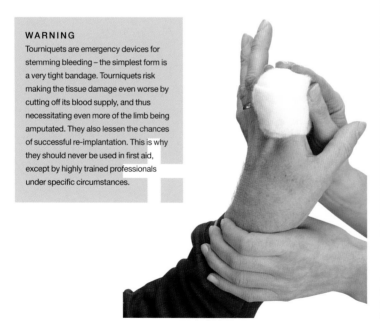

◁ Pressure and elevation are the key things for a first-aider to remember when trying to stop bleeding after an amputation.

Managing crush injuries

SEE ALSO

➤ Full resuscitation sequence, p34

➤ Dealing with shock, p68

➤ BONE AND MUSCLE INJURIES, p147

Someone who has suffered a crush injury requires the urgent attention of paramedics, and ambulance transfer to the hospital. Crush injuries occur in automobile accidents, for example when someone is crushed against the steering wheel, in buildings that suffer structural damage, and in industrial and agricultural accidents when someone is crushed by heavy machinery. The injury may result in serious complications, so it is essential to call the emergency services as quickly as possible, and to control any external bleeding.

In all cases in which people are trapped victims or suffer crush injuries, call the emergency services immediately. As well as paramedics, the fire service may be needed to release people: generally it is safer to leave this to the professionals.

CRUSHED HANDS, FINGERS, FEET AND TOES

If these are caught in machinery or tricky to release, wait for professional help. If the crushed part has already been released:

• Deal with any bleeding, and apply a sterile dressing.

• Treat as for fractures, with padding, immobilization, and elevation.

CRUSHED LIMBS

The offending object may be just bulky enough to cut off the blood supply, or a hard impact or very heavy object may have caused fractures and severe tissue damage.

If left too long, toxins, waste products, and blood clots can develop in crushed limbs. These may lead to fatal kidney and heart failure on release. However, this usually takes over 30 minutes to occur, by which time emergency personnel should be in control. Where a crushed limb has been released, treat it as a fracture.

CRUSHED ABDOMEN AND PELVIS

Any crushing or the impact of a blunt object on the abdomen can cause severe internal bleeding and damage. The injured person may show no outward signs at first, so the accident history could be the only clue to a potentially severe condition.

The ideal first-aid position to use is the "shock" position, with legs raised – unless this might worsen damage, in which case keep the person still. If they need to vomit, you may need to turn them on their side. Do not sit them up. Treat a crushed pelvis as a fracture, and get help very quickly.

CRUSHED CHEST

A heavy weight on the chest can cause breathing to stop. Check that nothing under the object is penetrating the chest and then carefully lift the object off, if you can. If breathing has stopped, prepare to resuscitate. If conscious, a person may find it easier to breathe sitting up, but keeping them in their current position until help arrives will often prevent further damage.

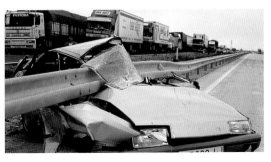

◁ **Automobile accidents** are a major cause of crush injuries. They also have potential for further disaster. Never enter a dangerous environment or try to release anyone if you are risking your own safety or could cause them further harm.

FIRST AID FOR CRUSH INJURIES

Call the emergency services. Make any threatening objects stable, **if this will not endanger yourself or the injured person.**

Check the person's level of response, breathing, and circulation. Only try to release them if vital (e.g. crushed chest) or if it will be 30 minutes or more before emergency aid arrives. **Do this only if you will not endanger yourself or further endanger the injured person.**

Control any bleeding and dress wounds; support suspected fractures. If injuries involve the head or neck, make sure that these are kept still (to avoid worsening any possible spinal injury).

Look for any signs of internal bleeding and shock and treat appropriately.

Reassure the person and keep them warm and still. Continue to monitor and record their vital signs until help arrives.

Controlling severe bleeding

SEE ALSO
➤ Dealing with head injury, p80
➤ Dealing with major wounds, p134

Stemming blood flow from a large wound is a life-saving procedure. The main method used combines pressure and elevation. Apply direct pressure to the site of the blood loss with your own or the injured person's hand, unless the wound contains foreign matter such as glass. In this case, squeeze the edges of the wound together. Elevating the wounded area also helps to stem blood loss – even if a limb is fractured, your priority is to stop the bleeding, especially if it is heavy, and then worry about the fracture. However, try to handle fractured limbs gently.

Injury to an artery can lead to a life-threatening loss of blood in a very short time. Stemming the blood flow may save the injured person's life and is your main priority as a first-aider once you have dealt with their ABC.

With more superficial wounds, bleeding may sometimes seem profuse without, in fact, being too dangerous. Head wounds are a good case in point here. The scalp has a very rich blood supply, so head wounds often bleed profusely, even if they are quite superficial. Do not, however, automatically go to the other extreme and assume that it is not serious. Always try to assess any underlying damage – this is especially important with head wounds.

CONTROLLING BLEEDING ON A HEAD WOUND

Dealing with bleeding from a head wound varies slightly from tackling heavy bleeding from other sites. Follow the treatment for head injury if this is suspected.

1 If the person is unconscious, follow DRSABC before dealing with the wound – airway and breathing are top priority. Try to find the source of the bleeding – remember that there may be more than one site. If the person is conscious, ask them to tell you all they can about what happened, to help your assessment.

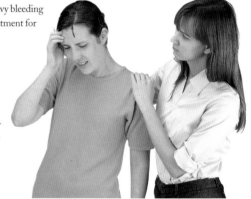

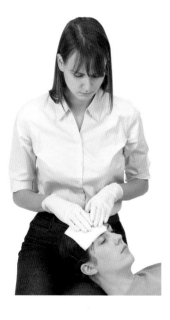

2 Wear protective gloves if possible. Replace any flaps of skin over the wound and place firm pressure directly to the injury using a sterile dressing or other clean pad. Use gentle pressure if you suspect a fracture. Get the injured person to lie down with their head and shoulders raised to help to reduce pressure in the head. Send for emergency help, if you have not already done so.

3 Secure the dressing with a roller bandage or equivalent. Make sure that the dressing covers the whole wound. If blood starts oozing through the bandage, don't take the original dressing off but place another one on top. If the injured person's general condition seems good, sitting them up may reduce the bleeding. Continue to monitor and record their vital signs.

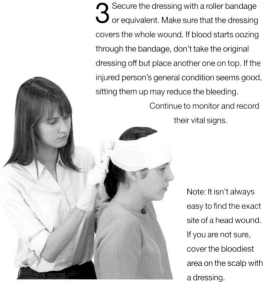

Note: It isn't always easy to find the exact site of a head wound. If you are not sure, cover the bloodiest area on the scalp with a dressing.

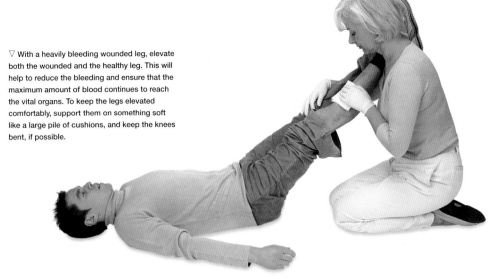

▽ With a heavily bleeding wounded leg, elevate both the wounded and the healthy leg. This will help to reduce the bleeding and ensure that the maximum amount of blood continues to reach the vital organs. To keep the legs elevated comfortably, support them on something soft like a large pile of cushions, and keep the knees bent, if possible.

FIRST AID FOR CONTROLLING SEVERE BLEEDING

Look for the source of the bleeding. Wearing gloves if possible, remove clothing to expose the wound.

Lay the person down. Elevate their legs in case of shock, and the bleeding part if possible. Place firm pressure over the wound using a sterile dressing or other clean pad (the injured person may be able to apply pressure themself). Call the emergency services.

Secure the pad with a bandage or equivalent; make sure that the dressing covers the whole wound.

If blood starts oozing through the dressing, don't take the original dressing off but place another dressing on top.

STEMMING BLOOD FLOW

The most effective method is applying direct pressure to the wound and, where possible, keeping the body part elevated – gravity naturally lessens the flow. If an object is embedded in the wound, compress the edges on either side of the object. Stemming blood flow by applying pressure to main arteries is not advised for the average first-aider – this can be tricky.

Bleeding may be copious in a head injury, and you may be hampered by the person's hair. Apply a dressing larger than the wound, bandage it in place and get medical help rapidly. If a limb is bleeding heavily, elevate it to reduce the blood flow to

THIGH INJURIES

A cut on the thigh can easily sever an artery with life-threatening results.
The use of very sharp knives by butchers can lead to an injury known as "butcher's thigh". The artery running down the front of the thigh is close to the skin's surface. If the butcher's knife slips and cuts through this artery, rapid and sometimes fatal blood loss follows. Many butchers have bled to death in this way over the centuries. These days, however, the injury is more likely to be caused by craft knives and construction tools.

TYPES OF BLEEDING

From arteries
➤ Blood spurts rhythmically with the beat of the heart.

➤ Blood is bright red.

➤ Blood loss is rapid and quickly leads to shock.

From veins
➤ Blood is darker red with a bluish hue.

➤ Blood oozes steadily.

➤ Blood loss is slower but can eventually cause shock.

the area. If the wound is on a leg, lift both legs to maximize blood flow to the person's vital organs, especially their brain. Even a fractured limb should be carefully elevated if it is bleeding very profusely.

AVOID TOURNIQUETS

Tourniquets should never be used to control serious bleeding except by fully trained medical professionals, and only by them as an absolute last resort. The scenario in which use of a tourniquet is most likely to occur is when a limb has been partially or wholly severed, when it has very little chance of survival anyway.

Recognizing internal bleeding

SEE ALSO

➤ Dealing with shock, p68

➤ Bleeding from orifices, p142

It is vital that the first-aider is able to recognize the signs of internal bleeding and take appropriate action. Internal bleeding can be caused by stabbing or shooting, which also cause external bleeding, or by a fall, a crush injury, a punch or kick, a fractured bone, or an ulcer, which may not. The signs include cold and clammy, pale skin, weakness, thirst, and blood coming from an orifice. The injured person needs urgent medical assistance, so the most effective action you can take is to call the emergency services immediately.

Unlike external bleeding, internal bleeding is a difficult condition to assess. It may be unclear what is happening until the problem is at a late stage, when the person has already bled a great deal and is going into shock. Detecting internal bleeding early on, and getting rapid expert assistance, is by far the most helpful action you can perform under these circumstances.

CAUSES OF INTERNAL BLEEDING

Stabbing and shooting are obvious causes of internal bleeding, and the size of an external wound is often no indicator of the extent of the internal damage. Internal blood vessels and organs can tear and rupture without any obvious external damage.

An injury caused by an object that is not sharp enough to penetrate the skin is called "blunt trauma". This may be due to many different causes – from a fall, a motor vehicle accident, or crush injury to direct punches or kicks. A warning sign of possible internal damage would be bruising on the skin, especially if it is over the abdomen or chest.

Another common cause of internal bleeding is fractured bones, especially the femur and pelvis, which quickly lead to serious blood loss. Conditions such as duodenal and gastric ulcers may lead to profuse internal bleeding. People with blood-clotting abnormalities such as hemophilia, or who are on anti-clotting treatment such as warfarin, may bleed heavily after relatively minor injuries. Many diseases affecting the liver may adversely affect the blood's ability to clot, and may also cause varices, which are like internal varicose veins – these can bleed catastrophically.

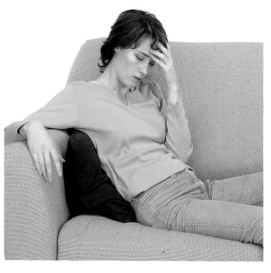

◁ Internal bleeding could be indicated if a person has just had a fall or a period of abdominal pain and exhibits the following symptoms: cold, clammy, pale skin, weakness, and inability to stand up.

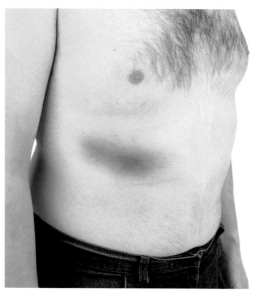

◁ Bruising on the skin, especially if it is over the abdomen or chest, may indicate internal bleeding.

SIGNS AND SYMPTOMS OF INTERNAL BLEEDING

➤ If someone shows signs of shock. This is indicated by: cold, clammy, pale skin; loss of consciousness on sitting or standing up; thirst and general weakness; a fast, weak pulse.

➤ If the victim coughs up blood or vomits blood or anything that looks like blood (bits of gritty brown vomit that look like coffee grounds are a classic sign of a bleeding duodenal ulcer).

➤ If they have passed blood from their rectum (back passage), especially black tar-like stools that smell strongly. This is likely to be due to a bleeding ulcer in the stomach or duodenum.

➤ If they have been in an accident where they fell from a height, or stopped suddenly, as in a motor vehicle accident, or fell off a bike onto the handlebars.

➤ If there is bleeding from the vagina with no obvious cause.

➤ If the person has bruising, tenderness and/or swelling, especially if it is over the abdominal area. The kidney, spleen, and liver may bleed after an accident.

➤ If a woman is in the early stages of pregnancy, particularly between 6 and 8 weeks. A pregnancy in the fallopian tube (known as an ectopic pregnancy) may cause profuse internal bleeding that is life-threatening. The woman may have warning pains low in her abdomen, but not invariably.

➤ If there is blood coming from the nose or mouth after a head injury. This may be due to a fracture of the skull.

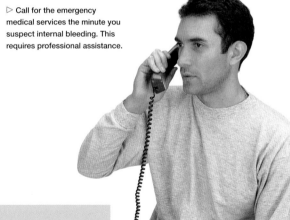

▷ Call for the emergency medical services the minute you suspect internal bleeding. This requires professional assistance.

WARNING
Signs of internal bleeding may not appear for some time after the incident that caused it, and after considerable blood has been lost from the circulation. This is why, if there is any risk that an accident or condition could cause internal bleeding, the injured person should be checked over promptly by a medical professional.

FIRST AID FOR SUSPECTED INTERNAL BLEEDING

If the injury is caused by an object that is still penetrating the skin, do not try to take the object out. You could do as much damage as occurred when it went in, and it may be "plugging" the wound.

Call the emergency services immediately.

Lay the person flat. To maximize blood flow raise their legs significantly and support them comfortably (on a pile of cushions, say), with knees bent.

Do not let them eat or drink anything.

Loosen any tight clothing and keep them warm.

Monitor and record their vital signs. If they lose consciousness, place them in the recovery position but still keep their legs elevated. Note the amount and source of any blood lost from orifices.

Bleeding from orifices

SEE ALSO

➤ Dealing with shock, p68
➤ Recognizing internal bleeding, p140
➤ Tackling skull and facial fractures, p152

Bleeding can occur from the mouth, nose, ear, rectum and vagina (menstrual bleeding is normal, obviously). These will require first aid to staunch the flow if possible, and you should also check for signs of shock. Bear in mind that dealing with another person's body fluids puts you at risk of infection, so always wear protective gloves if they are available and wash your hands thoroughly both before and after dealing with injuries. Bleeding from orifices with no obvious cause may indicate internal bleeding, which requires urgent medical attention.

VAGINAL BLEEDING

There can be many reasons for non-menstrual vaginal bleeding, including pregnancy problems and sexual assault.

Bleeding in early pregnancy is a warning that miscarriage may be imminent or might already have occurred, and the bleeding can be very heavy, including clots that look like lumps of liver. When the bleeding is this heavy, you must get medical aid urgently.

BLEEDING FROM ORIFICES – POSSIBLE SITES

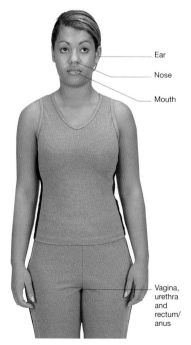

Ear
Nose
Mouth

Vagina, urethra and rectum/anus

In cases of sexual assault, the woman is likely to be very distressed, so use great tact and care. Ideally, she should not undress, go to the bathroom, or shower until she has been seen by the police. Your priorities are to staunch the flow, reassure the victim and contact the emergency services.

RECTAL BLEEDING

Bleeding from the rectum can be divided into two types. Bright red blood is usually due to problems lower down in the gut, most commonly piles or a small tear after passing a hard stool, although there may be more sinister causes. Dark, sticky, black stools indicate old blood from higher up in the gut. It is the dark blood that requires the most urgent action, as it signifies heavy bleeding that could be life-threatening.

VOMITING BLOOD

Bleeding from the stomach and upper digestive system may be bright red or resemble coffee grounds (it may also be swallowed blood from a nosebleed). The person may appear to be in shock, or seem almost normal. All vomiting of blood should be treated as serious. Sit the person down, or if pale or shocked lay them on their side, and seek urgent medical help.

COUGHING UP BLOOD

This usually appears as small spots mixed in sputum, and causes include lung disease and lung damage. Sit the person up, supported and quiet. If their breathing is distressed, or their history suggests lung damage, get help quickly. Anyone who coughs up blood must be seen by a medical professional.

FIRST AID FOR BLEEDING FROM THE VAGINA

Take the woman somewhere private and make her comfortable. Male first-aiders may need to enlist female help.

If the bleeding is very heavy, lay her down and treat for shock.

A towel may be better for soaking up the blood than a sanitary pad.

Call the emergency services if bleeding is very heavy, and not stopping.

FIRST AID FOR RECTAL BLEEDING

Check the person for signs of shock and act accordingly, then seek urgent medical attention.

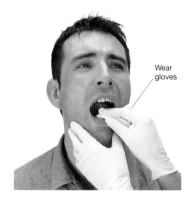

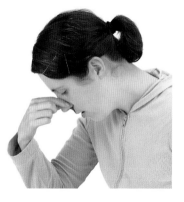

Wear gloves

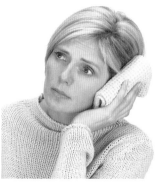

△ Bleeding from the mouth: place a wad of sterile gauze in the mouth and ask the person to bite down on it to control the bleeding.

△ Nosebleed: the victim should breathe though the mouth and pinch the soft end of the nose. If bleeding continues, they should pinch harder.

△ Bleeding from the ear: place a sterile pad or clean towel over the ear and tilt the head to drain out the blood. Call a doctor immediately.

BLEEDING FROM THE MOUTH

This may arise from biting the inside of the mouth, or after a tooth has fallen out or been extracted. It can occur after violent impact, along with concussion and jaw fracture. The main concern should be keeping the airway clear of blood, especially if the person is unconscious.

BLEEDING FROM THE NOSE

Nosebleeds usually start at the lower end of the nose, although in older people with very high blood pressure, they may come from the back of the nose and be harder to stop. Nosebleeds often occur during or after a cold when the lining is inflamed. Other causes are a direct impact (which may also have caused concussion and head or facial fractures), violent nose-blowing, and nose-picking. Watery blood from the nose may arise from a fracture at the base of the skull.

BLEEDING FROM THE EAR

Like a nosebleed, watery blood from the ear may be a sign of a fracture of the base of the skull if it happens after a head injury. However, it is usually due to local causes – often a foreign body has been inserted into the ear and has perforated the eardrum. Other causes of a perforated eardrum are loud explosions, blows to the head, and, most commonly, an infection in the middle ear. The person always has severe ear pain when this happens, after which those with middle ear infections will often feel a relief of their symptoms. Ear infections often need antibiotics.

FIRST AID FOR BLEEDING FROM THE MOUTH

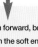

Wear gloves. If the person has lost a tooth or had one extracted, place a wad of sterile gauze against the tooth socket and get them to bite down on it. Change it if it becomes soaked. Place a gauze pad on a mouth wound and ask the person to apply pressure with their finger and thumb for 10 minutes, until bleeding stops.

Tell the person to spit out the blood – it may make them vomit if they swallow it. They should avoid hot drinks.

If bleeding persists for more than 30 minutes, take them to hospital or a dentist.

FIRST AID FOR A NOSEBLEED

The person must lean forward, breathe through the mouth, and pinch the soft end of the nose. If bleeding persists, they must pinch harder. Pinch for at least 10 minutes, then see if the bleeding has stopped. Place a bag of ice or frozen peas wrapped in a towel, over the nose.

Get the person to rest for several hours, and avoid sniffing, blowing, or picking their nose. If bleeding continues for 30 minutes, take them to hospital (lots of swallowing may indicate blood still going down the back of the throat). If it is very heavy and shock sets in, call the emergency services.

FIRST AID FOR BLEEDING FROM THE EAR

Help the person into a half-sitting position. Put a sterile dressing or clean pad over the ear, and get them to tilt their head to the injured side to allow the blood to drain out.

Send or take the victim to the hospital.

Miscellaneous foreign bodies

SEE ALSO

➤ Tackling embedded objects, p130
➤ Treating infected wounds, p132
➤ Bleeding from orifices, p142

As well as becoming embedded in wounds, foreign bodies of all kinds – from an insect flying into the ear to a piece of grit caught under an eyelid – can become lodged in the body's orifices. Such objects may cause injury, bleeding, infection, and other problems. Children are notorious for putting things in their mouths and ears and up their noses, as they explore the world around them, when they are too young to realize the potential danger. Foreign bodies must be removed safely and cleanly, to avoid the risk of damage or infection.

It is usually children and people with psychiatric problems who place foreign bodies inside their orifices deliberately. But foreign bodies can become lodged in part of the body accidentally as well.

SWALLOWING OBJECTS

Children often put things in their mouths and then swallow them – plastic toys, pen lids, money, and paper clips, to name a few. If this occurs, the child may have a choking episode and then fully recover – but with a noticeable absence of the object that was in their hand. Adults may also accidentally swallow small, whole items of food, such as peanuts or sweets, if they are eating while talking or laughing.

If, instead of being swallowed, the object sticks in the windpipe, it may cause partial or complete choking. Because this will impede breathing, it is an acute emergency. If the object sticks in the esophagus, the upper gullet leading down to the stomach, the person may drool, gag, or be unable to eat or drink anything – also a medical emergency.

Once in the stomach, inedible objects usually pass through the gut and out in the feces with no problems. Unless a child develops acute stomach pain or vomiting, or stops opening their bowels, nothing needs to be done. However, if they have swallowed a battery or a sharp object such as a pin, these can damage the digestive tract and must be removed; they will show up on an X-ray.

GENITALS AND RECTUM

People may end up with objects lodged in the penis, the female urethra, the vagina, or the rectum. In any of these cases, never try to retrieve the object, as this can cause damage to these delicate areas. Take the person to an emergency department for treatment by a doctor or nurse.

NOSES

Children often put small objects up their noses. The child may develop a foul-smelling or bloody discharge from one nostril if an object has been lodged in the nose for some time. They may also be having difficulty breathing, and the nose may become swollen. There is a danger that the child will inhale the foreign body into their airway, so you should take them to hospital immediately.

EYES

People often get things in their eyes – dust on a windy day, a speck of ash from a fire or a small fragment of metal hammered off a metal object. They can often feel the object in the eye, or the eye may feel irritated and painful, and it will usually water profusely and look red. An X-ray may be needed if any metal hits the eye at speed, as it may end up at the back of the eye.

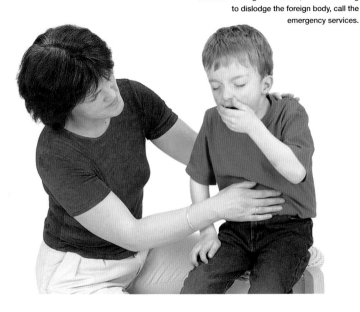

▽ If a swallowed object makes a child or adult continue to cough and choke, while still failing to dislodge the foreign body, call the emergency services.

HOW TO EXAMINE THE EYES

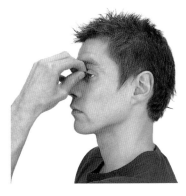

1 Examine the person's eye either in natural daylight or under direct light from a lamp. Stand behind them, so that you are looking down on the eye. Keeping their head very still, ask them to look from side to side and then up and down. While gently pulling the eyelids apart with your finger and thumb, have a good look at the white of the eye, then at the colored part, the iris. If anything is penetrating the eyeball, or resting on the iris or pupil, you should not try to remove it yourself but seek medical help.

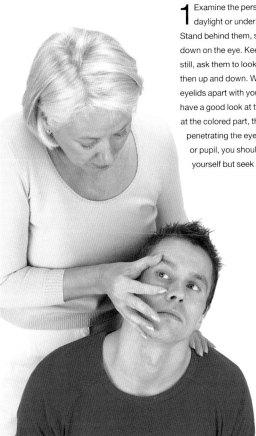

2 Ask the person to look down and then gently pull out the upper lid by the lashes. Look on the underside of the upper lid – specks of grit often lodge here.

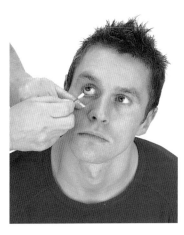

3 To remove an object you can see on the white of the eye, flush the eye with clean, tepid water or an eye-wash solution, or try to brush it off with a cotton bud moistened with water (try this only once). If all this fails, cover the eye with an eye pad and take the person to a doctor.

EARS

Insects flying into ears is a fairly common occurrence, and can be alarming. Deafness is the main symptom of a foreign body in the ear, or there may be a loud buzzing from a trapped fly. Whatever the culprit, do not try to prise it out. Try filling the ear with tepid water: insects and small foreign bodies may float out. Ask the person to turn their head so that the ear containing the foreign body points downward – this may lead to the foreign body dropping out. If the object is lodged in the ear, take or send the person to a doctor.

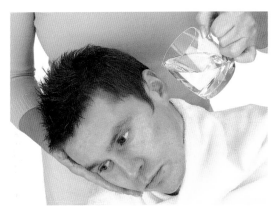

◁ Flush out an insect or foreign body in the ear with tepid water. Never try to dig or poke it out as you may damage the ear or push the object further in.

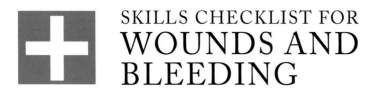

SKILLS CHECKLIST FOR
WOUNDS AND BLEEDING

KEY POINTS

- The basic issues of wound-care are stemming blood loss and preventing infection. For major wounds, the priorities (after assessing ABC) are stopping bleeding and getting help. ☐

- Heavy blood loss leads rapidly to body shut-down. ☐

- Foreign objects can cause severe damage and infection and must be dealt with promptly. ☐

- Any infected wound must be closely monitored. ☐

- Wounds may mask underlying damage – which is why getting help fast is so vital. ☐

- It is usually best to leave the release of those who are crushed or trapped to professionals. ☐

- Stem heavy blood loss by using pressure and elevation. ☐

- Internal bleeding often shows few clear outward signs. Urgent medical help is vital. ☐

SKILLS LEARNED

- How to recognize different types of wound and follow appropriate treatment. ☐

- How to control bleeding and deal with infection. ☐

- What to do with severe wounds and injuries. ☐

- When to suspect internal bleeding. ☐

- How to tackle embedded and lodged foreign bodies. ☐

BONE AND MUSCLE INJURIES

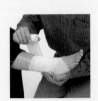

It is not always easy to distinguish a fracture from a dislocation or a sprain.
This chapter explains how to help the injured in the event of various types
of fracture, sprains, dislocations, and back pain. It is essential, if there is
any possibility of a neck or spinal injury, that the victim is not moved,
unless not moving them would put them in further danger. The main
priorities in dealing with bone and muscle injuries are to immobilize the
affected limb, cover any open wounds, and alert the emergency services.

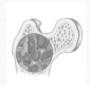

CONTENTS

Understanding the skeleton 148–149

Dealing with broken bones 150–151

Tackling skull and facial fractures 152–153

Managing spinal injuries 154–155

Coping with neck injuries 156–157

Tackling upper limb fractures 158–159

Managing rib fractures 160–161

Coping with pelvic and upper-leg injuries 162–163

Handling knee and lower-leg injuries 164–165

Coping with dislocations 166–167

Managing sprains and strains 168–169

Controlling back pain 170–171

Skills checklist 172

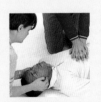

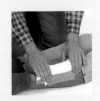

Understanding the skeleton

SEE ALSO

➤ Removing clothing and helmets, p18
➤ Moving and handling safely 1 and 2, pp20, 22
➤ Dealing with broken bones, p150

The body's bones come in all shapes and sizes, and it is the muscles that are attached at multiple points all over the skeleton that enable us to move about. If any of the 206 bones in the body are injured through fracture (a clean break, a messy break, a chip, a splinter, or a crack), our ability to move properly can be substantially diminished, and pain and swelling may occur around the site of the injured bone. Initial first aid, followed by professional treatment in a hospital, is vital for optimum healing of all such bone injuries or fractures.

Bone is a living tissue that continuously builds, degrades, and rebuilds itself throughout life. The skeleton's bony framework has many functions: bones protect the organs from damage; muscles attach to bones so that we can move; many types of blood cell are produced in the bone's marrow; and bone acts as a store of the minerals calcium and phosphate.

As we grow older, the strength of our bones – bone density – declines as bones lose calcium, so they become easy to break. Many elderly people break bones after minor bumps or falls.

WHAT IS BONE MADE OF?

Bone is made of a meshwork of a protein (collagen) into which calcium is deposited to give hardness and strength. Although bone is extremely strong it is not completely solid. The outer layer is hard and compact, but beneath it lies a center of spongy bone. The spaces within the spongy bone allow room for the skeleton's immense blood supply and nerves.

INSIDE A TYPICAL BONE

▽ The circle section shows a close-up view of the internal meshwork of the spongy bone.

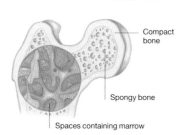

Compact bone

Spongy bone

Spaces containing marrow

THE SKELETON

▷ The many bones of the skeleton give the body shape and structure. Bones that are commonly fractured are named on this illustration.

Scapula (shoulder blade)
Humerus
Radius
Ulna

Calcaneus (heelbone)

Skull
Mandible (jaw)
Sternum (breastbone)
Clavicle (collarbone)
Rib
Vertebral column
Ilium
Pubis ⎤ (all three together known as the pelvis)
Ischium ⎦
Femur (thighbone)
Tibia
Fibula

WHAT HEALTHY BONES NEED

➤ Calcium – The diet should include plenty of calcium-rich foods such as milk, cheese and yogurt. At certain stages of life, such as childhood and during pregnancy and breastfeeding, a higher calcium intake may be needed so that the body does not raid the skeleton's stores of this mineral.

➤ Vitamin D – The body makes vitamin D in the skin when it is exposed to sunlight. This vitamin allows the body to absorb calcium and phosphorus from food.

➤ Exercise – Weight-bearing exercise, such as walking or skipping, promotes bone growth and bone densiity.

HOW BONES CAN FRACTURE

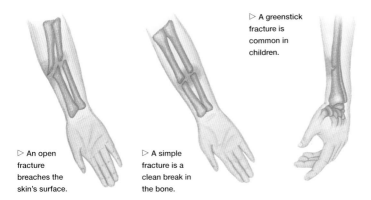

▷ An open fracture breaches the skin's surface.

▷ A simple fracture is a clean break in the bone.

▷ A greenstick fracture is common in children.

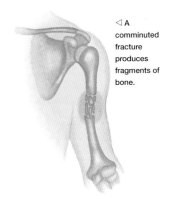

◁ A comminuted fracture produces fragments of bone.

WHAT CAUSES A FRACTURE?

A bone may break because of a direct blow, such as a punch or kick, or from indirect forces. Bones fracture indirectly when, for example, a person falls onto a hand that they have stretched out to break their fall. The forces from the fall travel up the arm (which remains unharmed) and cause the collarbone to break. Bones may also fracture from rotating movements – when someone twists an ankle, for example.

OPEN OR CLOSED FRACTURES?

There are two basic types of fracture, known as open and closed. Open fractures (also called compound fractures) occur when the broken ends of the bone stick out through the skin. In open fractures, the risk of developing an infection is much higher, as are the chances of nerve or blood vessel damage. Closed fractures are fractures in which the skin is not broken over the fracture site. Such fractures may however, damage internal tissues.

HOW BONES HEAL

Different bones heal at different rates, so while a fractured collarbone may heal fully in 6 weeks, a broken thighbone (femur) may take up to 6 months before it is mended completely. The rate of bone regeneration in children is much faster than in most adults, and so broken bones in children tend to heal much more quickly.

Bone-healing has several stages:
• From 6 to 8 hours after injury – In this inflammatory period, blood seeps out of the broken bone ends and forms a clot.
• After 2 days – Bone-making cells migrate to the blood clot and start to form new bone, called callus, to bridge the gap between the bones.
• A few weeks to several months – The original shape of the bone is restored.

COMMON FRACTURE TYPES

Bones fracture in different ways in different people and depending on how an incident came about. Common types of fracture are:

➤ Greenstick fracture – Children sometimes fracture only one side of a bone. The other side bends like a new tree branch.

➤ Comminuted fracture – The bone is splintered at the fracture site, and smaller fragments of bone are found between the two main fragments.

➤ Fracture-dislocation – This type of fracture occurs when a bone breaks or cracks near an already dislocated joint.

➤ Avulsion fracture – When a ligament or muscle attached to a bone is ripped off, it often takes a piece of bone with it.

➤ Pathological fracture – Certain medical conditions, such as osteoporosis and osteogenesis imperfecta, make bones more likely to break.

WHAT DELAYS HEALING?

Although infection increases the blood supply to a fracture site, it brings the wrong kind of cells, so healing is delayed. Also, if the bones are not in alignment with one another, they are not going to heal well. This is one reason why splinting, or at least immobilization, of a fracture is vitally important for proper and speedy bone healing.

HOW BONE HEALS

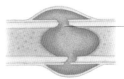

Blood clot fills the gap between the broken bones

△ Six to eight hours after the injury.

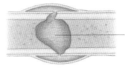

New spongy bone (callus) starts to form

△ Two days after the injury.

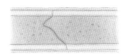

△ A few weeks or months after the injury.

Dealing with broken bones

SEE ALSO

➤ What is first aid?, p12
➤ Dealing with shock, p68
➤ Fixing slings, p206

Bones tend to break as the result of a huge impact or force. Someone with a fracture may be able to tell you that they heard or felt a crack when the accident occurred and that they can feel bones grating over one another when they try to move. These are important clues for the first-aider. Bear in mind that the injured person could be in great pain, and also watch for signs of shock – this may develop, for example, if the fracture causes heavy internal bleeding. Never move someone unless you have to in order to remove them from other serious dangers.

When managing someone with a fracture, monitor ABC before dealing with possible fractures and always assess the person as a whole – there could well be other injuries.

In the short term, the various methods used to deal with fractures focus on preventing the fracture from becoming worse, and they all achieve this by immobilization – keeping the fracture still. The general idea is to immobilize the fracture and the joints above and below the fracture. Movement of a fracture can cause increased pain, damage to surrounding tissue and structures, and possibly even severe complications such as shock from increased bleeding or from bone penetrating through skin, nerves, or blood vessels. In the long term, a broken bone needs to be left clean and undisturbed for proper healing.

SHOULD SPLINTS BE USED?

Using splints (rigid supports) for a fracture is little used by most first-aiders today, unless in very remote locations, or where the first-aider is forced to transport the victim to help. Improvised examples of splints include umbrellas and broom handles. Except for simple, undisplaced arm fractures, transporting a splinted fracture victim is not recommended unless you have proper training and practice, and a suitable vehicle.

IMMOBILIZATION STRATEGIES

There are two major types of immediate first aid for fractures:
• Basic hand immobilization. Try to imagine the break that has occurred in

BASIC CARE FOR A CLOSED FRACTURE

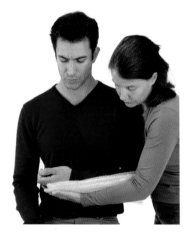
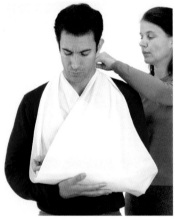
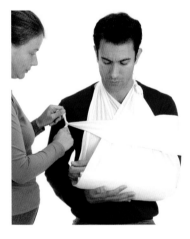

1 Having assessed the injury, ask the person to keep the fracture area still. Support the fracture and apply light padding, such as some folded bubble wrap or a small towel (nothing too bulky).

2 Depending on the part of the body involved, you should usually attempt to immobilize the area. Do this here by applying a broad arm sling, as shown, keeping the light padding in place within the sling.

3 Immobilize the arm further by tying a triangular bandage (folded into a long strip), or equivalent, across the chest. This will prevent movement when the person is in transit to the hospital. Call for medical help.

the normally rigid bone. Use your hands and arms to cradle the limb in order to stop all movement. This method is most appropriate when help will arrive fairly quickly, or where no other equipment or materials of any kind are available.

• Using padding and boxes. These first-aid props are used mostly for leg fractures or for arm fractures where bending the elbow to put the arm in a sling would cause further damage. For this method, hold the limb still. Roll large, loose sausages from objects such as blankets, coats, or towels and place these carefully against the fractured limb. Any gaps beneath the limb, such as under a bent knee, should be carefully filled with just enough padding material to provide support for the area without moving the limb at all. Boxes or other weighted items are now placed either side of the limb to hold the padding in place.

The padding and boxes method is ideal in most populated areas with good emergency response times. It frees the first-aider to concentrate on taking care of the person and simply minimizes any movement. It also means that paramedics arriving on the scene do not need to waste time removing a first-aider's bandages in order to replace them with their own, superior, equipment.

COMMON SIGNS AND SYMPTOMS OF A FRACTURE

➤ There may be a history of impact or trauma at the site.

➤ Swelling, bruising, or deformity at fracture site.

➤ Pain on moving.

➤ Numbness or tingling in injured area.

➤ Wound site at or near fracture site.

➤ The injured person may have heard the bones grating on one another.

FIRST AID FOR FRACTURES

First, assess the situation and reassure the injured person.

Prevent movement at the injury site and stem bleeding if an open fracture.

Phone the emergency services and arrange transport to hospital.

Monitor the person's condition, paying particular attention to the circulation beyond any tied bandages.

FIRST AID FOR AN OPEN FRACTURE

When you are dealing with an open fracture, it is important to prevent blood loss and infection at the injury site as well as immobilizing the area.

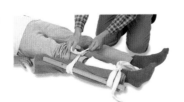

▷ Call the emergency services urgently. Carefully place a sterile dressing or pad over the wound site, and apply hand pressure either side of the protruding bone to control the bleeding. Never press on the protruding bone itself. Build up padding alongside the bone if it is sticking out of the skin. You may want to secure the dressing and padding firmly with a bandage, but do not do so if it causes any movement of the limb, and never bandage too tightly. Monitor the person's condition, specifically their ABC, as there may be a risk of shock. Check circulation in the limb beyond any bandages every 10 minutes.

▷ In more extreme circumstances – if you are in a very remote location, emergency help is seriously delayed, or you are forced to take the person to a doctor/hospital yourself – you may need to splint the fracture. Add extra padding around the limb and tie with bandages or equivalent. Keep any movement to a minimum.

WARNING

In most cases, a first aider must never straighten or move the fractured limb. If a foot looks blue or bloodless, tell the paramedics; they may manipulate the fracture in order to restore circulation.

Tackling skull and facial fractures

SEE ALSO

➤ Responsiveness and the airway, p28

➤ Dealing with head injury, p80

➤ Dealing with broken bones, p150

Suspected head injury is always a serious situation. The spinal cord, brain, or organs within the head, such as the eye or ear, may also be damaged – not only by the impact of the injury but also by the potential bleeding into the brain that such an injury can cause. It is vital to monitor someone with a suspected skull fracture as they may lose consciousness and/or may have a neck or spinal injury. The main point to bear in mind with any facial fracture is that swollen tissues, blood, and saliva may impair breathing by obstructing the airway.

Skull fractures are worrying because an impact large enough to fracture skull bones might also injure the delicate brain beneath. The fracture itself may cause no damage, but if a slab of skull bone is crushed inward (a "depressed fracture") it may put pressure on the brain. Skull fractures may also cause internal bleeding into the brain area.

Call the emergency services as promptly as possible. Be aware of anything that might suggest a neck or spinal injury – if there is any chance of these injuries, treat the injured person with extreme care and keep them totally still.

SKULL FRACTURES

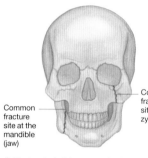

Common fracture site at the mandible (jaw)

Common fracture site at the zygoma

A depressed fracture puts pressure on the brain beneath

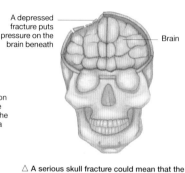

Brain

△ The tough skull bones can be fractured; common injury sites are shown above.

△ A serious skull fracture could mean that the vulnerable tissues of the brain directly beneath are also damaged. If there is also a wound over the fracture site, then the brain may become exposed to the possibility of infection.

SIGNS OF A SKULL FRACTURE

➤ A soft swelling or egg-shaped bruise on the head.

➤ Bruising around eye and/or ear area.

➤ A noticeably lopsided appearance to the head – very serious sign.

➤ A deteriorating level of consciousness (remember AVPU) – very serious sign.

➤ Any blood visible in the whites of the eyes – very serious sign.

➤ Clear or blood-stained fluid leaking from the nose or ears – very serious sign.

Signs of possible internal bleeding:

➤ One-sided, worsening headache; headache that worsens with lying flat/making any effort.

➤ Any visual problems.

➤ Change in/loss of consciousness.

➤ Vomiting.

FIRST AID FOR SUSPECTED SKULL FRACTURE

CONSCIOUS VICTIM

Help the person lie down, with the head and shoulders raised and supported. Control bleeding and dress any open scalp wounds. Look for and treat any other injuries. Call the emergency services. Monitor and record breathing, circulation and response level until help arrives.

UNCONSCIOUS VICTIM

Check DRSABC and begin CPR if needed. If the person is breathing, with signs of circulation, place in the recovery position and dress any open head wounds. Look for and treat other injuries. Call the emergency services and continue to monitor vital signs until help arrives.

FRACTURES TO THE FACE

Facial injuries are not often fatal, but they are worrying because of their potential to obstruct the airway and result in breathing problems. The wearing of seat belts can dramatically reduce facial injuries due to motor vehicle accidents, but these are still a main cause, together with sports, falls, and assaults. Heavy force is needed to fracture a bone in the face, and there will often be other injuries of the neck, chest, and skull to look out for.

Suspect a facial fracture if:

• The face looks asymmetrical or deformed in any way.

• There is bruising and/or a black eye.

• There is bleeding from the teeth or nose.

• The person cannot clench their teeth.

• There is difficulty breathing, or the person is snoring if unconscious.

FIRST AID FOR FACIAL FRACTURES OR INJURIES

Ensure that the person's airway is clear. If necessary, remove any debris from the mouth.

If there is a possibility of a spinal or neck injury, hold the head still. Cover any wound with a sterile dressing or clean pad and use direct pressure over the dressing to stem bleeding.

Call the emergency services promptly. Place an ice pack on any facial swelling.

FRACTURES TO THE JAW

The jaw is a common bone to break. Any blow to the chin may break one or both sides of the jaw. If both sides fracture, then the tongue can become unstable and may block the airway. Suspect a fractured jaw if:
- There is pain, nausea and/or swelling of the jaw area.
- The person cannot bite and is dribbling.
- The person has difficulty swallowing, breathing or speaking.

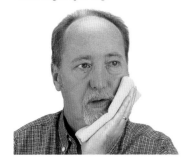

△ With a suspected jaw fracture, ask the person to hold a soft cloth against the injured site to protect it, and then transport them to hospital without delay.

FIRST AID FOR A FRACTURED JAW

If the person is seriously injured treat as for a facial fracture. If not, help them to sit up with their head forward to allow blood and saliva to drain out of the mouth. They should spit out any loose teeth.

If only one side of the jaw is painful and swollen, get them to hold a soft cloth against the area to keep it still.

Take or send them to the hospital, keeping the jaw supported.

NOSE AND CHEEKBONE FRACTURES

Fractures of the nose and cheekbone are generally not serious unless the cheekbone injury involves the eye socket. A direct blow to the eye, especially common in squash games, may cause what is called a "blow-out fracture", making it impossible for the person to look upward.

If you suspect either a nose or cheekbone (or eye socket) fracture, do not let the person blow their nose. This is because it may cause air to track through broken bones into the skin or into the brain.

Action to take if you suspect a fracture of a cheekbone or nose is to:
- check carefully to see whether the airway is clear and that it is not obstructed by swollen tissues
- apply a cold compress to the injured site to reduce pain and swelling
- get the person to the hospital.

If the injured person has a nosebleed, you should try to stop the bleeding; if the liquid is either clear or yellow, then treat as you would for a skull fracture.

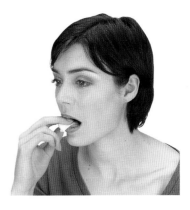

△ A dislodged tooth should be held in its socket either by keeping the mouth shut or by pressing on it with a gauze pad.

KNOCKED-OUT TEETH

Tooth injuries are especially common in children, and any loose first teeth should be taken out by a dentist, to avoid possible inhalation. Adult teeth can be damaged permanently by fracture or by being dislodged from a socket. If the tooth is not put back into its socket within 24 hours, the tooth dies and the socket shrinks, so that even false teeth cannot be used.

FIRST AID FOR A KNOCKED-OUT TOOTH

Pop the tooth back into its socket and ask the injured person to hold the tooth in place.

If they cannot hold it firmly in place, put the tooth in a cup or plastic bag of water or milk to prevent it drying out.

Take them to the hospital or dentist within 24 hours.

Managing spinal injuries

SEE ALSO

➤ LIFE-SAVING
PRIORITIES, p25

➤ Coping with neck
injuries, p156

The golden rule with spinal injuries (and neck injuries) is that the injured person must not be moved unless it is vital to do so. People with head injuries of any kind often have spinal injuries as well. The spinal cord, housed within the vertebrae, is commonly damaged at the mobile parts of the backbone such as the neck and lower back. Motor vehicle accidents, contact sports, and diving are notorious causes of spinal injuries; other causes include falling from a height, being thrown from a horse, and impact to the head and/or face.

The term spinal injury can refer to damage to the bones of the spine (vertebrae), the spinal cord, the disks between the backbones, or any muscles and ligaments attached to the spine. The most serious type of injury is to the spinal cord, as a partial or complete break can result in permanent paralysis. If a splinter of bone or swollen tissue compresses a nerve, a person may suffer a temporary paralysis, but sensation and movement return once the injury is treated.

THE BACKBONE

There are 24 moving vertebrae in the spine, and these form a column between the skull and the pelvis. The spinal cord travels down through a channel formed by the vertebral arches. Nerves supplying the arms pass out at the highest level, then those to the trunk, and then those to the legs. Between each vertebra and the next is a disk, which cushions force or pressure on the vertebrae. Ligaments and muscles also protect and strengthen the spine.

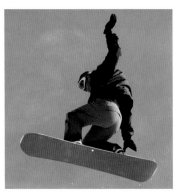
◁ Sport and recreational pursuits are common causes of spinal injury.

THE SPINE OR VERTEBRAL COLUMN

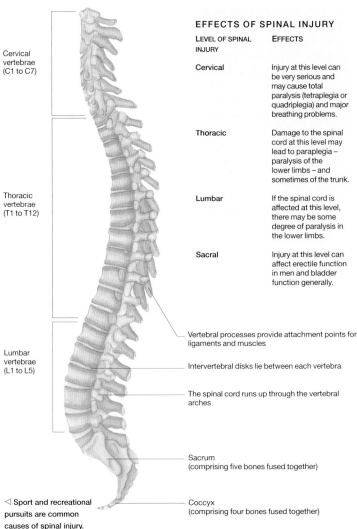

Cervical vertebrae (C1 to C7)

Thoracic vertebrae (T1 to T12)

Lumbar vertebrae (L1 to L5)

EFFECTS OF SPINAL INJURY

LEVEL OF SPINAL INJURY	EFFECTS
Cervical	Injury at this level can be very serious and may cause total paralysis (tetraplegia or quadriplegia) and major breathing problems.
Thoracic	Damage to the spinal cord at this level may lead to paraplegia – paralysis of the lower limbs – and sometimes of the trunk.
Lumbar	If the spinal cord is affected at this level, there may be some degree of paralysis in the lower limbs.
Sacral	Injury at this level can affect erectile function in men and bladder function generally.

Vertebral processes provide attachment points for ligaments and muscles

Intervertebral disks lie between each vertebra

The spinal cord runs up through the vertebral arches

Sacrum (comprising five bones fused together)

Coccyx (comprising four bones fused together)

FIRST AID FOR SPINAL INJURY IN AN UNCONSCIOUS PERSON

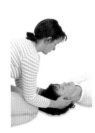

1 Keep the person still, in the position in which they are found. Hold the head still, as shown here, in its current position. Ask other people to support the rest of the body using hands and blankets, coats, or towels. Continue to keep the person as still as possible. If the injured person is already on their back, and their airway is clear, with nothing in the mouth and no signs of possible bleeding or vomiting, keep them in that position. If the tongue is falling back and blocking the airway, bring it forward by pushing up at the angles of the jaws, as already explained elsewhere. Do not use a head tilt to clear the airway.

2 With both unconscious and conscious victims, blood, vomit, or other substances in the mouth or throat can block the airway (listen for gurgling). Only if this is a risk, make sure that they are in a position that allows fluids to drain out of the mouth. If you need to move them for this, be gentle, keep movement minimal, and keep the head still as you do so. Use a "log roll" if turning them from their back to their side.

▽ Using the "log roll" – for draining the mouth or resuscitation.

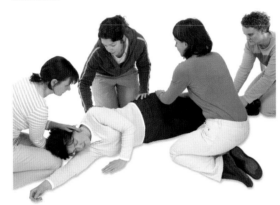

3 If the breathing or heartbeat stops, and the person is not already on their back, you must turn them onto their back to perform rescue breaths or CPR. Use the "log roll" technique, so that there is no change in the head position relative to the spine.

4 To resuscitate, one person holds the head still while another performs resuscitation.

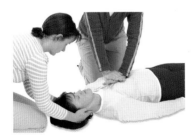

WARNING
Move a person with a suspected or certain spinal injury only if you really need to: to remove them from further serious danger; carry out resuscitation techniques (for which they must be on their back); or drain the mouth (for which they need to be on their side). Any moving needs at least four people – to make sure that the spine and the head do not change position.

SIGNS AND SYMPTOMS OF A SPINAL INJURY
Suspect a spinal injury if a person:

➤ Has suffered a significant impact/fall.

➤ Is unconscious after a head injury.

➤ Has fallen from a height and injured their face or head.

➤ Says that their neck hurts.

➤ Holds their neck in an odd position.

➤ Has any paralysis (loss of movement and sensation), loss of sensation, or tingling or numbness in their arms and/or legs.

➤ Is confused and uncooperative.

➤ Has lost bowel and bladder control.

➤ Has difficulty breathing, with only small amounts of movement in the abdomen.

➤ Is lying flat on their back with arms stretched above the head, or with arms and hands curled to the chest.

FIRST AID FOR A CONSCIOUS SPINAL INJURY VICTIM

Reassure the person. Unless there is an urgent reason to move them, such as breathing difficulties, do not do so. Call the emergency services promptly.

Ask the person to keep absolutely still. Kneel behind their head and hold their head still, in the position in which you found it.

Support their head at all times and ask someone to help monitor their breathing and circulation until medical help arrives.

Coping with neck injuries

SEE ALSO

➤ Removing clothing and helmets, p18
➤ Full resuscitation sequence, p34
➤ Managing spinal injuries, p154

The most important rule for dealing with a person with a suspected neck injury is that they are not to be moved, unless they would be in great danger, for example lying in the middle of a road or in the path of a spreading fire. A first-aider's priorities in such accidents are to prevent any further injury and phone the emergency services for urgent assistance. If an injured person has to be moved, the "log roll" technique, which requires a team of at least four people, must be used to keep the spine straight and supported at all times.

Fractures of the bones in the neck may be life-threatening injuries because the nerves that supply the main breathing muscle (the diaphragm) pass out of the spinal cord here; if these nerves are damaged by a fractured vertebra, breathing stops. The bones in the neck are more vulnerable than other vertebrae in the backbone, and are easily damaged.

BREATHING IS VITAL

Keeping the neck still is extremely important in a neck injury, but the ability to breathe is even more important. If a person is not breathing, then you must breathe for them. It is perfectly possible to do mouth-to-mouth on a person with a suspected neck injury. Ideally, you should get someone else to keep their head steady and supported, while you perform resuscitation techniques.

FIRST AID FOR A NECK INJURY

In any injury affecting the spine, but especially the neck, it is vital to keep the head still. Another helper should phone for help while you deal with the victim. You may well find the person on their back, as shown here. If not, do not move them onto their back unless you need to in order to deal with ABC problems.

IF YOU ARE ALONE...

If you are a lone first-aider, and have to leave the injured person to get help, immobilize their neck before you go with something like rolled-up towels, held in place by heavier objects. Tell the person to stay still and reassure them that you will return as soon as possible.

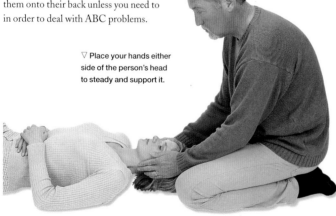

▽ Place your hands either side of the person's head to steady and support it.

HOW A NECK INJURY CAN DAMAGE BREATHING

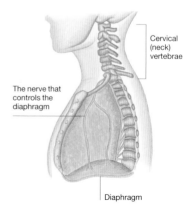

Cervical (neck) vertebrae

The nerve that controls the diaphragm

Diaphragm

▷ The nerve that controls the diaphragm exits the spine in the neck area. If this is damaged by a neck injury, breathing could cease.

THE "LOG ROLL" TECHNIQUE

If you absolutely must move someone with a spinal injury you should only use the "log roll" technique. By moving them "as one piece", with everyone in synchronicity, you avoid the head twisting on the shoulders or the body rotating on the pelvis. This minimizes the chances of any of the spinal vertebrae moving and causing more damage. There should be a minimum of four people present to carry out this technique. One person should be in charge of the head and should dictate everyone else's movements. There should always be one helper at the injured person's feet. The other helpers are positioned along the body at close intervals and act as a team. To be absolutely safe, the log roll needs training and team practice.

FIRST AID FOR A SUSPECTED NECK INJURY

Don't try to straighten or pull on the neck. Keep it in the position found, and as still as possible.

Ask a helper to get some towels or clothing and place these rolled-up items either side of the neck, all the time keeping it still.

Monitor and record their breathing and circulation and be prepared to start resuscitation procedures. If they vomit, "log roll" them onto their side.

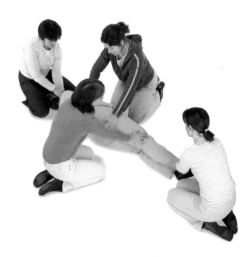

1 To move someone from their back onto their side (if they want to vomit or if blood, vomit, or other substances are blocking their mouth/throat): cross their arms over in front. Then, while one person supports the head, the other people stagger themselves along the body, gently straighten out the limbs and prepare to make the "log roll".

2 The head is supported all the time, and the helpers must hold the body, legs, and feet steady. The person's head, body, and toes must align and all face in the same direction. Once turned onto their side, keep them there, perfectly still, until professional help arrives. Move them (onto their back again) only if they stop breathing or their heart stops and resuscitation becomes necessary.

PREVENTING NECK/SPINAL INJURIES

Most spinal injuries occur in men aged 18 to 30 – the "risk-takers". Certain simple measures can prevent many such injuries:

➤ Always wear proper protective clothing when participating in a sport.

➤ Never dive into water until you know the depth, especially in tidal waters.

➤ Never dive into a swimming pool unless the water is at least 9 ft deep.

➤ Wear a seat-belt in any vehicle, and a padded jacket on a motorbike.

Tackling upper limb fractures

SEE ALSO

➤Fixing slings, p206

The bones of the shoulder, upper arm, forearm, wrist, and hand can all be fractured, and such fractures are relatively common. An outstretched hand or wrist often takes the brunt of forces from a fall but such forces can also travel up the arm and fracture one of the collarbones. With any upper limb fracture, the first-aider's main aims are to immobilize the injured limb (as it may well be unstable) and arrange transport to the hospital. Skill in applying various types of slings and bandages is crucial for dealing with such injuries.

When you arrive at an accident scene, watch out for these common signs of a potential fracture:
• Pain and tenderness at the site of injury, which is worse on moving.
• Swelling and deformity.
• Attempts by the person to support the injured arm by holding it in a certain way.

A FRACTURED COLLARBONE

The collarbones, also known as the clavicles, are one of the commonest bones to break, especially among young people doing sports. Sometimes the broken ends of the collarbone can pierce surrounding tissues and result in bleeding and swelling.

Most collarbone fractures knit together well simply by fixing the arm in a sling, which uses the weight of the arm to pull the fractured bones slowly back into line.

▽ By immobilizing the arm in a high (or "elevation") sling, pain and discomfort from collarbone fractures can be minimized until arrival at the hospital.

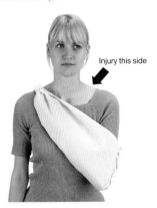

Injury this side

FIRST AID FOR A FRACTURED COLLARBONE

⬇

Ask/help the injured person to sit down.

⬇

Holding the upper arm (on the fracture side) still, carefully raise that forearm until the fingertips just touch the opposite collarbone. Ask the person to support the elbow with their other hand.

⬇

Place a triangular bandage over the affected arm, and tuck it under to form an elevation sling. If this causes pain, secure the arm in whatever position is comfortable.

⬇

Arrange transport to the hospital.

FRACTURES OF THE UPPER ARM

The long bone that joins the shoulder to the elbow – known as the humerus – fractures most frequently at the top end nearest the shoulder, which is its weakest part. This form of fracture may go unnoticed by an observer as it is usually a stable fracture (the bone ends are jammed together). The injured person may well be feeling some pain but may not seek medical assistance for some time.

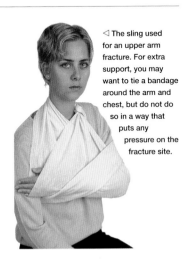

◁ The sling used for an upper arm fracture. For extra support, you may want to tie a bandage around the arm and chest, but do not do so in a way that puts any pressure on the fracture site.

FIRST AID FOR AN UPPER ARM FRACTURE

⬇

Ask the person to hold the injured arm across their body with their good hand.

⬇

Place a triangular bandage between the arm and the chest and tie a sling.

⬇

Tie a broad-fold bandage around the chest and arm to secure the sling before transporting the person to the hospital. Do this very low down the bent arm, so no pressure is put on the fracture site.

HUMERUS FRACTURE

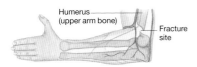

Humerus
(upper arm bone)

Fracture
site

△ Fractures of the humerus above the elbow are common in children. This unstable fracture may damage nearby blood vessels and nerves.

AN INJURED ELBOW

Elbows are highly sensitive when injured, even without fractures, and may be painful and stiff for weeks after an injury.

Dealing with elbow injuries depends on whether or not the elbow can be bent. For elbows that can bend, follow the advice for an upper arm injury. Non-bending elbows need completely different first aid.

FIRST AID FOR AN INJURED FOREARM, WRIST, OR HAND

Ask the injured person to sit down and help them if necessary.

Place the arm gently across their body keeping it steady and supported.

↓

Slide a triangular bandage in between the chest and the arm. Cradle the forearm in a well-padded support, such as a large padded envelope or a small pillow.

Finish tying the arm sling and arrange transport to the hospital.

DEALING WITH AN ELBOW THAT CANNOT BEND

1 Help the injured person to lie down. Position soft padding to support and cushion the arm, as shown below. Now add weighted boxes or objects at the side to hold the padding in place. Phone the emergency services. (Note: If you are in a remote location and are forced to transport the person to the hospital yourself, use broad bandages tied around the body to secure and immobilize the limb. However, never do this under normal circumstances, as it causes pain and potentially harmful further movement.)

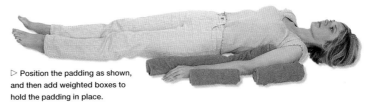

▷ Position the padding as shown, and then add weighted boxes to hold the padding in place.

FRACTURES TO THE FOREARM, WRIST OR HAND

It may be obvious when there is a fracture of the radius and ulna bones of the forearm, as there can be swelling and extreme tenderness. In children, whose soft, new bones often bend rather than break, there may only be a small crack called a greenstick fracture, and minimal swelling in the forearm.

A Colles fracture – a break of the radius bone near the wrist – is a common wrist fracture, often affecting older women.

The most common type of hand fracture affects the knuckle, often from a punch, but the hand can also be crushed, resulting in open fractures with profuse bleeding and swelling. As with any fracture, always compare the suspected injured side with the healthy side.

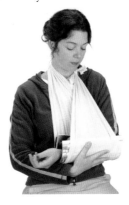

SIGNS AND SYMPTOMS OF A HAND INJURY

➤ An uninjured hand has a natural look called the "cascade" when it rests palm upward on a flat surface. Each finger curls naturally just under the larger finger next to it. If one finger lies straight or is very bent, serious tendon, bone, or nerve injury is likely.

➤ Ask the injured person to make a fist. Do all the fingers work together or do any seem to be out of line? If so, a bone may be broken.

➤ Numbness of any part of the hand beyond a wound is an ominous sign of nerve damage, as is lack of sweating.

FRACTURES TO THE FINGERS

For fractured fingers, apply padding around the hand, elevate in a high sling and take to the hospital. Avoid taping fingers together to splint them, as the tape will only have to be removed by hospital staff, causing pain and possible movement. Only splint if help will be delayed for more than 12 hours.

◁ Fractures to the forearm or wrist require supportive padding and a secure sling. Make sure that the support is lightweight – you must not use anything that will strain the neck.

Managing rib fractures

SEE ALSO

➤ Dealing with shock,
   p68
➤ Dealing with major
   wounds, p134
➤ Fixing slings, p206

While a cracked rib usually constitutes a relatively minor accident, multiple rib fractures can lead to a collapsed lung (a pneumothorax) or later to pneumonia. If part of the chest wall caves in completely an injury known as a "flail chest" may occur, which may cause severe breathing difficulties and is potentially life-threatening. If ribs lower down the rib cage are fractured they may damage internal organs nearby, such as the liver and spleen, causing internal bleeding, which could cause the injured person to go into shock.

A human rib cage has 12 pairs of ribs. All ribs connect with the spine at the back, and all but the lowest pair attach to the sternum at the front. The ribs are joined together by muscles, which expand and contract in order to move the rib cage. This movement, along with the movement of the diaphragm muscle, allows us to breathe.

The upper ribs protect the heart, lungs, and vital blood vessels in this area. The lower ribs help to protect internal organs such as the liver, stomach, and spleen.

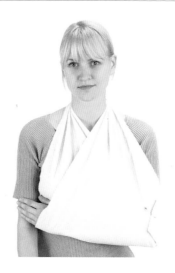

▷ For a fractured rib, use this type of sling to support the arm on the injured side. This prevents certain muscles (the ones that are attached to the chest and help to move the arm) from pulling on the ribs.

TYPES OF RIB FRACTURE

There is a difference between a cracked rib caused by a badly aimed kick during a football game, and the sort of fractures that might result from the impact of a steering wheel on the driver's chest in a motor vehicle accident. Although a single rib fracture can be excruciatingly painful and may remain so for up to 10 days after the injury, there is little chance that it could cause serious internal damage. Sometimes, although it is unusual, the jagged edge of a

SIGNS AND SYMPTOMS OF A FRACTURED RIB OR RIBS

As fractured ribs can cause a collapsed lung, possible internal bleeding, and/or breathing difficulties, it is vital to know the symptoms that indicate the severity of the injury so that the right help can be given.

Signs of fractured ribs:

➤ Sharp pain at the site of fracture.

➤ Painful breathing, especially when taking a deep breath in.

➤ Shallow breathing or breathlessness.

➤ Swelling or bruising over the fracture site.

➤ A crackling sensation affecting the chest wall.

➤ "Sucked in" air sounds through an open wound over the fracture site.

Signs of internal bleeding:

➤ Bright red, frothy, coughed-up blood in the mouth.

Signs of shock (due to internal bleeding):

➤ Pale skin, and/or a blueness just inside the lips.

➤ Dizziness.

➤ Nausea, possibly vomiting.

➤ Rapid shallow breathing or gasping for air.

➤ Any degree of deteriorating level of consciousness.

FIRST AID FOR A FRACTURED RIB

YOUR AIMS:
For a minor rib fracture you need to prevent further damage, such as from bending forward. For rib injury with possible complications (e.g. lung damage), call the emergency services and sit the person up, supported and relaxed, so that they can breathe more easily and oxygen demand is reduced.

For all cases: keep the person comfortable and supported and apply a broad arm sling to support the arm on the injured side.

For more minor cases, get them to hospital, keeping the chest supported.

fractured rib may penetrate a lung and cause it to collapse.

Multiple rib fractures are a different matter. These not only indicate the greater forces involved (and thus an increased chance that internal organs may be damaged) but also pose a potential danger in that the damaged section of the chest wall may lead to a pneumothorax and later to pneumonia. If damaged ribs become detached from the chest wall, part of the chest wall can cave in completely and form what is known as a "flail chest". Such a condition can cause serious breathing problems and is a potentially life-threatening situation.

In cases of rib fracture, especially if the person has been crushed, there is increased chance of internal bleeding and, in turn, of developing shock. Be aware of such events, monitor the injured person's ABC and be prepared to give first aid accordingly until medical help arrives.

PARADOXICAL BREATHING

This is a condition that occurs with some cases of flail chest. Usually, as a person breathes in, the rib cage moves up and out, and as they breathe out it returns to a lower position. If part of the chest wall is damaged, then it will move in a paradoxical way – in on inspiration and out on breathing out.

FIRST AID FOR FLAIL CHEST

When two or more consecutive ribs on the same side of the chest are fractured in two places, the injured part of the chest wall is known as a "flail segment". The injured person will display all the symptoms of a rib fracture, and may have paradoxical breathing.

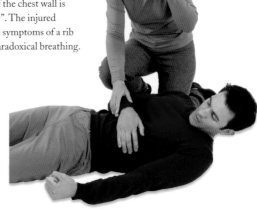

1 First assess the injured person, including their ABC. Whatever their condition, phone the emergency services promptly.

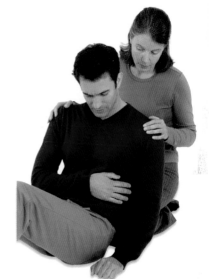

2 ▷ IF THE PERSON IS CONSCIOUS: Keep them sitting up as much as possible, relaxed, and supported from behind. This means they can breathe more easily and reduces the body's oxygen demand.

▽ IF THE PERSON IS UNCONSCIOUS: Place them in the recovery position, injured side down. This allows the uninjured side of the rib cage to expand. Place padding, in the form of folded blankets, towels, or clothes, either side of the flail area, to take pressure off the flail site itself. Avoid moving the person to tuck padding underneath them: you should place the padding on the floor first and then roll them very carefully onto it.

OPEN CHEST WOUNDS
If there is a deep chest wound at the fracture site, call the emergency services promptly. Apply a sterile dressing and a layer of plastic, secured with a firm bandage or adhesive tape on three sides. The person should be sitting up, preferably leaning toward the injured side. Apply a sling as for a simple rib fracture, keep the person supported, and await medical help.

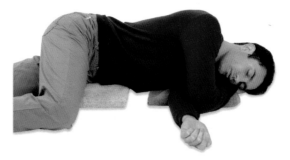

Coping with pelvic and upper-leg injuries

SEE ALSO
➤ Full resuscitation sequence, p34
➤ Dealing with shock, p68
➤ Recognizing internal bleeding, p140

The pelvis, hips, and thighbones all have a huge nerve and blood supply, and the pelvis contains many vital organs. Damage to any of these regions is an emergency. If fractured, the pelvis and/or thighbone can bleed profusely; multiple pelvic fractures are often fatal. Pelvic fracture may be caused by a crush injury, such as from a steering wheel in an automobile accident, or by indirect forces of the type occurring during vehicle collisions. A horse rider may suffer pelvic injury if they are thrown off, and/or are then kicked by, their horse.

PELVIC FRACTURES

Injuries to the pelvis must be taken seriously. Major blood vessels might be damaged, leading to profuse and even life-threatening internal blood loss. The bladder and urethra may be damaged by the fractured bones, as may the reproductive organs.

Pelvic fractures tend to result from high-speed accidents, and so there will often be other injuries too, including internal damage and spinal injuries. All of these factors may quickly lead to signs of shock developing.

SIGNS AND SYMPTOMS OF A FRACTURED PELVIS

➤ Pain and tenderness in the pelvis, groin or hip, especially on moving.

➤ Inability to walk or stand or to lift the legs while lying flat on the floor.

➤ An obviously deformed pelvis.

➤ Blood seeping from the penis or urethra (urinary outlet).

➤ Signs of shock or internal bleeding.

THE PELVIC REGION

▽ The pelvis comprises the ilium, pubis, and ischium bones. The head of the femur (thighbone) fits into the pelvis at the hip.

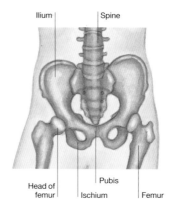

Ilium | Spine

Head of femur | Ischium | Pubis | Femur

WARNING

You should never attempt to move a person if you suspect a fractured pelvis unless they are in immediate danger – you could risk further serious damage.

STABILIZING A FRACTURED PELVIS

▷ To immobilize the legs while waiting for the emergency services, place padding either side of the body, extending above the pelvis, held in place by weighted objects. Make sure the feet cannot rotate – this rotates the head of the femur in the pelvis.

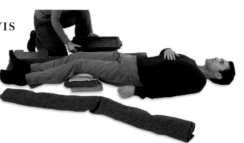

FIRST AID FOR A FRACTURED PELVIS

Call the emergency services urgently.

Move the injured person as little as possible; try to keep their feet in the position found. Place padding beneath the knees if this is more comfortable.

Stabilize the pelvis by immobilizing the legs: bandage the legs together, placing padding between the bony points at knees and ankles.

Do not bandage the legs if it is intolerably painful. Keep them still by placing rolled blankets or clothes either side of the legs, held in place by weighted objects.

Monitor the victim's condition, and keep a close watch for signs of shock.

FRACTURES TO THE THIGHBONE

The thighbone (femur) forms a large ball and socket joint – the hip – where it meets the pelvis. Any fracture to the thighbone is a serious emergency as it can lead to profuse bleeding if the broken bones pierce the large blood vessels nearby. Shock, then, is a distinct possibility and the injured person should be monitored closely for any such signs that appear.

The thighbone can fracture anywhere, but common sites include the long shaft and the neck (top) of the bone, near the hip joint. Fractures to the long shaft would occur after the considerable force involved in traumas such as motor vehicle accidents; fractures of the neck of the bone (that is, at the hip) are common in elderly people simply because their bones become much weaker and more brittle with age. If such a fracture is stable, an elderly person may hobble about on the injured leg. When combined with confusion or dementia, such a fracture may go unnoticed for some time as the person may forget that they have fallen or are in pain.

FEMUR FRACTURES

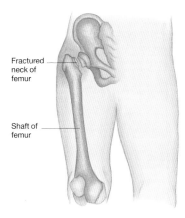

Fractured neck of femur

Shaft of femur

△ The thighbone (femur) commonly fractures at the top or along its shaft.

FIRST AID FOR A FRACTURED THIGHBONE

Call the emergency services promptly.

Keep the area still by using your hands or by placing padding (such as blankets or towels) around the hip, leg, and body, held in place with weighted objects. Ideally, padding should extend above the pelvis and below the knee.

Monitor the victim's vital signs and keep a close watch for signs of shock.

Only if you are in a very remote location and need to move the injured person yourself, splint the body (ideally from armpit to below the feet) on the injured side and secure the body and limb to the splint with bandages, tied at regular intervals.

SIGNS AND SYMPTOMS OF A FRACTURED THIGHBONE

➤ Pain and tenderness at the site of injury or at the knee.

➤ An inability to walk or put weight on the affected leg.

➤ Deformity in the affected leg, making it look shorter than the unaffected one.

➤ An awkward-looking leg that is noticeably bent at the knee and also turned outward at the ankle.

➤ Signs of shock.

FIRST AID FOR A FRACTURED THIGHBONE

▷ If someone with a fractured thighbone is found on their side, keep them in that position (always try to treat in the position found), but support their back in some way. Essentially, a fractured thighbone is treated in the same way as a fractured pelvis, using support and padding. This picture shows an alternative manual method of support, where the first-aider's arm is being used as a splint – this would be suitable for fracture cases where help will arrive quickly or there are few materials to hand.

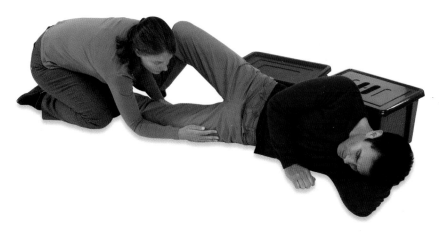

Handling knee and lower-leg injuries

SEE ALSO

➤ Managing sprains
and strains, p168

The knee is the body's largest joint. It can perform complex movements and is structured so that it remains stable while bearing the body's weight. The knee has sets of ligaments to hold the bones in place, including the patella (kneecap) at the front. Broken bones, tears, or impacts to the knee joint can produce incredible pain and swelling. Any fracture or tear requires immobilization, and open wounds should also be dealt with. Your first-aid aims are to immobilize limbs, minimize swelling, and arrange for urgent transport to the hospital.

INJURIES TO THE KNEE

There are two cruciate ligaments in the knee joint, so called because they cross over each other as they pass diagonally down from the thighbone to the shinbone. These ligaments are most commonly damaged in accidents when the knee is twisted. Other tissues in the knee that can suffer injury include the cartilage and the bony kneecap.

SIGNS AND SYMPTOMS OF A LOWER-LEG INJURY

➤ Pain deep within the knee or localized pain to the injury site, often made worse by trying to move the limb or put weight on it.

➤ Swelling and/or bruising around the knee or injury.

➤ Great pain when trying to straighten the leg (gently) if the knee has "locked".

➤ Broken bones protruding through the skin at the fracture site.

➤ Inability to bear weight on the affected side.

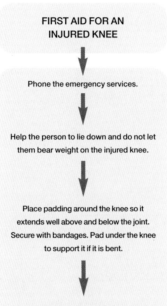

FIRST AID FOR AN INJURED KNEE

Phone the emergency services.

↓

Help the person to lie down and do not let them bear weight on the injured knee.

↓

Place padding around the knee so it extends well above and below the joint. Secure with bandages. Pad under the knee to support it if it is bent.

↓

If you are in a very remote location, you may need to transport the injured person to the hospital yourself. In this case, apply thick bandages well above and below the knee joint.

INJURIES TO THE LOWER LEG

The fibula is a spindly bone that fractures easily without necessarily stopping a person from bearing weight. Fractures of the fibula, therefore, may not be initially obvious. However, if the larger, load-bearing tibia (shinbone) is broken, a person cannot usually stand up or bear weight. A fracture of the tibia may cause bleeding and circulation problems in the area beyond the fracture site. Other injuries include tears to muscles, tendons and ligaments of the lower leg.

LOWER-LEG FRACTURES

▷ Any of the lower leg bones – patella, tibia or fibula – may be fractured in an accident. This illustration shows a fracture site in the thinner fibula.

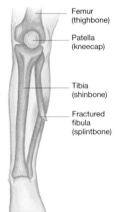

Femur (thighbone)

Patella (kneecap)

Tibia (shinbone)

Fractured fibula (splintbone)

FIRST AID FOR AN INJURED KNEE

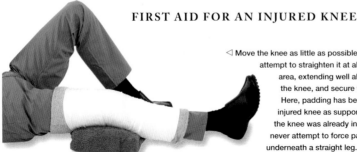

◁ Move the knee as little as possible, and never attempt to straighten it at all. Pad a wide area, extending well above and below the knee, and secure with bandages. Here, padding has been slid under the injured knee as support only because the knee was already in a bent position; never attempt to force padding underneath a straight leg.

FIRST AID FOR A LOWER-LEG FRACTURE

1 Help the injured person to lie down while supporting the injured leg. Feel the foot and lower leg for warmth and to check that the person can sense your touch.

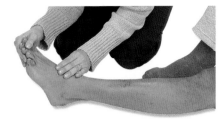

WARNING
Do not try to straighten the knee, as injuries within the knee joint may worsen as a result. With any lower-leg injury, do not let the victim bear any weight on the affected leg.

2 Phone for the emergency services. Place some soft padding on both sides of the legs, extending well above the knees and held in place by weighted boxes. Ensure that the foot is supported in the position found.

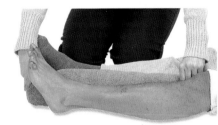

▷ If the paramedics are delayed, splint the injured leg to the uninjured one. Place padding between the legs and tie the bandages well above and below the site of the fracture.

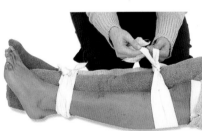

ANKLE INJURIES

By far the most common ankle injury is a sprain, which is dealt with elsewhere using the RICE guidelines (RICE stands for rest, ice, compression, and elevation). Any fracture to the ankle bone should be treated as for a lower-leg fracture.

A BROKEN FOOT

There are many small bones in the foot, any of which could be broken during an accident, most often one of a crushing nature. A fracture of the calcaneum (heelbone) is particularly common after a fall from a height onto the feet.

Individual toes may also suffer injury, but unless a toe is twisted right out of its usual alignment, even broken toes generally heal extremely well after professional medical treatment.

FIRST AID FOR A FRACTURE OF THE FOOT

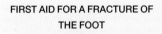

Help the injured person to sit down. Elevate and support the injured foot immediately to minimize swelling.

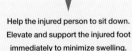

Applying a cold compress may further reduce swelling, but do not use if painful.

Get the person to the hospital by either car or ambulance.

▽ Elevate and comfortably support a fractured foot. Apply a cold compress (such as ice wrapped in a towel) to reduce swelling, but only if this does not cause pain. Raise the leg above horizontal if possible and comfortable, and try to keep it elevated during transportation to the hospital.

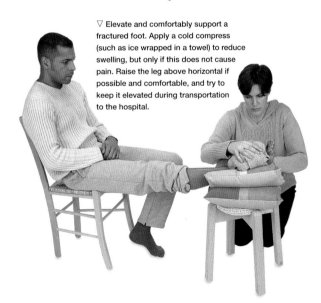

Coping with dislocations

SEE ALSO

➤ Moving and handling safely 1 and 2, pp20, 22

➤ Understanding the skeleton, p148

Any joint may become dislocated due to a violent wrenching action. When a joint is dislocated, surrounding muscles, ligaments, tendons, and blood vessels may be disturbed or damaged as a result. The force of dislocation can sometimes also produce a fracture nearby.

The dislocated joint looks misshapen and soon becomes swollen, discolored, and immobile, and the person experiences extreme pain. First-aiders should try to immobilize the injured joint, to prevent further injury and reduce pain, and seek emergency medical help.

Dislocations may occur within any joint, when the end of a bone is pulled or pushed out of place and thus out of the joint. It can be a very distressing experience as the muscles around a dislocated joint often go into spasm, causing intense pain. Nerves and blood vessels around the joint may also be damaged.

It is not always possible to distinguish between a fracture and a dislocation, and both may occur within a joint at the same time. If in doubt, treat a dislocation as if it were a fracture.

The most common joints for dislocation are the shoulder, hip, elbow, jaw, and joints of the thumbs and fingers.

WARNING

Never try to relocate the bone of a dislocated joint or attempt any strategies to get the bone to "pop" back in again. It is easy to inflict further serious damage.

SIGNS AND SYMPTOMS OF A DISLOCATED SHOULDER

➤ It may be possible to feel the "popped out" rounded head of the humerus (upper arm bone) in front of the shoulder joint.

➤ Distortion in the shoulder joint; the upper arm may look flat.

➤ Severe pain in the shoulder, which is also difficult to move.

➤ Swelling and/or bruising in the joint.

FIRST AID FOR A DISLOCATED SHOULDER

Get the person to sit down and make them as comfortable as possible. Let them hold their arm in whatever position is least painful. Calm and reassure them – dislocations can be sudden and acutely painful and so may be highly distressing.

Slide a triangular bandage between the arm of the affected shoulder and the chest, as for an arm sling. Very gently place some padding under the affected arm.

Tie the arm sling so that the affected arm is well supported.

Arrange transport to the hospital. In transit, the person should stay seated.

SHOULDER DISLOCATION

Some people are unlucky enough to suffer from this common injury recurrently. For these unfortunate few, the condition is often just as painful as for one-off or occasional cases, but the shoulder does "pop" back in much more easily.

IMMEDIATE HELP FOR A DISLOCATED SHOULDER

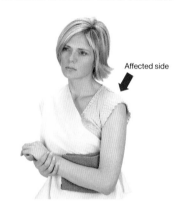

Affected side

1 Carefully place a sling and some soft padding between the arm of the affected shoulder and the body.

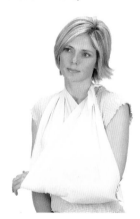

2 Once the padding is in place, tie the sling so that the joint is supported. Get the person to the hospital right away.

HOW TO DEAL WITH A DISLOCATED HIP

The hip joint may dislocate, for example, when the knee hits the dashboard in a motor vehicle accident. This often results in a fractured pelvis and damage to nearby nerves as well, resulting in paralysis. The head of the thighbone usually moves backward, and the leg rotates outward and is bent at the knee. The bony end of the thighbone may be easily felt or seen sticking out under the skin at or near the hip.

▽ Treatment for a dislocated hip is essentially the same as for a fractured pelvis or thighbone. Treat the person in the position found and do not move them if at all possible. Immobilize the immediate and surrounding area by padding and supporting it – using rolled blankets, towels, or clothes located under the knees and either side of the body and secured by weighted objects such as boxes and briefcases.

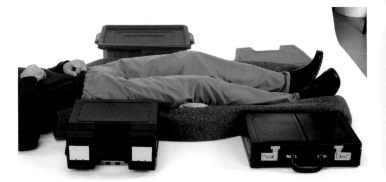

A DISLOCATED ELBOW

Children very easily stretch ligaments. In the elbow, the top of one of the forearm bones (the radius) sometimes "pops out" of the elbow joint, especially if a child's arm is yanked suddenly as might happen in a fall. Suspect a pulled elbow if:
- The child suddenly stops using the affected arm.
- The child cries when the arm is moved or touched at all, especially in the elbow area.

HOW TO DEAL WITH A CHILD'S PULLED ELBOW

Reassure the child and allow them to hold their arm in whatever position they find comfortable.

Do not try to "pop" the lower arm back into place. Phone the emergency services or take the child to the hospital.

A DISLOCATED JAW

This is a fairly common occurrence and may be caused by an everyday action of the jaw, such as yawning. In cases of a dislocated jaw, a person will not be able to move the jaw at all so they will be unable to close their mouth or speak properly. The jaw will have to be relocated in hospital, after which it will have to be kept completely immobile for 24 hours.

HAND DISLOCATIONS

Contact sports, such as martial arts, and skiing accidents can often lead to the dislocation of one of the many joints in the hand, especially the thumb. The best action to take is to pad up the hand and elevate it in a high sling before taking the person to the hospital for medical treatment. Never attempt to change the position of any damaged fingers.

HOW TO DEAL WITH A DISLOCATED HAND

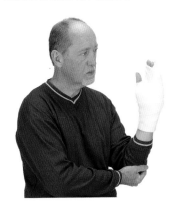

1 Remove any rings before the hand starts to swell, but only if you can avoid bending affected fingers. Ask the person to support their arm while you wrap the hand in padding.

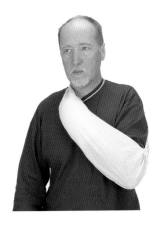

2 Once the hand is comfortable and the arm supported, immobilize the joint using a high sling (and more padding if necessary). Firmer support could be given by tying another bandage around the sling to attach it to the body. Get the person to the hospital.

Managing sprains and strains

SEE ALSO

➤ Moving and handling safely 1 and 2, pp20, 22

➤ Applying dressings & bandages, p200

➤ Applying bandages 1, p202

The soft tissues – muscles, tendons, and ligaments – that attach to or support the bones of the skeleton can also be injured or damaged in an accident. Such injuries are generally called sprains and strains and happen most often during sporting activities. The first-aid aims of treating such soft-tissue injuries are to reduce pain and swelling and to seek medical help if necessary. It can sometimes be tricky to distinguish between a sprain and a fracture, and so medical advice should be sought if there is any doubt about the injury.

For your skeleton to be able to move your body about, it needs the help of essential soft tissues – muscles, tendons and ligaments. Muscles attach to bones via tendons, while ligaments are the tough fibrous cords that hold bones together at joints and allow joints to function properly. Together the bones, muscles and joints are known as the musculoskeletal system.

When there are no broken bones, the injury is called a soft-tissue injury. These are perceived to be less serious than fractures but can still cause a great deal of pain and disability. If they are not dealt with properly in the initial stages, they may lead to long-term weakness and malfunction in a muscle or joint.

SPRAINED ANKLE

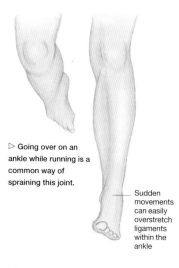

▷ Going over on an ankle while running is a common way of spraining this joint.

Sudden movements can easily overstretch ligaments within the ankle

TORN LIGAMENTS

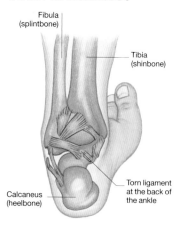

Fibula (splintbone)

Tibia (shinbone)

Calcaneus (heelbone)

Torn ligament at the back of the ankle

△ In a sprained ankle, one or more of the ligaments are partially or completely torn.

SIGNS AND SYMPTOMS OF A SPRAIN OR STRAIN

Bear in mind that it can be difficult to distinguish between a sprain or strain and a fracture. There are a few clues, though, to watch out for.

Symptoms of a sprain or strain include:

➤ Pain and tenderness. (If the injured person heard or felt a crack at the time of the incident, the injury is more likely to be a fracture.)

➤ Inability to use the injured part. (However, an immediate inability to bear weight on the injured part points to a fracture.)

➤ Swelling and bruising. (If the swelling takes several hours to appear it is more likely to be a soft-tissue injury; swelling after a fracture is immediate.)

DIFFERENT TYPES OF SOFT-TISSUE INJURY

➤ Sprain – A common form of ligament injury resulting in tearing or overstretching of the ligament.

➤ Strain – The tearing or overstretching of a muscle. Strains often happen near the junction of the muscle and its tendon, which tethers the muscle to the nearby bone.

➤ Rupture – The complete tearing of a ligament or a muscle.

➤ Bruise – The swelling, pain and bleeding below the skin that result from a direct blow to the body. A large amount of blood that collects as a result of damage is known as a hematoma.

HOW TO TREAT SPRAINS AND STRAINS

After following the RICE guidelines (opposite), you may decide to seek medical attention. After following RICE, minor soft-tissue injuries should be followed by gentle, controlled exercise as soon as symptoms allow. Many sprains remain stiff, swollen, and painful even after 48 hours of RICE treatment. This is normal, and it is important to start using the joint or muscle, as it can easily stiffen up and recover slowly. If not properly treated in the first few weeks after injury, a sprain can cause recurrent problems in the long term – even more so than a simple fracture in the same area.

HOW TO DEAL WITH A SPRAINED ANKLE

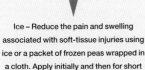

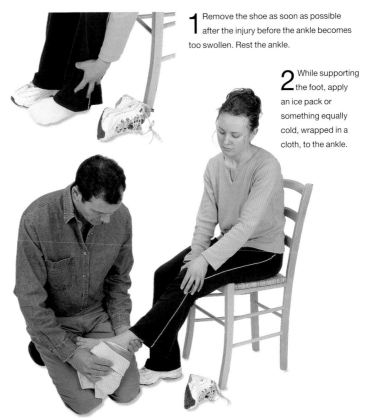

1 Remove the shoe as soon as possible after the injury before the ankle becomes too swollen. Rest the ankle.

2 While supporting the foot, apply an ice pack or something equally cold, wrapped in a cloth, to the ankle.

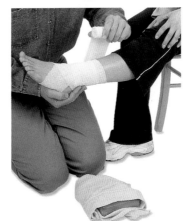
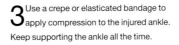

3 Use a crepe or elasticated bandage to apply compression to the injured ankle. Keep supporting the ankle all the time.

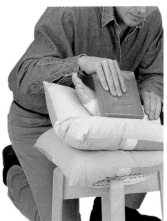

4 Carefully place the injured ankle in a position that keeps it rested, comfortable, and elevated. Apply a cold compress regularly.

Controlling back pain

SEE ALSO

➤ Moving and handling safely 1 and 2, pp20, 22

➤ Managing spinal injuries, p154

Back pain varies enormously from person to person. Even an excruciating bout of back pain can resolve itself in a matter of a few weeks. However, anyone who is worried about what is causing the pain in their back should consult their doctor. When approaching an incident where someone complains of back pain, be alert to the danger signs that could indicate some form of spinal injury. Much back pain resolves with painkillers and, contrary to popular opinion, staying active – resting can make the back stiff and immobile.

Most people suffer from back pain at some point in their lives. In the vast majority of cases, the pain is in the lower back, or lumbar region. The lumbar spine has to be strong as it bears the weight of the body as well as any other loads it has to carry.

It is reassuring to know that back pain is not usually due to any serious disease. Most cases of low back pain resolve quickly, although they may take up to 6–8 weeks to settle down completely. Upper back pain is more unusual.

▷ Pain in the mobile regions of the spine – the neck and lower back – is the most common form of back pain.

COMMON PAIN SITES

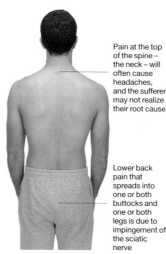

Pain at the top of the spine – the neck – will often cause headaches, and the sufferer may not realize their root cause

Lower back pain that spreads into one or both buttocks and one or both legs is due to impingement of the sciatic nerve

CAUSES OF BACK PAIN

Frustratingly for the sufferer, the exact cause of most back pain is rarely discovered. Back pain tends to originate in the muscles, ligaments, and joints of the back, but pinpointing exactly which ones is often impossible. Rarely, there is an underlying cause, such as a tumor, kidney problems, a collapsed vertebra due to the bone-thinning condition osteoporosis, scoliosis (loss of the natural curvature of the spine), or a slipped intervertebral disk.

SPINAL COMPRESSION

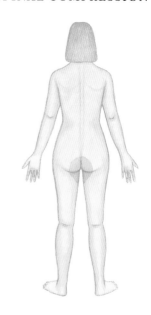

△ People with numbness in this "saddle" area may have spinal compression and should see a doctor immediately. (Sphincter disturbance and lower limb weakness are other signs.)

SIGNS AND SYMPTOMS OF BACK PAIN

Signs of back pain:

➤ Pain, which may vary from dull to severe, across the lower back is particularly common. Sometimes this pain spreads into the buttock and shoots down the leg (sciatica); such pain is due to pressure on the sciatic nerve.

➤ Inability to move the back, especially bending and leaning back.

➤ Muscle spasm in the back muscles, causing a rigid or stiff neck.

➤ Tenderness in the back muscles themselves.

Seek medical help if there is also:

➤ Pain in the buttocks, legs, or arms.

➤ Any numbness or tingling in the limbs.

➤ Weight loss.

➤ Fever.

➤ Any loss of sensation or movement.

➤ General feeling of being unwell.

➤ Incontinence or inability to open bowels. Urinary problems such as low output, pain on urinating, unusual color, smell, or cloudiness.

➤ Unremitting/increasing back pain.

➤ If the person is under 20 or over 50.

WHAT YOU CAN DO AT HOME

Most people find it useful to use pain-controlling medication of some kind but a doctor may prescribe a muscle relaxant if the pain is not relieved by painkillers alone. Many physical activities can also be modified in order to avoid potential problems in the first place:

• Lifting – Never twist the back, but turn with the feet instead. Always bend at the knees to grasp the object and use the legs to help you lift rather than relying solely on the strength of your back. Keep the heaviest side of the object close to your body and get help if needed.

PAIN IN THE OVER-50S

The sudden onset of severe and unremitting back pain in anyone over 50 should be taken seriously, especially if it is not in the lower back, but higher up. The bones of the back are a common place for various cancers to spread to, and there are also cancers that develop in the bones of the back.

• Sitting – Sit in an upright chair for no longer than 20–30 minutes at a time. Also, a lumbar support helps to keep you sitting "tall" rather than slumping.
• Driving – Traveling of any kind can make back pain much worse, especially when undertaking long-distance journeys.
• Sleeping – Get a good night's sleep and lie on a fairly firm, flat surface. Too soft and too hard are both bad for the back.
• Working – Make sure all working surfaces are at a good height for you, so that you are not straining.

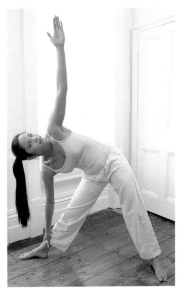

△ When trying out a new activity, such as yoga, take it easy on your back and stretch slowly and gradually.

STAY ACTIVE AND AT WORK

People who are physically fit suffer from less back pain and generally recover faster than those who are unfit and overweight. Regular gentle activity helps to strengthen a painful back, and the sooner this exercise is started the better. Swimming, walking, and cycling are all good low-impact exercises that will not damage the back.

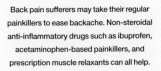

HOW TO DEAL WITH BACK PAIN

Back pain sufferers may take their regular painkillers to ease backache. Non-steroidal anti-inflammatory drugs such as ibuprofen, acetaminophen-based painkillers, and prescription muscle relaxants can all help.

In the first 24 hours, apply an ice-pack or bag of frozen peas wrapped in a towel to the back for regular periods of 10 minutes. Then try alternating this with a soak in a hot bath or a hot-water bottle (but be aware that heat can worsen inflammation).

Back manipulation – Physical therapies such as osteopathy and chiropractic can help relieve back pain and solve many back-related problems.

Alternative therapies – Acupuncture and reflexology are just two of the alternative treatments available for easing back pain.

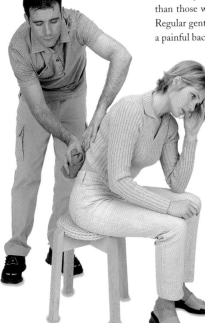

◁ To ease back pain, apply an ice pack or bag of frozen peas – wrapped in a towel – to the site of the pain.

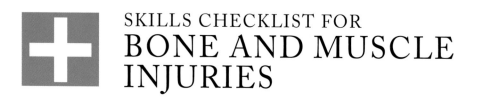

SKILLS CHECKLIST FOR
BONE AND MUSCLE INJURIES

KEY POINTS

- Take great care over how and when to move someone with a bone or muscle injury, especially if they have a definite/suspected spinal injury; keeping affected parts still and supported is key ☐

- Splinting is best reserved for extreme situations where you are forced to take the injured person to the nearest hospital yourself ☐

- Be alert to the possibility of a spinal injury after any accident ☐

- Do not try to relocate a dislocated joint ☐

- Back pain usually resolves itself within 6–8 weeks ☐

SKILLS LEARNED

- How to tackle both "open" and "closed" fractures ☐

- How to deal with the many different types of fractures, all over the body ☐

- How to recognize and manage potential spinal problems ☐

- How to "log roll" an injured person ☐

- How to deal with dislocations, strains and sprains ☐

- How to relieve back pain ☐

11

BURNS AND SCALDS

First aid is of paramount importance for the burn victim. The first-aider can significantly limit the pain, damage, and trauma caused by the burn by cooling the area as quickly as possible. Reducing the skin's temperature in this way helps to limit the depth and severity of damage to underlying tissues. Burns range from a straightforward, relatively superficial injury to a very deep injury that penetrates muscles, nerves, and bone. Many burns are associated with electrical faults and with smoking and alcohol. Home safety has a major part to play in preventing such accidents. Burns are the third largest cause of accidental deaths in the home.

CONTENTS

Understanding and assessing burns 1 174–175

Understanding and assessing burns 2 176–177

Managing burns 178–179

Chemical, electrical and inhalation burns 180–181

Coping with facial burns 182

Tackling sunburn 183

Skills checklist 184

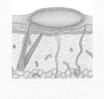

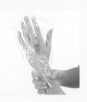

Understanding and assessing burns 1

SEE ALSO

➤ Assessing burns 2,
  p176

➤ Safety in the home,
  p224

➤ Safety in the
  kitchen, p226

Initial action with any burn, however severe, is the same – having dealt with any danger, remove the source of the burn and cool the burned area. Cooling the skin as quickly as possible reduces any pain and swelling and also helps to prevent damage to underlying tissues.

Burns weaken and damage the skin, so when you flood the burned area with water do not turn on a faucet to full power. Remove any constricting articles, such as jewelry. If a burn is larger than 1in square, the injured person should be taken to the hospital.

The skin is the body's largest organ, covering its entire surface. It forms a barrier against infection and also helps protect against injury and maintain body temperature. Burns to the skin cause instant damage but quick thinking and rapid first-aid action can make all the difference to the outcome. If deep layers of the skin are damaged, they will not heal easily and may even require skin grafts.

COMPLICATIONS OF BURNS

When giving first aid for a serious burn, bear in mind the following life-threatening burn-related complications:

• If the victim's airway becomes burned it may swell, resulting in potentially fatal breathing problems.

• The victim may have other injuries (if they have jumped to escape a fire or have been in an explosion, for example).

• If the entire circumference of the chest is burned, they will not be able to move their chest in order to breathe.

• Severe burns lead to large amounts of fluid loss and therefore can lead to shock.

GIVING ALL THE DETAILS

When speaking to the emergency services, it is essential to tell them anything you know about the cause of the burn. If there was an explosion, for example, the person may have other injuries. And if there was burning material, or the fire was in an enclosed space, there is a risk of inhalation poisoning and airway swelling. Knowing how long the victim was exposed to the material will help paramedics to assess the extent of any damage.

THE SKIN'S STRUCTURE

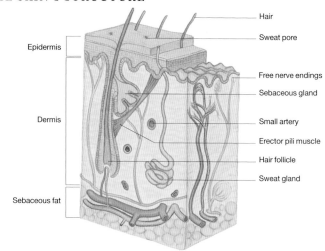

- Hair
- Sweat pore
- Free nerve endings
- Sebaceous gland
- Small artery
- Erector pili muscle
- Hair follicle
- Sweat gland

Epidermis

Dermis

Sebaceous fat

DIFFERENT TYPES OF BURNS

➤ Dry burns – Such injuries are caused by any form of flame or hot surface, such as lighted cigarettes, hot irons and hobs, bonfires and hot barbecue coals.

➤ Wet burns – Also called scalds, these are caused by boiling liquids, steam, and hot cooking fat or oil.

➤ Cold burns – The skin can also be burned by extreme cold, such as contact with ice-cold metal.

➤ Friction burns – These are the result of a surface (especially of a synthetic material) rubbing against the skin at speed. A moving rope or wire, revolving brushes, and machine belts are common culprits.

➤ Radiation burns – Most commonly from over-exposure to ultraviolet light, such as in sunburn.

➤ Chemical burns – Many common home and industrial chemicals (such as bleach, ammonia, dishwasher products, oven cleaners, sodium hydroxide, dry lime, and sulfuric acid) cause burns if they come into contact with skin. Appropriate safety gloves should be worn when using such products in the home, and protective clothing should be worn by anyone dealing with industrial chemicals.

➤ Electrical burns – These burns are caused by contact with electricity in any form, including lightning.

ESSENTIALS OF BURN MANAGEMENT

Cooling and covering the burned area are the major principles to remember when dealing with burns and scalds. Cooling the area is vital – not only will this reduce pain but it will also limit the extent of the burn and any damage.

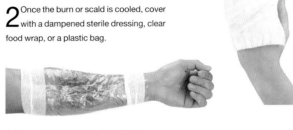

▽ Loosely wrapped damp gauze placed around a finger burn.

2 Once the burn or scald is cooled, cover with a dampened sterile dressing, clear food wrap, or a plastic bag.

△ To use clear food wrap, discard an initial length of wrap (it will be dirty). Place a piece of wrap around the area fairly loosely, with the edges folded into pleats; this allows room in case the burn swells. Secure with bandages.

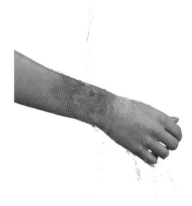

1 Cooling the burned or scalded area is a top priority. Hold the affected area under a stream of cold water for at least 10 minutes. You should cool only the burned area; do not overcool the injured person.

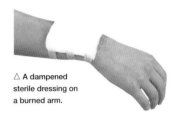

△ A dampened sterile dressing on a burned arm.

ASSESSING BURNS

One important aspect of dealing with burns is deciding how severe the problem is. You need to assess whether a burn is minor or major. Factors affecting this include the depth, extent, and site of the burns. For example, burns in the neck and head area can compromise the airway, while burns in the genital area may lead to large amounts of swelling and serious problems with urination.

MINOR AND MAJOR BURNS

Use the following summary when assessing whether a burn is minor or major and deciding what to do. (However, if you are at all unsure, always seek expert help.)

Minor/superficial burns

If the burn seems relatively small and superficial and there is no risk of infection or scarring, you should give appropriate first aid and advise the injured person to see their doctor if they are concerned.

Superficial/mild partial-thickness burns

(Note: thickness of burns is dealt with in more detail on the following pages.) If the burn is of this type, and there are other symptoms present – such as dizziness, headache or fainting – the casualty should be seen by a doctor or emergency department without delay.

Serious burns

These include:
- Non-superficial burns with an area greater than 1in square.
- Burns in young children and the elderly.
- Electrical and chemical burns.
- Deep/full-thickness burns of any size.
- Burns that go all around a limb or the chest ("circumferential" burns).

WARNING

Do not touch the burned area. Do not break blisters or remove loose skin. Never use adhesive, dry, or fluffy dressings. Do not apply anything (lotions, ointments, or grease) to the burned area.

- Burns to either the palms of the hands or the genitals.

Potentially life-threatening burns

These include:
- Burns to the airway, face, or neck.
- Anyone who has inhaled smoke, fumes, or flames.
- A burn over a large area (more than 1 percent of the body; see following pages), if deeper than superficial.

You must get these burns seen by emergency medical help immediately.

Understanding and assessing burns 2

SEE ALSO

➤ Understanding and assessing burns, p174

➤ Safety in the kitchen, p226

It can be hard to judge exactly how severe burns are, but understanding a little more about burn depth and area will help. If you are in any doubt about the severity of any kind of burn, seek medical help as fast as possible. If the injured person is clearly in distress and some pain, call the emergency services immediately, or take the victim to the nearest emergency room yourself. If the burns are severe or over a large surface area, then the victim may go into shock, so watch for shock signs and be prepared to resuscitate if necessary.

ASSESSING A BURN'S DEPTH

The depth of a burn depends upon the intensity of, and length of exposure to, the burn agent (such as heat, cold, or chemicals). The skin has two layers: a surface layer called the epidermis and a deeper layer called the dermis. How deeply a burn has damaged the skin is an indicator of potential complications – fewer such events occur with superficial burns compared with partial- or full-thickness burns.

SUPERFICIAL BURNS

Formerly known as first-degree burns, this type of burn involves only the very uppermost layer of the skin – the epidermis. Typical features of a superficial burn include:

- Red-looking skin that may be a little puffy but with no blistering; it will feel very sensitive and painful.
- Blanching of the skin when pressed.
- Fairly fast healing – usually within 10 days and without leaving a scar.

PARTIAL-THICKNESS BURNS

Burns of this kind used to be called second-degree burns. They destroy areas of the epidermis and result in blistering. Large amounts of fluid may be lost from partial-thickness burns if they cover a large area of the body.

- The skin is red or white, blistered, and extremely painful.
- The burn may heal within 21 days and cause little scarring, but very deep burns may take up to 60 days and leave more extensive scars.

DEPTHS OF BURN

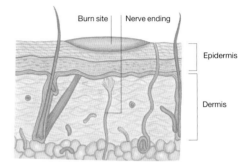

▷ Superficial burns involve only the outermost layer of skin – the epidermis. Underlying layers and the structures they contain, such as nerve endings, are unaffected.

Burn site | Nerve ending

Epidermis

Dermis

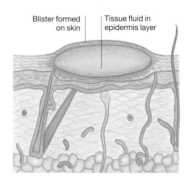

▷ A partial-thickness burn is again limited to the epidermis layer. The skin will look red and raw and will be blistered because tissue fluid from damaged tissues accumulates.

Blister formed on skin | Tissue fluid in epidermis layer

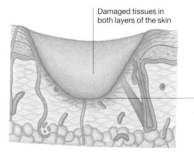

▷ A full-thickness burn affects both layers of the skin. Because of the burn's severity, fat, nerves, muscle, and blood vessels may also be damaged.

Damaged tissues in both layers of the skin

Pain sensation may be lost as nerve endings are damaged

FULL-THICKNESS BURNS

This type of burn was previously known as a third-degree burn. Such serious burns extend into the skin's dermis and beyond. Hair follicles, nerves, and sweat glands, which lie within the dermis, may never recover if they are badly burned. Fluid is unable to ooze through the damaged dermis but is lost internally. In a full-thickness burn:

• The skin is white, black, or brown.
• The skin appears leathery or waxy (do not touch it to see how it feels).

• The burned area is numb and therefore, paradoxically, less painful than a less serious burn.
• The affected skin will never heal on its own and requires a skin graft.

THE EXTENT OF THE BURN

When assessing burns, it is vital to judge how much of the body's surface area is affected, as this will indicate likely fluid losses. When tissue is damaged by burns, tissue fluid leaks from tiny capillaries in the skin as a response and forms blisters or

seeps out of the skin blood vessels. The bigger the burn, the bigger the fluid loss and thus the higher the risk of shock.

When trying to assess just how serious a victim's burns are, it can be helpful to think of the palm of the person's hand (including their fingers) as representing 1 percent of their total body surface. As a good general guide, any partial-thickness burn of 1 percent or more should be seen urgently by a doctor. Any suspected full-thickness burn, no matter what size, is an emergency and must be seen immediately.

ASSESSING THE BURN AREA

▽ Professional medical personnel have traditionally used the "rule of nines" as a way of accurately assessing the area, and therefore the potential severity, of a burn. Under this rule, parts of the body can be assigned 9 percent or multiples of 9 percent. However, the average first-aider should never waste valuable time trying to make such a detailed assessment. Instead, they can quickly compare it to the size of the inner surface of the hand (see right).

▽ Using the burn victim's hand as a guide is now a common way for first-aiders to assess a burn area. The area of the inner surface of their hand, including the fingers, represents about 1 percent of their body area. If a burn is deeper than superficial and has an area of 1 percent or more, the victim must be seen urgently in hospital.

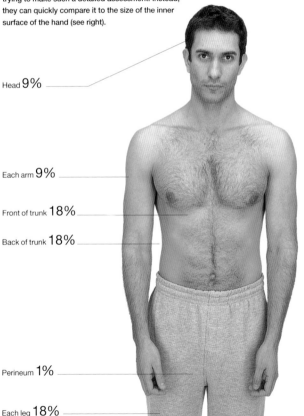

Head 9%

Each arm 9%

Front of trunk 18%

Back of trunk 18%

Perineum 1%

Each leg 18%

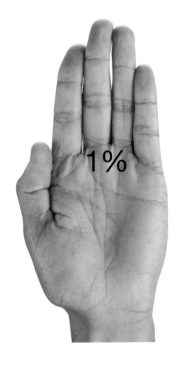

1%

Managing burns

SEE ALSO

➤ Dealing with shock, p68

➤ Understanding and assessing burns, p174

➤ Assessing burns 2, p176

Time is of the essence when giving first aid to a person with burns. You must ensure that they are no longer in danger of further burns and then cool the affected area of skin. Do not turn the faucet on full as a powerful jet of water may cause further damage to the delicate skin of the burned area. Reassure the victim and phone the emergency services if necessary. If you think the burns are deep or cover a large proportion of the injured person's body, watch them carefully and be ready to deal with signs of further problems, such as shock.

As already mentioned, a major priority in all burn cases is to cool the skin. This not only eases much of the pain, but also ultimately reduces the amount of damage done to the skin, so that it heals faster and scars less. However, be careful about making the person too cold and causing hypothermia. If in doubt, cover them with a coat or light blanket.

COVERING BURNS

Skin damage allows potential infection to enter, so burns must be covered. Dry dressings, even non-fluffy ones, tend to stick to burns, so the best options are: wet sterile dressings of various kinds (or dampened clean handkerchiefs or clean cotton pillowcases), clean plastic bags, or clear food wrap.

PUTTING OUT FLAMES

If someone's clothing is on fire, drop them to the ground and, if possible, wrap them from head to toe in a heavy, non-synthetic material (for example, a cotton or wool rug, coat, or curtain) to exclude air. Roll them on the ground to smother the flames, then douse their burns in plenty of water.

WHAT TO DO WITH SMALL BURNS AND SCALDS

BURNS: BASIC PRIORITIES

⬇

Follow the "Danger" step of DRSABC. Protect yourself and the victim from any further danger and further burns.

⬇

Check the victim's RABC; monitor for noisy or difficult breathing.

⬇

Cool down the burned skin. For serious burns, call the emergency services.

⬇

Cover the burn, to prevent infection.

⬇

Minimize shock and check for any other injuries.

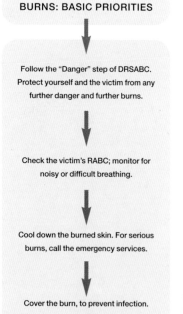

1 Run cold water over the burn site for at least 10 minutes. If the burn is on a hand or arm, remove any watches, rings, or bracelets while you are cooling the skin, as the burn may cause some swelling of tissues.

2 After cooling, help prevent infection by wrapping the area with a damp sterile bandage, clear food wrap, or a small plastic bag (for hands and feet). When using a plastic bag, fill it with air (do not blow into it, as that will introduce germs), gently place the hand or foot in the open bag, then hold loosely in place at the wrist or ankle with a length of dressing, a bandage or similar – never use rubber bands.

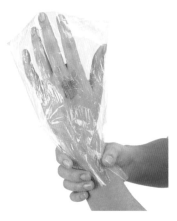

FIRST AID FOR ALL MAJOR BURNS AND SCALDS

1 Having controlled or eliminated any dangers, put the
victim into a safe position. This is usually lying flat, unless
there is breathing difficulty, in which case they should sit
upright and supported. Send for the emergency services.
Now cool the burned area with cold water for at least
10 minutes. While cooling, remove any constricting items
such as rings, watches and bracelets before swelling cuts off
the circulation. See box for advice on clothing removal.

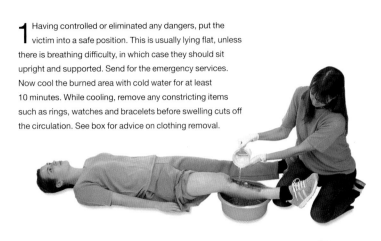

2 If the paramedics have not arrived after 10 minutes of
cooling, cover the burned area to prevent infection.
Observe the victim for breathing problems or worsening
shock. Carefully check for other injuries.

▷ Raising a burned limb may
help to minimize swelling;
raising both legs may help to
reduce any shock symptoms.

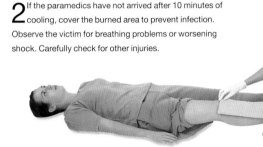

REMOVAL OF CLOTHING

Dry burns (from flames, for example):
Douse any smoldering clothes with water. Try to cool burns by
pouring water directly onto the skin, but do not remove the clothing
unless it is impeding the cooling (in this case, cut around any adhered
clothing, leaving the adhered material in place).

Wet burns (scalds from boiling water, for example):
Flood water under the clothing to start cooling and separate it from
the skin. Scalded skin is often fragile, so remove clothing carefully by

first cutting it some distance away from the scalded area. Continue
to cool the affected area gently.

Chemical burns (caustics, acids or alkalis, for example):
Use a shower or hose to drench the area. Remove affected clothing in
the shower. In the absence of water, use scissors to remove affected
clothing quickly. At any stage, avoid contact with the chemical, the
contaminated area, or with "run-off" water used for dousing. Wear
suitable protective gloves/clothing – if you can find them quickly.

Chemical, electrical and inhalation burns

SEE ALSO

➤ Understanding and assessing burns, p174

➤ Assessing burns 2, p176

➤ Keeping yourself safe, p220

Chemical and electrical burns are especially hazardous, as further injury is possible both for victim and helper. With a chemical incident, make the area safe or remove the victim to safety and then get someone to inform the fire department about the chemical in question.

Electrical burns can look deceptively mild at skin level while underlying muscles, nerves, and organs may be badly burned. With both chemical and electrical burns, the victim could go into shock, so monitor and record their vital signs until medical help arrives.

BURNS FROM CHEMICALS

Corrosive chemicals will continue to damage the skin while in contact with it so dispersing the harmful chemical as soon as possible is a priority. Chemical burns tend to develop more slowly than those from other causes. They are also particularly hazardous for the first-aider, because you may easily be burned yourself and they may give off fumes that could be inhaled. If there is any doubt about the chemical, move everyone away from the injured person and summon expert help.

You may recognize an injury as a chemical burn because:
• The victim informs you what happened.
• There are containers of chemicals nearby.
• The victim is suffering intense, stinging pain around the burned area.
• After some time, blistering and discoloration may develop, along with swollen tissues in the affected area.

▽ While wearing protective gloves, flood the burned area with cold water to cool the skin and disperse the chemical.

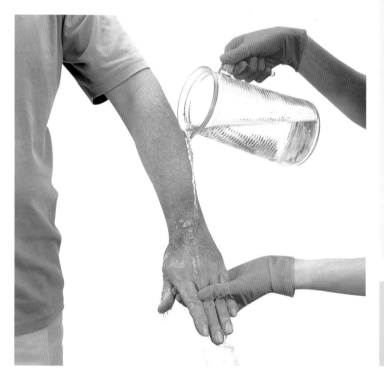

FIRST AID FOR CHEMICAL BURNS

Phone the emergency services or arrange urgent transport to the hospital.

⬇

Get the injured person out of the contaminated area as soon as possible, without exposing yourself to danger.

⬇

Protect yourself. Wear appropriate gloves/apron if readily available; open windows and doors for ventilation.

⬇

Flood the injured part with water, for at least 20 minutes or until help arrives. Pour the water so that contaminated water neither runs onto other parts of the injured person's body nor onto you.

⬇

Remove any contaminated clothing, unless it is stuck fast to the skin.

WARNING
Do not try to "neutralize" the chemical (by putting alkali on acid or vice versa) as the resulting reaction may produce heat or exacerbate the existing burn.

COMMON CAUSES OF CHEMICAL BURNS

Certain chemicals can irritate, burn or even penetrate the skin's protective layer. Many chemical-related accidents happen in industry, but the following corrosives are found in the home.

➤ Dishwasher products.

➤ Oven cleaners.

➤ Bleach.

➤ Ammonia.

➤ Caustic soda.

BURNS FROM ELECTRICITY

Electrical burns can occur from all kinds of electric current – from lightning strikes and overhead power cables to domestic current. There are three distinct types of electrical burn:

• A flash burn, caused by electricity arcing over a distance. It leaves a distinctive residue on the skin that is sometimes coppery in appearance.
• Burns from flames caused by electricity.
• Direct burning of the tissues by an electric current.

ELECTRICITY-RELATED DAMAGE

Electrical burns can look deceptively mild. Like chemical burns, the extent of the burn may not be immediately obvious and often looks quite innocuous. There may be entry and exit wounds, which give an idea of the path of the electric current, but these are often hard to find.

Underneath the fairly normal-looking skin, the muscle, blood vessels, and nerves may literally have "fried". In addition, the jolt of electricity could have affected the injured person's heartbeat.

If you arrive at an accident scene and find that a person is unconscious, first ensure they are not still connected to a live power source, and then check their ABC and be prepared to start resuscitation techniques immediately and to continue until emergency medical assistance arrives.

FIRST AID FOR ELECTRICAL BURNS

Do not touch the injured person unless and until you know they are no longer connected to a live electrical source.

If the person is unconscious, check their ABC and start resuscitation if necessary. Call the emergency services.

Treat as for a dry burn.

Watch for any signs of shock, or for any effects on the heartbeat.
Note: Anyone who has suffered more than a mild tingling sensation should be seen in the hospital – electricity can affect the heart some time after the initial exposure.

INHALATION BURNS

Breathing in dangerous fumes may affect the respiratory system – the trachea, bronchi and lung tissue – and can cause serious damage. Such fumes include car exhaust emissions (including carbon monoxide), smoke from a fire, fumes from faulty domestic appliances (such as a gas heater), and fumes from smoldering foam-filled upholstered furniture. Certain chemicals, including dry-cleaning solvents, may also give off toxic or irritant fumes.

Signs of inhalation burns are:
• Soot and singed hairs around the mouth and nose area.
• Breathing difficulties.
• Headache.
• Dizziness.
• Shock.

The best first-aid approach is to send for the emergency services immediately; get the victim to a safe place in clean air and do not expose yourself to fire, smoke, or fumes; position the victim sitting up and supported; monitor them for changes in consciousness or breathing; be prepared to resuscitate if necessary – however, if chemicals have been inhaled, this may be unsafe without special equipment.

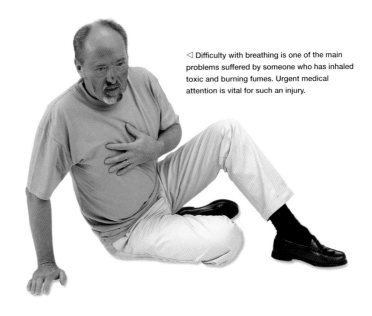

◁ Difficulty with breathing is one of the main problems suffered by someone who has inhaled toxic and burning fumes. Urgent medical attention is vital for such an injury.

Coping with facial burns

SEE ALSO

➤ Dealing with shock, p68
➤ Assessing burns 2, p176
➤ Managing burns, p178

Any type of facial burn is an emergency because it can result in possible blindness, breathing difficulties, and obvious scarring. The priorities are to cool the burned area with cold water and to convey the injured person to the hospital. Do remember to reassure the victim all the time and keep watch for any signs of shock. It is a good idea to gather any details you can on what has caused the burn in the first place: you can then relay this information to medical personnel so that they can take prompt and appropriate action.

Burns to the face can have further, very serious, implications. Because they strongly suggest that there may be other burns – to the victim's airway, nose, and

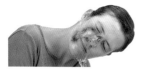
◁ Flood a facial burn with cold water and continue to do so for at least 10 minutes.

mouth – there is a danger they may compromise the person's breathing. Also, it is vital to take rapid action in order to minimize any scars from a facial burn, as significant scarring can cause psychological difficulties.

BURNS TO THE EYE

Facial burns to the eye area are especially painful and are prone to significant amounts of swelling, which can make it difficult for the victim to see and for you to examine the eyeball.

It is vital to get the person to a doctor or hospital very quickly as any burns to the

eyelid or cornea can lead to scarring that may cause blindness. Reassure the person throughout as they may think that they are going blind and panic. Keep them calm and remind them that it is just the swelling that is obstructing their vision.

CHEMICAL BURNS TO THE EYE

Chemicals can burn the delicate tissues of the eye and cause scarring, which may lead to blindness. The main first-aid priority is to irrigate the eye to remove as much of the chemical as possible. The eye may be very painful, red, and watery, making it difficult to prise open and flush out.

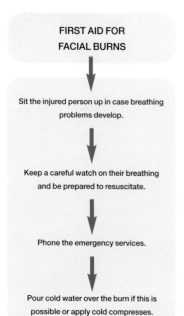

FIRST AID FOR FACIAL BURNS

⬇

Sit the injured person up in case breathing problems develop.

⬇

Keep a careful watch on their breathing and be prepared to resuscitate.

⬇

Phone the emergency services.

⬇

Pour cold water over the burn if this is possible or apply cold compresses.

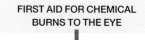
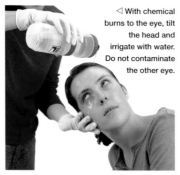
◁ With chemical burns to the eye, tilt the head and irrigate with water. Do not contaminate the other eye.

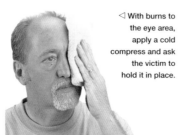
◁ With burns to the eye area, apply a cold compress and ask the victim to hold it in place.

FIRST AID FOR CHEMICAL BURNS TO THE EYE

⬇

Turn the person's head to one side with the affected eye below the good eye so that no chemical runs into the good eye.

⬇

Hold the eyelid open under a gently running faucet or pour water from a glass or bottle. Flush both sides of the eye; don't splash contaminated water into the good eye.

⬇

Cover the eye with a sterile eye pad and secure loosely. Try to find out what chemical has caused the burn and always take the person to the hospital.

Tackling sunburn

SEE ALSO

➤ Understanding burns, p174

➤ Assessing the severity of burns, p176

Burns caused by the ultraviolet rays of the sun can be as dangerous as those caused by anything else. The immune system reacts to the sun's assault to protect the body. First, the skin reddens and starts to itch; then it becomes swollen and painful, eventually blistering and flaking (and sometimes even scarring). Sunbeds and tanning lamps can inflict the same damage as natural sunlight, and so are best avoided. Taking sensible precautions when out in the sun can ensure that a holiday is a happy and healthy one.

Sunburn can not only cause severe skin damage but may also lead to the serious conditions of heat exhaustion or even heatstroke. The sun's ultraviolet radiation can be harmful to the eyes, and sunglasses should be worn when outside, especially in areas where there is a lot of reflected light such as on the sea or in snow. The effects of too much sun are not immediately obvious and can take 12–24 hours to develop.

Many people don't realize that you can get sunburn even on a cloudy day. There are also other factors that make sunburn more likely, including:

• High altitudes – The thinner the atmosphere, the greater the risk of even small amounts of sun causing burning.
• Reflective surfaces – Water, sand, wind, snow, and paved areas increase the sun's strength by reflecting its rays.
• Sweat and water on the skin – Such moisture increases the chances of the skin burning and stops sunscreens from working properly.

PREVENTING SUNBURN

A few sensible precautions can prevent sunburn in the first place. Take on board the following advice.

➤ Use a sunscreen on all exposed skin, especially when in open areas with little shade. Reapply regularly.

➤ Wear a wide-brimmed hat, ideally with a neck flap.

➤ Always wear sunglasses, especially near snow or expanses of water.

➤ Stay out of the midday sun altogether, especially when close to the equator. Make a siesta part of any holiday; resurface at around 3pm when the sun's rays are less damaging.

➤ Lacking a sun tan has to be better than risking skin cancer. If you must sunbathe, build up exposure to the sun very slowly, staying in the sun for no longer than 20 minutes on the first day. Never use low-factor sunscreens.

FIRST AID FOR SUNBURN

Remove the person from the sun and keep them in the shade or, preferably, indoors.

Apply cold compresses to the burned area to cool the skin or immerse the affected area in a cool bath for at least 10 minutes.

As the person may be dehydrated, encourage them to take frequent small sips of water.

If the sunburn is mild, apply some soothing after-sun lotion; if sunburn is severe take the person to see a doctor right away.

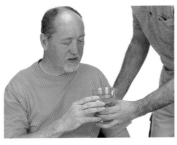

△ To prevent sunburn, wear a T-shirt and a hat and apply some sunscreen.

△ Encourage someone with sunburn to sip water frequently as they may be dehydrated.

USING A SUNSCREEN

All sunscreens have an SPF (Sun Protection Factor), which is measured by timing how long skin covered with the sunscreen takes to burn compared with unprotected skin. If your skin normally burns after 10 minutes, then an SPF 15 sunscreen should allow protection for 150 minutes; an SPF8 offers 80 minutes' protection. Even "waterproof" or "water resistant" sunscreens lose their effectiveness once you have been in the water for 40 minutes. The minimum recommended sunscreen is SPF15.

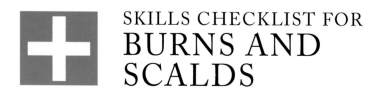

SKILLS CHECKLIST FOR
BURNS AND SCALDS

KEY POINTS

- Burns must be cooled – run cold water over a burn site for a minimum of 10 minutes in order to limit the internal damage ☐

- Do not touch burned skin, to avoid inflicting further injury ☐

- Use non-adhesive dressings (preferably dampened) – never adhesive or fluffy ones ☐

- Many burns occur in domestic house fires that could often have been prevented. They are the third largest cause of accidental deaths in the home ☐

SKILLS LEARNED

- How to treat minor burns and scalds ☐

- How to treat more extensive burns or scalding ☐

- Assessing the depth, extent, and seriousness of a burn ☐

- Recognizing the possibilities of breathing difficulties, shock, and internal injury as a consequence of burns ☐

- Avoiding sunburn ☐

ACTION ON POISONING

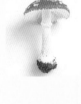

There are some substances that the human body cannot tolerate. These poisons – also known as toxins – include a wide variety of plants and fungi, homecare products and medicines (both prescribed medication and illicit drugs). The body's defense system recognizes such toxins as threats to survival and tries to get rid of the offending substance – by vomiting and/or diarrhea, for example. When encountering a poisoning incident, the first-aider is limited to calling for the emergency medical service and to gathering any evidence on what the poison could have been. Do not under any circumstances try to make the victim vomit up the poison.

CONTENTS

Understanding poisoning 186–187

Managing drug poisoning 188–189

Tackling alcohol and illicit drug poisoning 190–191

Dealing with food and plant poisoning 192–193

Managing poisoning in children 194–195

Skills checklist 196

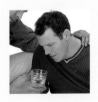

Understanding poisoning

SEE ALSO
➤ Managing drug poisoning, p188
➤ Managing poisoning in children, p194

The golden rule in giving first aid for a suspected poisoning is never to attempt to make the person vomit until you know what the poison is. Vomiting a poisonous substance back up the esophagus (gullet) can double the damage if the poison is a corrosive chemical.

Poisons can get into the body in many ways – via the skin, digestive system, lungs, or bloodstream. The mode of entry influences the speed of reaction; for instance, if a poison is injected into the bloodstream, it can reach all parts of the body within a minute or so.

A poison is any substance that can cause temporary or permanent damage to the body if taken in sufficient quantities. Poisoning may occur accidentally or intentionally. Suicide attempts often involve more than one poisonous agent, and the person may resist any help that is offered. Some drugs have no obvious immediate effects when taken in overdose but ultimately are fatal.

Accidental poisoning is most often seen in children and in the elderly. There are fewer deaths from such incidents in children, but some agents may wreak havoc in a child. Elderly people may get confused and take the wrong medication or the wrong amount.

There are many categories of poisons:
• Noxious gases or fumes.
• Cleaning products.
• Toxins in plants and fungi.
• Bacterial and viral toxins (in food).
• Drugs and alcohol.
• Toxins from bites and stings.

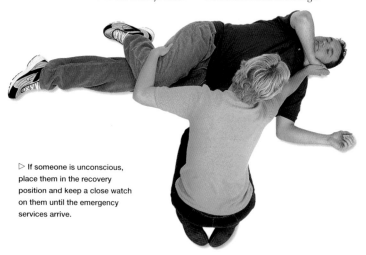

▷ If someone is unconscious, place them in the recovery position and keep a close watch on them until the emergency services arrive.

BASIC GUIDELINES FOR DEALING WITH POISONING

Assess the person's ABC. If they are breathing but unconscious, put them in the recovery position.

If they are not breathing, start resuscitation techniques once you have checked that there is no poison on the face or in the mouth area. If there is, rinse with cold water and use a face shield to protect yourself.

Call the emergency services.

If the person starts to have a fit, do not restrain them. Keep them out of danger and ensure a clear airway.

Look around to see if you can find any clues to the identity of the poison that has been taken. If the person has vomited, take a sample of the vomit to hospital as there is a good chance it will help doctors identify the appropriate treatment.

IDENTIFYING THE CAUSE OF THE POISONING

Once you have dealt with the person's immediate needs, try to gather information to help identify the poison.

➤ Look for empty containers or loose pills or capsules on the floor. Bag them and give to the paramedics.

➤ Search for codes on containers that will identify any chemical.
➤ Scan the area for a dead insect or snake to bag up and take to hospital.
➤ Look around for any potentially poisonous foods.

HOW POISONS AFFECT THE BODY

▷ Poisons can have wide-ranging effects on different parts of the body. Effects depend on how the poison gets into the system and how much poison has been taken.

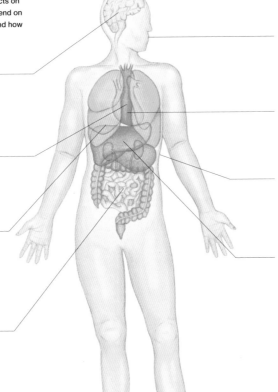

Brain
Once in the bloodstream, drugs can easily reach the brain causing confusion, drowsiness, fits and, at worst, coma. If the part of the brain that controls breathing is affected, a person's breathing can stop altogether.

Blood
Poisonous gases such as cyanide and carbon monoxide react with the blood, so that there is not enough oxygen in the circulation, leading to potentially lethal effects on the body.

Lungs
Inhaled fumes or drugs quickly reach the lungs and then travel in the bloodstream. Such poisons cause breathing difficulties (which can be fatal in people with asthma) and lead to blue skin (cyanosis) – a sign that there's too little oxygen in the body.

Digestive tract
Toxins from bacteria or viruses in contaminated food commonly cause nausea, vomiting and diarrhea.

Mouth
Corrosive substances such as bleach and dishwashing powder may burn the tissues lining the throat and esophagus (gullet) and cause nausea and vomiting.

Heart
Injected and swallowed poisons can result in an irregular heartbeat or in the heart beating too fast or too slowly.

Chest wall
Certain snake venom, certain garden fertilizers and botulinum toxin can lead to paralysis of the muscles in the chest wall and therefore cause suffocation.

Liver
This is the body's vital detoxifying center. Toxins from some wild fungi may cause severe liver damage and the painkiller acetaminophen can destroy liver cells if taken in excess (even relatively small amounts over the recommended dosage).

COMMON POISONS

Homecare products:

➤ Bleach, caustic soda, home cleaning products, perfume, aftershave, hair spray, nail polish remover, lighter fuel, turpentine, white spirit and all kinds of solvents, including dry cleaning fluids, mercury-filled thermometers, child's play "putty", shoe creams and polishes, slug pellets, tobacco, weedkiller, glues, wood preservative, lead paint (in old houses), antifreeze, bug and rodent killers.

Drugs and chemicals:

➤ Medicines in excess of stated dose (or if taken by someone who suffers from an allergic reaction to them), large amounts of vitamins A and D, large amounts of Epsom salts, iodine.

Fungi:

➤ Certain species of toadstools and mushrooms can be lethal – even if only tiny quantities have been eaten.

Bites and stings:

➤ From insects, jellyfish and snakes, among others.

Plants:

➤ For example, laburnum, foxglove, holly berries, monkshood and yew.

Gases:

➤ Carbon monoxide may leak from faulty gas heaters, boilers, and the vents of air conditioning systems.

Managing drug poisoning

SEE ALSO

➤ What is first aid?, p12
➤ Understanding poisoning, p186
➤ Tackling alcohol and illicit drug poisoning, p190

Each type of drug usually quickly produces specific signs and symptoms when taken in overdose; the exception here is excess acetaminophen, which can take a few days to produce recognizable symptoms. The effects of a drug depend on the type of drug and how it is taken (swallowed, inhaled or injected). The basic first-aid aims when dealing with drug poisoning are to maintain breathing, call the emergency services and look for any information at the scene that could provide vital clues for the medics treating the victim.

Drug poisoning can result from overdosage of prescription or over-the-counter medicines or from abuse of illicit drugs. Less commonly, it is caused by two or more drugs interacting.

It is often possible to identify what substances have been taken, as they each cause specific signs and symptoms. Such information may be incredibly helpful as the victim may be unconscious by the time they reach the hospital.

ACETAMINOPHEN-BASED PAINKILLERS

These painkilling medicines can easily be bought over the counter and are a basic ingredient of most home medicine cupboards. If acetaminophen is taken in overdosage, even just a relatively small amount, destruction of the liver can occur.

The person may feel fine for the first few days, until liver (or, less commonly, kidney) damage starts to take effect. Then,

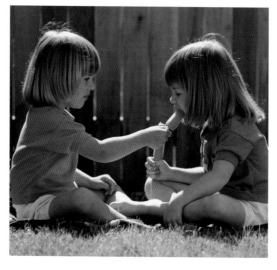

◁ Children love to experiment with tasting things, but if unsupervised, their natural curiosity may result in a poisoning incident. In the same vein, keep an eye on small children going through an adult's bag or a kitchen or bathroom cupboard.

the following symptoms may appear:
• Nausea and profuse vomiting.
• Pain in the upper right-hand abdomen after 24 hours (a sign of liver damage).

Irreversible liver damage can occur within 3–4 days so prompt recognition and transfer to hospital is vital.

ASPIRIN-BASED PAINKILLERS

If these common painkillers are taken in excessive amounts they can cause the following symptoms:
• Upper abdominal pain.
• Nausea and vomiting.
• Fever, with sweating and dizziness.
• Deep "sighing" breaths.
• Deafness and/or loud noises heard in the ears (tinnitus).
• Restlessness and confusion.
• Deterioration in consciousness or fitting.

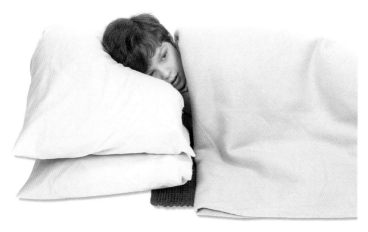

◁ Drowsiness followed by loss of consciousness can be a sign of poisoning. Seek immediate medical help.

FIRST AID FOR POISONING

⬇

If the person is conscious, let them rest in a comfortable position. Reassure them and ask if they can tell you what they have taken.

⬇

Phone the emergency services.

⬇

Monitor the person's breathing and talk to them until help arrives.

⬇

Keep samples of any vomit. Look for any clues as to the identity of poisons.

ANTIDEPRESSANT DRUGS

There are many different types of antidepressant medication available on prescription. If taken in excess, the older type of tricyclic antidepressants, such as amitryptyline, initially cause:

• Blurred vision.
• Dilated pupils.
• Dry mouth.
• An inability to pass urine.

They can then result in:

• Drowsiness.
• Drops in blood pressure and temperature.
• Fits, followed by cardiac arrest.

The newer-style antidepressants, such as fluoxetine and sertraline, have completely different overdosage effects – notably the tendency to cause an erratic heart rate.

TRANQUILIZERS

Tranquilizing drugs are often prescribed for anxiety and sleeping problems, and commonly include barbiturate and benzodiazepine drugs. If these are taken in overdose, they can result in the following:

• Slurred speech.
• Drowsiness and lethargy, leading to a loss of consciousness.
• Weak, irregular, or slow or fast heartbeat.
• Slow breathing rate (breathing may actually stop altogether).

If tranquilizers are taken in combination with excessive alcohol the situation is much more dangerous. Older people often take sleeping tablets; when taken in excess, these may produce hypothermia – a condition to which they are vulnerable.

IRON SUPPLEMENTS

Women often take an iron supplement (commonly as iron tablets) during pregnancy and while breastfeeding. Children can mistake such tablets for sweets and eat them. The signs of iron overdosage include:

• Stomach pain.
• Vomiting and diarrhea.
• Blood in the vomit or the stool.

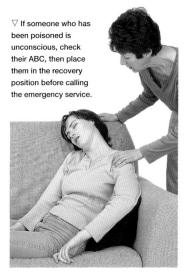

▽ If someone who has been poisoned is unconscious, check their ABC, then place them in the recovery position before calling the emergency service.

Excessive iron can cause severe damage to a child's liver and this is one of the few types of tablet that children accidentally take that can turn out to be lethal.

▽ Iron poisoning causes vomiting and severe stomach pain in children. They should be taken straight to the hospital.

Tackling alcohol and illicit drug poisoning

SEE ALSO
➤ Understanding
  poisoning, p186
➤ Managing drug
  poisoning, p188
➤ Managing
  poisoning in
  children, p194

Alcohol in moderate amounts is easily detoxified by the liver; but in very large quantities alcohol becomes a poison that the body can no longer deal with – and it can prove fatal. The same is not true, however, for many illicit drugs. Even relatively small amounts of a substance such as cocaine or fumes from glue can result in severe effects on the body. Emergency medical treatment is vital, especially if a child has taken alcohol or a drug because children absorb the toxins much more quickly than adults.

Taking illicit substances and drinking large quantities of alcohol is socially acceptable in some parts of society, but such practices are potentially dangerous and lead to medical crises and even fatalities.

ALCOHOL POISONING

Alcohol is a poison when drunk in sufficient quantities. Consumption of a pint of a spirit, such as vodka, is enough to cause severe alcohol poisoning. Alcohol-related risks include:
• Depression of the central nervous system, most seriously the brain.
• Widening of blood vessels, making the body lose heat and risking hypothermia.
• The inebriated person may choke on their vomit while unconscious.

SIGNS AND SYMPTOMS OF ALCOHOL INTOXICATION

It is usually fairly obvious when someone is intoxicated with alcohol, but similar symptoms may be caused by a head injury or a diabetic hypoglycaemic (low blood sugar) condition.

➤ A smell of alcohol on the breath.

➤ Empty bottles or cans nearby.

➤ Flushed and warm skin.

➤ Actions are aggressive or passive.

➤ Speech and actions are slow and become less coordinated.

➤ Deep, noisy breathing.

➤ Low level of consciousness; they may often slip into unconsciousness.

HOW TO DEAL WITH ALCOHOL INTOXICATION

1 Check that the person is rousable by shaking them and shouting their name, if you know it. If they respond but fall back into unconsciousness, watch them until they start to come around. If outside, insulate them from the ground and cover them to keep them warm.

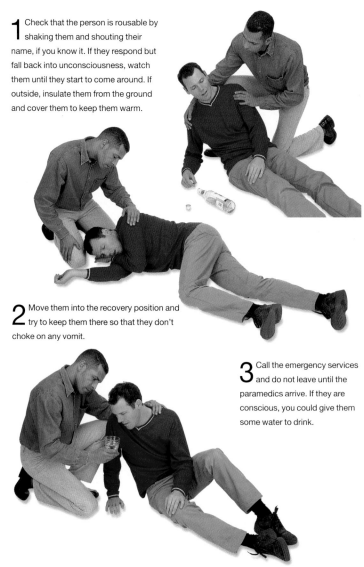

2 Move them into the recovery position and try to keep them there so that they don't choke on any vomit.

3 Call the emergency services and do not leave until the paramedics arrive. If they are conscious, you could give them some water to drink.

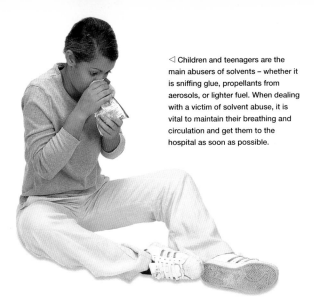

◁ Children and teenagers are the main abusers of solvents – whether it is sniffing glue, propellants from aerosols, or lighter fuel. When dealing with a victim of solvent abuse, it is vital to maintain their breathing and circulation and get them to the hospital as soon as possible.

ILLICIT DRUGS

Illicit stimulant drugs include Ecstasy, amphetamines, cocaine, and LSD. If you suspect someone has taken any of these drugs, watch out for the following signs:
• Excitable and hyperactive behavior.
• Sweating.
• Shaking hands.
• Hallucinations.

These drugs can occasionally be fatal. Ecstasy interferes with the brain's ability to control body temperature, which can rise to over 107.6°F and cause heat exhaustion. Ecstasy-takers often drink lots of water, which can cause kidney malfunction and abnormal heart rhythms. Cocaine's main effects are on the heart rate – with the potential to lead to abnormal rhythms and even cardiac arrest.

Opiate drugs such as heroin and codeine may depress the respiratory system, causing breathing to stop. Rapid recovery occurs if medication is given intravenously, but this must be done urgently, by trained medical personnel.

POISONING VIA SOLVENT ABUSE

Children and adolescents are the main solvent abusers – they may inhale fumes from glue, paint, lighter fuel, cleaning fluids, aerosols and nail polish to get a "high". All such solvents depress breathing and heart activity, and may cause respiratory and cardiac arrest.

FIRST AID FOR SOLVENT ABUSE POISONING

Check the person's ABC. If they have stopped breathing or their heart has stopped beating, start resuscitation immediately.

If unconscious but breathing, place them in the fresh air in the recovery position.

Call the emergency services.

Check their ABC regularly.

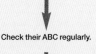

Often, the person starts to come around quickly and may seem normal after 20 minutes. Stay with them until help arrives.

SIGNS AND SYMPTOMS OF SOLVENT POISONING

➤ The person has a dry throat and cough.

➤ Their chest feels tight and they may be breathless.

➤ They have a headache.

➤ They feel nauseous and may vomit.

➤ They have hallucinations – they "hear voices" or "see things".

➤ Their breathing becomes faster and more labored as fluid builds up in their lungs.

➤ They become drowsy and confused and eventually may lose consciousness.

➤ They have episodes of fits (convulsions), which may lead to a coma and eventually to death.

FIRST AID FOR ILLICIT DRUG POISONING

Do not try to make the person vomit.

Place them in the recovery position.

Call the emergency services.

Check their ABC and monitor their breathing every 10 minutes.

Dealing with food and plant poisoning

SEE ALSO

➤ Dealing with shock, p68
➤ Understanding poisoning, p186
➤ Managing poisoning in children, p194

Potentially poisonous things to eat are all around us: in the garden, the kitchen, the bathroom, or a nearby wood. Make your garden safe if you have young children by ensuring that all plants are harmless or that any toxic plants are inaccessible. Never be tempted to try a mushroom of uncertain identity; it could give you severe, or even fatal, poisoning. Always practice good food hygiene to avoid food poisoning at home. If you have any worries or doubts at all about a potential poisoning incident, you should always call the emergency services.

Young children are the most likely group to eat poisonous plants as they find brightly colored seeds and berries attractive. Adults may eat poisonous fungi if they mistake them for an edible species. The effects of plant poisoning can be almost anything depending on the plant, while fungi tend to upset the digestive system. While many fungi are relatively harmless, a few are deadly. The death cap mushroom, for example, contains a toxin that destroys the liver after a delay of several days.

First-aid priorities for poisoning, whether it is from a plant or a fungus, are to:
• Identify the poisonous agent, if possible.
• Manage any fitting episodes.
• Call the emergency services.

MUSHROOM POISONING

Serious poisoning through eating poisonous mushrooms is rare. Some species of fungus may cause some less serious digestive symptoms, but eating a species such as the death cap can be fatal.

Suspect mushroom poisoning if you notice these signs and symptoms:
• Nausea and vomiting.
• Crampy abdominal pain and diarrhea.
• Episodes of fitting.
• Deterioration in level of consciousness.

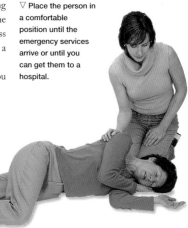

▽ Place the person in a comfortable position until the emergency services arrive or until you can get them to a hospital.

SOME COMMON POISONOUS PLANTS

➤ Autumn crocus (*Colchicum*) – all parts are very toxic and can prove fatal.

➤ Californian glory (*Fremontodendron*) – little hairs on the stem and leaves can cause skin irritation and itching.

➤ Castor oil plant (*Ricinus communis*) – all parts of this plant – especially the seeds – are very toxic if eaten and could be fatal.

➤ Daffodil (*Narcissus*) – if a bulb is eaten (a child can mistake it for an onion), it causes vomiting, stomachache, and diarrhea.

➤ Deadly nightshade (*Atropa belladonna*) – toxic if eaten and can irritate skin.

➤ Dumb cane or Leopard lily (*Dieffenbachia*) – eating any part of the plant, even a small quantity, can make the tongue, mouth and throat swell and interfere with breathing. Skin contact with the sap causes irritation.

➤ Foxglove (*Digitalis purpurea*) – all parts can be very toxic. As this bitter plant often causes vomiting first, poisoning is rare.

➤ Holly (*Ilex aquifolium*) – the red berries are poisonous.

➤ Hyacinth (*Hyacinthus*) – if the bulbs are mistaken for onions and eaten, they will make a person sick and can sometimes cause a skin rash.

➤ Laburnum (*Laburnum anagyroides*) – all parts are toxic, especially the seeds.

➤ Lantana (*Lantana camara*) – all parts of this plant are toxic. The unripe berries, in particular, are attractive to young children.

➤ Lupin (*Lupinus*) – the seeds and pods are poisonous but would have to be eaten in large quantities to do real harm.

➤ Monkshood (*Aconitum*) – all parts are highly toxic if eaten and contact with the sap can cause skin irritation.

➤ Spurge laurel (*Daphne laureola*) – all parts are highly poisonous if eaten.

➤ Umbrella tree (*Schefflera*) – any contact with cut stems or leaves causes skin irritation.

➤ Winter cherry (*Solanum capsicastrum*) – the fruit is poisonous but not fatally so.

➤ Woody nightshade (*Solanum dulcamara*) – the berries of this plant are poisonous and when eaten can cause stomachache, vomiting, and diarrhea.

➤ Yew tree (*Taxus*) – all parts of this tree are toxic if eaten.

FIRST AID FOR PLANT OR MUSHROOM POISONING

↓

If the person is conscious, ask them what they have eaten.

↓

If unconscious, check their ABC and be prepared to resuscitate if necessary. Place them in the recovery position.

↓

Try to identify what poisonous plant or fungus they could have eaten.

↓

Phone the emergency services or take the person to the hospital. Take a sample of the plant with you to the hospital.

SOME EXAMPLES OF POISONOUS FUNGI

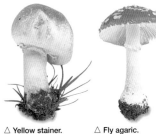

△ Yellow stainer.   △ Fly agaric.

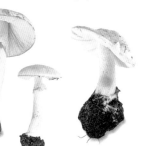

△ Death cap.   △ Destroying angel.

FOOD POISONING

Symptoms of food poisoning may develop within an hour after consuming tainted food, although it can sometimes take up to three days. Contaminated food often tastes and smells entirely normal. The commonest culprits of food poisoning are bacteria and viruses, including *E. coli*, *Salmonella*, and *Staphylococcus*. Foods that often become contaminated and give people food poisoning include shellfish and other protein-containing foods, such as meat or fish, that have been stored badly or inadequately cooked.

Food poisoning may cause such severe fluid losses, through vomiting and diarrhea, that dehydration develops. If the fluids that have been lost are not replaced quickly enough, then a further danger is the development of shock.

FIRST AID FOR FOOD POISONING

↓

Encourage the person to rest and drink plenty of water. Provide a container in case they vomit.

↓

Call a doctor for medical advice.

↓

If the victim's condition worsens, call the emergency services.

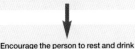

◁ Brown roll-rim.

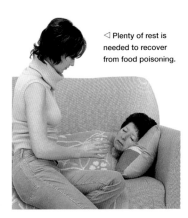

◁ Plenty of rest is needed to recover from food poisoning.

Typical signs of food poisoning are:
• Nausea and vomiting.
• Crampy abdominal pain.
• Diarrhea, which may be blood-stained.
• Fever and shivering and/or headache.
• Signs of shock.

PREVENTING FOOD POISONING

Take these sensible precautions to prevent food poisoning altogether.

➤ Fully defrost food before cooking.

➤ Cook meat, fish, poultry, and eggs very thoroughly.

➤ Always wash hands thoroughly after using the bathroom, and again before food preparation or cooking starts.

➤ Cooked food gathers bacteria fast, so store it in the refrigerator or freeze it.

➤ Be aware that raw eggs, used in recipes such as mayonnaise, may contain *Salmonella* bacteria.

➤ When visiting countries where the water supply could be dirty, never eat or drink anything that may be contaminated with local water, such as ice (in drinks), unpeeled fruit or vegetables, ice-cream, and salads (washed in water).

➤ When in a part of the world where the water supply is suspect, use bottled (or sterilized) water when brushing your teeth.

Managing poisoning in children

SEE ALSO
➤ What is first aid?, p12
➤ Understanding poisoning, p186
➤ Safety in the home, p224

Young children are naturally interested in searching through cupboards and boxes and generally exploring their environment. They will also put anything and everything into their mouths, including mothballs, dishwasher powder, and many other potentially fatal homecare products, liquids, and powders. Preventing poisoning in children is an essential part of safety in your home. As with all poisoning incidents, find out what has been taken so that the appropriate medical help can be given and keep a close watch on your child.

Children are naturally inquisitive and have no qualms about touching, inhaling, or ingesting anything – all pills are sweets, powders are sugar, and liquids are drinks. Parents are often taken by surprise by what is dangerous for young bodies – alcohol is lethal even in tiny quantities, an excess of iron can kill a child, and dishwashing powder can corrode a child's digestive tract in seconds.

Poisons are absorbed faster in children than adults, so their effects can be seen fairly quickly. Suspect poisoning in a child if:
• You observe unusual behavior such as slurred speech, giggling inappropriately, staggering, drowsiness.
• You find a child playing near an empty pill or chemical container.
• You can see scalds, stains, or bits of tablet around their mouth.

HOW TO POISON-PROOF YOUR HOME

The best cure is, of course, prevention. Take on board the following advice to ensure your children are never allowed access to potentially deadly poisons.

➤ Never leave unattended glasses full of alcohol around, especially overnight. Children are early risers and may decide to drink up all the dregs while you are sleeping.

➤ Never decant substances from their original containers into unlabeled bottles as it may lead to confusion.

➤ Do not use empty food containers such as soda bottles to store hazardous substances.

➤ The best place for all potential poisons is out of reach and out of sight in a cupboard that is secured with a childproof catch.

➤ Do not store food and non-food items in the same place.

➤ Make sure all medicine containers have child-resistant lids.

➤ Keep a close watch on visitors, especially older people, who may take regular medication and may inadvertently leave pills in an open handbag or overnight bag. Almost all adult medicines can have devastating effects on a child. For example, diabetic pills that lower blood sugar can reduce a child's blood sugar to such an extent that they fall into a coma and die.

FIRST AID FOR ALCOHOL POISONING IN A CHILD

⬇

If they are unrousable, check their ABC and be prepared to resuscitate if necessary.

⬇

If they are breathing, place in the recovery position. Call the emergency services.

⬇

If the child is awake, try to keep them awake. Provide a bowl in case they vomit. Stay with them until the paramedics arrive.

SYMPTOMS OF ALCOHOL POISONING IN CHILDREN

➤ Strong smell of alcohol.

➤ Flushed skin.

➤ Staggering about.

➤ Slurring of speech.

➤ Nausea.

➤ Noisy breathing.

WARNING
Even a small amount of alcohol can be very harmful to a child.

▷ If you suspect alcohol poisoning, place a bowl nearby for any vomit and call the emergency services.

FIRST AID FOR CHEMICAL POISONING IN A CHILD

Try to find out what chemical has been taken. Look for obvious clues nearby.

Do not make the child vomit; the chemical may do more damage on its way back up.

Call the emergency services.

If they complain of a sore mouth, rinse it with cold water (they should drink nothing).

To soothe burned lips, keep moistening frequently with water.

FIRST AID FOR FUME INHALATION IN A CHILD

Remove the child from the source of danger, making sure you don't put yourself in danger as well.

Check their breathing. If they are not breathing, start resuscitation immediately. If they are breathing, place them in the recovery position until help arrives.

Call the emergency services.

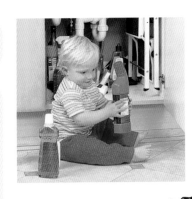

△ All low cupboards should have childproof locks so that homecare products can be stored safely away from inquisitive children.

FIRST AID FOR DRUG POISONING IN A CHILD

If the child is unconscious, check they are breathing. If breathing seems normal, place them in the recovery position. If they are not breathing, start resuscitation immediately.

Call the emergency services, who may be able to advise you over the phone.

Look for any signs that the child has swallowed drugs – bits of tablet on the tongue or dye around the mouth.

Try to work out what drug has been taken and how much and how long ago, if possible.

Continue to watch ABC until help arrives. Take the drug container with you to the hospital or give to the paramedics.

△ Search the child's mouth for any foreign matter. Moisten the lips with water, especially if they are burned (nothing should be drunk).

FIRST AID FOR PLANT POISONING IN A CHILD

If the child is unconscious, check that they are breathing. If they are not breathing, start resuscitation immediately. If breathing seems normal, place them in the recovery position.

Call the emergency services or take the child to the hospital.

Ask the child what they have eaten.

Use your finger to search the child's mouth and remove any unswallowed pieces of plant – keep these to hand over to medical personnel.

SKILLS CHECKLIST FOR
ACTION ON
POISONING

KEY POINTS

- Never encourage someone to vomit back up any poison ☐

- Keep a sample of the suspected poison ☐

- Call the emergency services immediately ☐

SKILLS LEARNED

- Prevention of home poisoning accidents ☐

- How to deal with poisoning in children ☐

- Recognizing the dangers of medication in excess ☐

- How to deal with food poisoning ☐

- How to cope with illicit drug excess ☐

- How to deal with alcohol poisoning ☐

13

FIRST-AID KIT

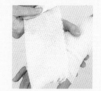

It is immediately reassuring to an injured child or anyone else if you can produce a well-equipped first-aid kit, and it will probably help you to approach any situation confidently if you have certain essential items to hand. An injured person will certainly feel calmer if you show you can dress and bandage an injury professionally and you know how to apply a sling. However, in an emergency, nothing in a first-aid kit is as important as you and your ability to think on your feet and improvise with materials at hand. Communication with the outside world is also very important, so make best use of telephones, neighbors, or passersby, if you are able to.

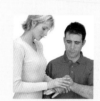

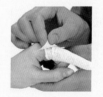

CONTENTS   Assembling a first-aid kit 198–199
Applying dressings and bandages 200–201
Applying bandages 1 202–203
Applying bandages 2 204–205
Fixing slings 206–207
Skills checklist 208

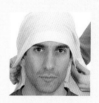

Assembling a first-aid kit

SEE ALSO
➤ What is first aid?, p12
➤ Safety in the home, p224
➤ Traveling safely, p246

A clean and fully equipped first-aid kit in the home, in the car, and in the workplace is very important. It should be easily accessible in a kitchen or bathroom cupboard but out of the reach of children. Some items are essential to a first-aid kit, but you may find that you'll want to supplement the basic kit with items that you know you use a lot, such as ibuprofen tablets, acetaminophen syrup for children or antihistamine cream. Such medications do not form part of the first aid offered in emergencies and should be for personal use only.

As well as making sure that you have a first-aid kit in the home and the car, you should be aware that all workplaces, recreation establishments, and other public places are required to have first-aid kits on the premises. So an incident at such a location should prompt a call for their kit. First-aid kits for public use are not supposed to contain any kind of medication (including painkillers) or ointments, in case people have an adverse reaction to them – what you have in your box at home for private and family use is entirely your affair, of course.

WHAT SHOULD GO IN THE KIT?

The first-aid kit must be kept clean and dry. A large plastic box is ideal for storage, as it is light, durable, and easy to open. The following are essential kit items:

• Adhesive dressings – A good selection of different sizes, shapes, and types, for example waterproof, digit-shaped, and fabric-backed. However, note that very minor cuts and grazes are often better left uncovered.

• Non-adhesive dressings or sterile gauze pads – Usually sealed in protective wrappers, these are easy to use to protect an open wound from possible infection and do not stick to wounds. Have plenty of gauze pads – the best dressing to stop bleeding from a small wound and to dress most small to medium-sized wounds. (Note: in wounds that are bleeding heavily, you may find that a dish cloth or towel is the most helpful impromptu dressing.)

• Bandages – Various sizes and types, especially a triangular bandage (for slings/head wounds), elasticated tubular bandages for joints, and roller bandages for securing dressings, stopping bleeding and immobilizing limbs.

• A thermometer, either mercury or digital, to determine body temperature.

• A pair of scissors – Choose a sharp pair that has one blade with a rounded end for the safe cutting of dressings and clothing (for example when treating burns) without the risk of cutting the skin.

• Safety pins – To fix slings and bandages.

• Disposable gloves – Put on gloves before attending to cases with blood or open wounds – to ensure that a wound is kept ultra-clean and your hands are protected.

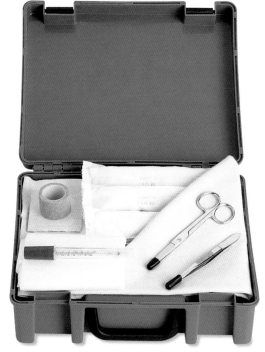

◁ When assembling your own first-aid kit, make sure the box is large enough, watertight and easily identifiable as a first-aid kit.

ESSENTIAL ITEMS FOR A FIRST-AID KIT

Your kit should contain:

➤ Adhesive dressings in various sizes.

➤ Sterile dressings in various sizes; about 30 gauze dressings and 1 large sterile dressing; plenty of gauze pads.

➤ 1 triangular bandage, tubular bandages and roller bandages.

➤ A thermometer.

➤ A pair of scissors.

➤ Safety pins.

➤ Disposable gloves.

➤ Emergency numbers.

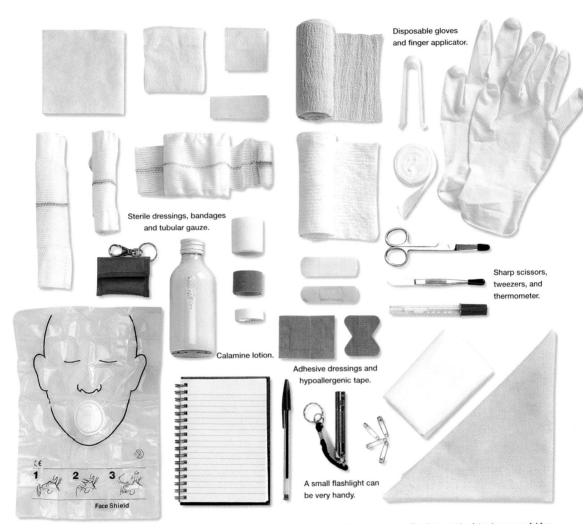

Disposable gloves and finger applicator.

Sterile dressings, bandages and tubular gauze.

Sharp scissors, tweezers, and thermometer.

Calamine lotion.

Adhesive dressings and hypoallergenic tape.

A small flashlight can be very handy.

Face Shield

A plastic face shield for protection during mouth-to-mouth resuscitation.

A notepad and pen for emergency numbers and to record your observations during treatment.

Bandages and safety pins are useful for securing dressings and restricting movement.

- List of emergency telephone numbers – Include your doctor, pharmacist, the nearest hospital with an emergency room, neighbors and cabs.

Make a note if you use any item from your kit so that you can replace it swiftly.

USEFUL FIRST-AID EXTRAS

In a kit for personal/family use, you may want to keep some basic medications such as acetaminophen, calamine lotion or antihistamines, and medicine spoons.

- Tweezers – Keep some in your kit for removing splinters of glass and wood.
- Cotton padding or alcohol-free cleansing wipes – Either can be used to clean the skin around a wound but should not be used to dress open wounds, as the fluff will stick to, and clog up, the wound.
- Face protection – A mask or face shield offers protection to you and the injured person when giving mouth-to-mouth.
- Adhesive tape – Waterproof tape can be

△ These are some of the items you may want to keep in your first-aid kit. Select the items you know you may need and that you feel confident about using.

useful when bandaging areas such as the hands, which often get wet. Some people are allergic to such tape; try to check first.

- Cold packs – These gel-filled packs can be warmed up or cooled down. They are useful for easing sprains, cooling a child with a fever, bringing down swelling, or cooling superficial burns.

Applying dressings and bandages

SEE ALSO

➤ Assembling a
first-aid kit, p198

➤ Applying bandages
1 and 2,
pp202, 204

All first-aiders should be able to produce a makeshift dressing at the scene of an emergency if none is available. Improvising is a key part of giving first aid, and this can apply to bandages, too. Correct methods of bandaging are easy to learn and are invaluable in many first-aid situations. It can take time to become the perfect "bandager", so practice on friends, or on children (when they are well) if you have them. To be effective, bandages should be applied with a certain amount of pressure and be neither too tight nor too loose.

A dressing is any material held over a wound to stop it from bleeding and protect it from contamination, whereas a bandage is what holds the dressing in place.

APPLYING DRESSINGS

Common basic guidelines apply to the use of any dressing, whichever type is used.

• If possible, wear disposable gloves when applying dressing, except for adhesive dressings. Wash your hands thoroughly before and after dressing a wound, and cover any cuts on your hands with waterproof adhesive dressings.

• Choose the right size dressing so that it covers all of the wound and its edges.

• Avoid touching the dressing where it will come into contact with the wound; hold it at the sides so that it stays sterile.

• Ensure that the dressing sits over the entire surface of the wound and the area immediately surrounding it. Never slide a dressing around on top of a wound and reposition any dressing that slips off.

• Never take off a dressing, even if a wound continues to bleed through it. Instead, apply more dressing material on top of the first until the bleeding is controlled.

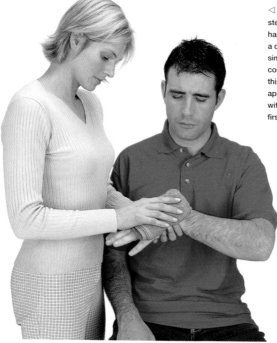

◁ If there aren't any sterile dressings at hand, improvise using a dish towel or similar. If the bleeding continues through this dressing, then apply another on top without removing the first one.

TYPES OF DRESSINGS

Ideally, pre-packed sterile dressings should be used in any incident so that the wound site is free from all germs. However, these dressings are not always at hand, and it is useful to know the other types you can use or how to improvise if you have no first-aid kit at all.

Some different types of dressings include the following:

• Sterile dressings – These are made up from a sterile gauze pad that is covered with a layer of cotton padding and then a bandage. Some sterile dressings come pre-packed and ready to use.

• Adhesive dressings – These come in a variety of shapes and sizes (some are specifically designed to fit a finger or

▽ You should aim to wrap a large area of the injured limb in such a way that you are not impeding the circulation.

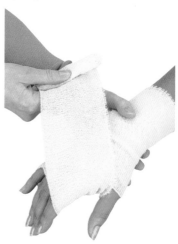

particular body part). Some people have an allergy to certain types of adhesive dressing, so check with the injured person before you apply one.

- Non-adhesive dressings – These non-fluffy dressings can be applied directly onto a wound and won't stick.
- Makeshift dressings – As is often the case in first-aid situations, improvisation is key. When sterile dressings aren't available, use the cleanest (non-fluffy) material available – dish towels, head scarves, or torn-up sheets are all ideal. Sanitary napkins make good dressings as they are clean (but not sterile) and bulky.

BANDAGING CORRECTLY

Effective bandaging has several roles – it controls bleeding, aids the return of blood from the wound site, ensures that any dressing stays firmly in place, and immobilizes and supports injured limbs. The three basic types of bandage are:

- Roller bandages, for securing dressings and supporting limbs.
- Triangular bandages, for making slings or securing large dressings.
- Tubular bandages, for supporting injured limbs and holding dressings on digits.

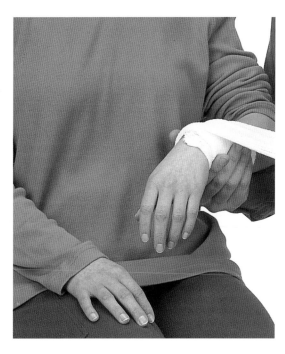

◁ Start from the bottom of the limb and roll the bandage up the arm. Make sure the injured person is comfortable and work from the injured side.

The pressure applied when putting on a bandage is crucial. If a bandage is too tight, fingers or toes will feel cold, the skin will look blue, and the limb will be painful. Later on, the skin may look pale and feel cold, and the person will tell you that their fingers or toes feel tingly and stiff. Conversely, a loose bandage won't control bleeding or protect a wound site from contamination. Practice makes perfect.

▽ To check that a bandage isn't too tight, press hard on an area downstream of the bandage, a finger in this example. If it takes more than 3 seconds to turn pink again, after being pressed, the bandage needs to be redone more loosely.

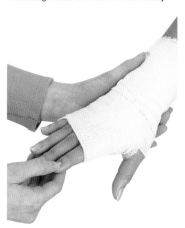

THE BASIC RULES OF DRESSING AND BANDAGING

To bandage and apply dressings effectively, follow these simple rules:

DO

➤ Start bandaging from the bottom of a limb and work toward the top.

➤ Bandage firmly; it shouldn't be too loose, but also not so tight that it cuts off the person's circulation.

➤ Secure the bandaging with adhesive tape, and guard against loose ends that might get caught when the person is being moved.

➤ Use uniform pressure when bandaging, and wrap a large area of the limb, which lessens the chance of impeding the circulation.

DO NOT

➤ Use an elasticated bandage to hold a dressing in place, as it may be too tight and cut off the blood flow.

➤ Bandage over toes or fingers, unless they are damaged, so that you can check the bandaging is not too tight.

➤ Use the wrong-sized bandage – too big and it will be baggy, too small and it will be potentially too tight.

➤ Secure a dressing with adhesive tape before first asking the person if they have an allergy to such tape.

➤ Apply adhesive tape all the way around a limb or a finger or toe, as it could cut off the blood flow.

Applying bandages 1

SEE ALSO

➤ Applying dressings and bandages, p200

➤ Applying bandages 2, p204

The only way to become proficient at bandaging is to practice; joints, such as ankles or elbows, can be especially tricky to master. You may find it easiest to watch someone else first and repeat it while you have a chance for some feedback. Make sure that the bandage overlaps on each turn and that you roll it out firmly but not too tightly. If your finished bandage looks floppy within an hour, unwind it and reapply using slightly more pressure. Bandages can become stretched with use but washing quickly restores their elasticity.

The first decision to be made when bandaging an injury is to choose the correct-sized bandage for the affected body part. If the bandage you use is too small or too big, it won't do its job efficiently and could cause more damage. As a guide, these widths fit the following body parts: 1in finger; 2in hand; 3–4in arm; and 4–6in leg.

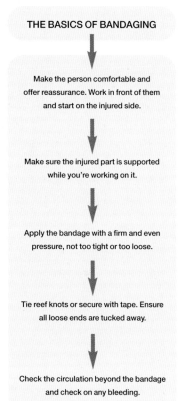

THE BASICS OF BANDAGING

Make the person comfortable and offer reassurance. Work in front of them and start on the injured side.

⬇

Make sure the injured part is supported while you're working on it.

⬇

Apply the bandage with a firm and even pressure, not too tight or too loose.

⬇

Tie reef knots or secure with tape. Ensure all loose ends are tucked away.

⬇

Check the circulation beyond the bandage and check on any bleeding.

HOW TO APPLY A ROLLER BANDAGE

The tip of a roll of bandage is called the "tail", while the roll is called the "head". Keep the head of the bandage uppermost, so that if you drop it, it does not fall on to the ground. Think about how the finished bandage will look before starting.

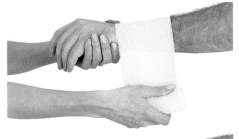

1 Place the tail of the bandage below the injury and work from the inside to the outside, and from the furthest part to the nearest.

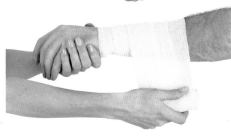

2 Roll the bandage around the limb and start with two overlapping turns. Cover two-thirds of the previous turn with each new one. Finish with two overlapping turns.

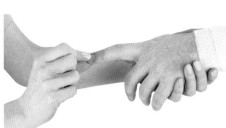

3 Once you've finished, check the circulation; if the bandage is too tight, unroll it and reapply it slightly more loosely.

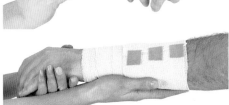

4 Secure the end with adhesive tape or tie the ends of the bandage using a reef knot.

BANDAGING A HAND OR FOOT

The bandaging method below for a hand also applies to a foot, although the heel should be kept clear unless injured. When working on a foot, start bandaging at the big toe.

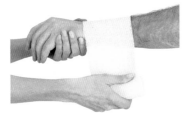

1 Start at the wrist and make two straight turns, working from the inside to the outside of the wrist.

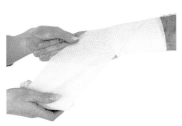

2 From the thumb side of the wrist, take the bandage diagonally across the back of the hand until it is touching the nail of the little finger.

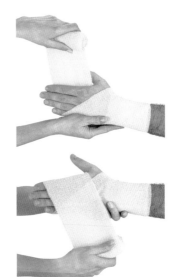

3 Leave the thumb free and take the bandage across the front of the fingers, also keeping the fingertips free.

4 Now, take the bandage across the back of the hand to the outside of the wrist, then around the wrist and back up to the little finger.

5 Repeat these turns, and cover about two-thirds of the previous turn with each new turn.

BANDAGING AN ELBOW OR KNEE JOINT

Bandaging these joints can be tricky, especially if you try to bandage while the joint is fully flexed. So, bandage in a partly flexed position so that it stays in place. For maximum support, these bandages need to be applied using figure-eight turns.

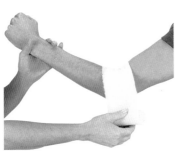

1 Put the tail of the bandage on the inside of the elbow; wind the bandage around the joint twice.

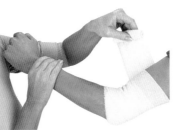

2 Now move the head of the bandage above the joint and wind two turns diagonally, making sure that you have covered half of the previous turn.

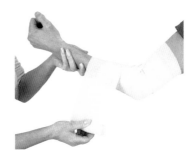

3 Now move the head to below the joint, cover half of the initial straight turns and do two diagonal turns.

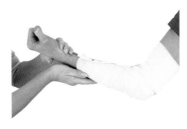

4 Continue doing two diagonal turns above and then below the joint in a figure-eight and then finally finish off the bandage with two straight turns.

Applying bandages 2

SEE ALSO

➤ Applying dressings and bandages, p200

➤ Applying bandages 1, p202

The head and fingers or toes are probably the trickiest areas to perfect in terms of bandaging technique. Apart from being difficult areas in which to make bandages stay in place, they may cause other problems for someone new to bandaging. Tightly wrapped adhesive tape, for example, around a finger can act as a tourniquet. Scalp wounds often bleed profusely and bandages need even but firm pressure to be effective. Here you'll learn how to use a tubular gauze bandage and a triangular bandage, which are included in most first-aid kits.

Tubular bandages come in two types: tubular elasticated bandages for supporting injured joints and tubular gauze for covering a finger or a toe.

Tubular gauze bandages help to stem the bleeding and also protect a digit from others nearby without impeding its blood flow. They are usually supplied with a special applicator to help you slip the bandage into place, but if this is not available you can improvize by bending a piece of card in two.

HOW TO APPLY A TUBULAR BANDAGE TO A FINGER

These elasticated bandages allow sufficient pressure to stop the bleeding but do not impede blood flow.

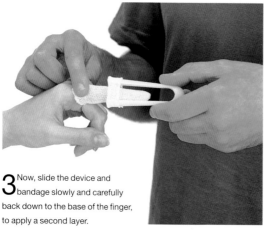

1 Load a piece of bandage, at least two to three times the length of the finger, onto an applicator. Push the applicator over the finger.

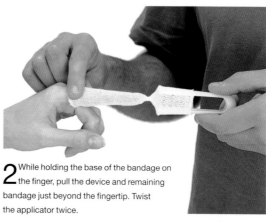

2 While holding the base of the bandage on the finger, pull the device and remaining bandage just beyond the fingertip. Twist the applicator twice.

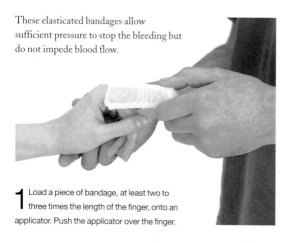

3 Now, slide the device and bandage slowly and carefully back down to the base of the finger, to apply a second layer.

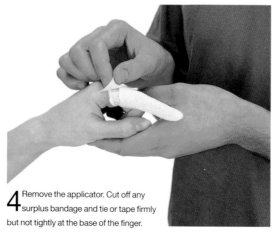

4 Remove the applicator. Cut off any surplus bandage and tie or tape firmly but not tightly at the base of the finger.

HOW TO BANDAGE A HEAD

Initially, apply a gauze wad to a head wound, especially if it is bleeding heavily. The wad helps to apply firm but even pressure across the whole scalp. If blood soaks through the bandage, apply another on top to avoid disturbing any blood clots. A strip bandage could be used, but is harder to keep in place.

1 Apply the triangular bandage with the folded longest edge over the forehead.

2 Take the two long "tails" at the back of the head and, using firm pressure, cross them over one another.

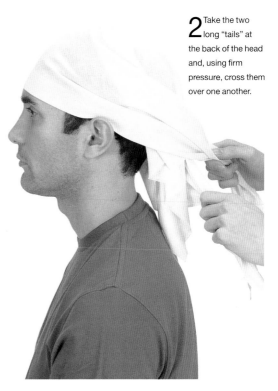

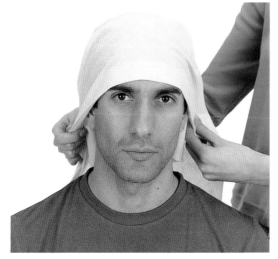

3 Bring the two tails around to the front and tie in the middle of the forehead.

4 Draw up the spare end to the top of the person's head, and then secure with a safety pin or tape.

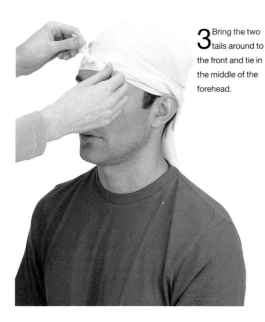

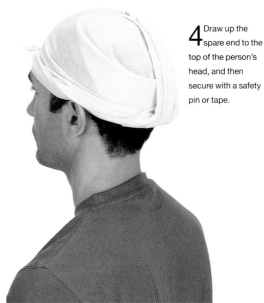

Fixing slings

SEE ALSO
➤ Wounds and wound healing, p128
➤ Treating infected wounds, p132
➤ Dealing with broken bones, p150

Triangular bandages are first-aid kit staples and most kits will contain quite a few. Usually a large triangular bandage is used for making a sling. If there is not one available at the scene of an emergency then you can improvise with the upturned hem of a jacket or shirt, or the sleeve of a shirt or jumper. The important functions of a sling are to support and immobilize an injured part of the body, and, in some cases (called high-arm or elevation slings), to stem bleeding from a wound. Here, you'll learn how to tie both types of arm sling.

Slings usually support the arm and can be classed as either a "broad-arm" sling, which supports the arm horizontally, or a "high-arm" sling, which both supports the limb and helps to reduce swelling and bleeding. High-arm slings also support rib fractures.

HOW TO TIE A HIGH-ARM SLING

This high-arm or elevation sling is used to stop the bleeding in a finger or forearm injury and also helps to reduce pain and prevent further injury by immobilizing the limb. This sling can also be used in burn victims to minimize swelling.

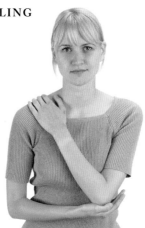

1 Place the injured arm so that the fingers touch the opposite collarbone.

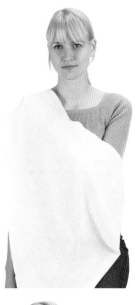

2 Place the triangular bandage to lie over the injured arm with the long edge against the uninjured side and the point to the injured side.

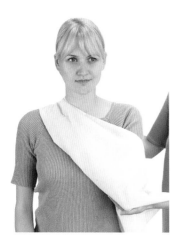

3 Tuck the bandage behind the elbow and forearm. Pass the free end behind the back.

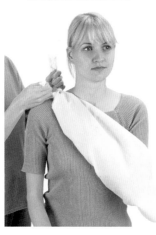

4 At the collarbone, tie the two ends of the bandage together on the uninjured side.

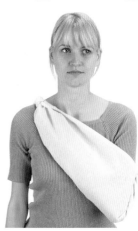

5 To secure the bandage at the elbow, tuck in the fabric or fold and use a safety pin.

FIXING A BROAD-ARM SLING

This type of sling is used for an arm or hand injury, such as a fracture or a sprain. Such a sling immobilizes the limb and can be improvised in many ways.

1 Ask the person to support their injured arm so that the hand lies just above the uninjured elbow. Now place the bandage between the body and arm, so that the straight edge lies on the uninjured side.

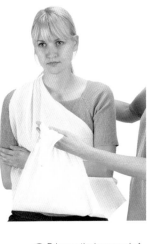

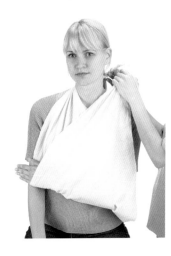

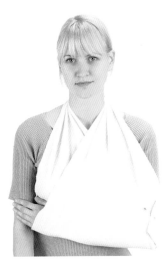

2 Bring up the lower end of the bandage to meet the other end at the shoulder. Tie (or pin) to secure and tuck both ends under the knot.

3 The person can let the arm go once you have secured the ends.

4 Finish the sling by folding over the pointed end of the fabric at the elbow and pinning. This is how the sling should look.

SOME IDEAS FOR IMPROVISING SLINGS

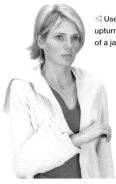

◁ Use the upturned hem of a jacket.

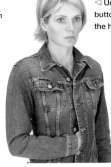

◁ Undo a jacket button and tuck the hand inside.

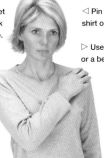

◁ Pin the sleeve of a shirt or sweater.

▷ Use a pair of tights or a belt.

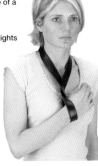

SKILLS CHECKLIST FOR
FIRST-AID KIT

KEY POINTS

- Always have a first-aid kit available at home and in your car □

- While a first-aid kit is important the ability to improvise is an essential skill for a first-aider □

- Practice your bandaging skills on a friend □

SKILLS LEARNED

- How to dress and bandage a wound or injury □

- How to improvise dressings and bandages if necessary □

- How to bandage an elbow and knee □

- How to bandage a finger □

- How to cope with scalp bandaging □

- How to make slings □

14

COMPLEMENTARY THERAPIES

Complementary health therapists believe that their practices encourage the body's natural defenses to heal injury – whether that injury is physical or emotional or a combination of the two. Of course, complementary techniques will not be appropriate in most emergencies, where conventional medicine is vital. Where they come into their own is in working alongside conventional medicine, especially for more minor complaints, such as cramps, stings, and constipation. As with any first-aid treatment, safety must always be your watchword. Use only safe techniques, sterile dressings, and medications you feel very well informed about. Always ask for a medical opinion before using complementary therapies on children.

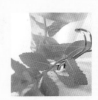

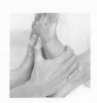

CONTENTS

Understanding complementary therapies 210 – 211

Complementary first-aid kit 212 – 213

Using complementary therapies 1 214 – 215

Using complementary therapies 2 216 – 217

Skills checklist 218

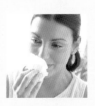

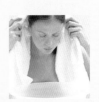

Understanding complementary therapies

SEE ALSO

➤ Complementary first-aid kit, p212

➤ Using complementary therapies 1 and 2, p214, p216

The complementary therapies frequently referred to in the context of natural first aid are aromatherapy, herbalism, acupuncture, reflexology, and homeopathy. You may find that a number of other therapies – such as Alexander technique, reiki, massage, color therapy, meditation, or yoga – also have a part to play in calming someone with minor injuries and in helping them to convalesce. Be sure to seek conventional medical assistance first, and then choose from the many natural therapies to soothe, calm, and heal after an emergency.

It is not so long ago that people had only natural remedies to turn to when dealing with illness or injury. In very recent times, these types of treatment have made a comeback, and new "complementary" approaches have been developed. Many people perceive them to be safer, gentler, and more natural than conventional medication, preferring their holistic approach over modern medicine's emphasis on the disease rather than the person.

Some first-aid scenarios demand life support skills and complementary tactics are not appropriate, but there are many minor cases where alternatives are fine to use. Some of these have been proved effective in clinical trials, while others may not have been formally tested, but are commonly accepted as useful and effective alternatives.

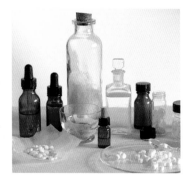

△ A wide range of homeopathic remedies are now widely available from conventional drugstores, where expert help is on hand to advise about their use.

▽ Herbal remedies can be used for all kinds of conditions, but seek advice before using.

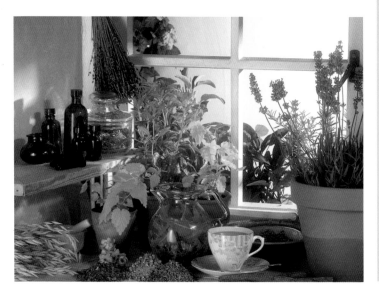

BE SAFE!

➤ **Seek conventional advice first**
Before embarking on the use of a complementary therapy, you should have the person checked out by a conventional doctor. (Using homeopathy to treat meningitis, or acupuncture for acute asthma, is downright dangerous – sadly, deaths have resulted from such scenarios.) In fact, always seek conventional advice whenever considering complementary treatments. This advice applies especially strongly if you have any medical condition at all.

➤ **Use herbal remedies carefully**
Herbal remedies work because they contain chemicals that interact with the receptors in the body. We should be wary of seeing all herbal and related treatments as "naturally safe" – aspirin, for example, was originally a herbally derived drug, and it has both good and bad effects. Herbal remedies can interact with conventional medicines or may contain unknown or toxic substances, or steroids. Unlike prescribed medication, they are rarely tested properly, if at all.

➤ **Using aromatherapy oils**
Always seek expert help before using these. Many natural oils are highly potent, and specific ones can be dangerous if taken by those with certain conditions – pregnant women must be especially careful which oils they use. In most cases, never apply oils directly to skin (lavender and tea tree are notable exceptions), but dilute – for example in a carrier oil. Before applying oils to the skin, always do a patch test.

AROMATHERAPY

What is it? This literally means "treatment using scent". The term "aromatherapy" was first used by a French chemist called Gattefosse in 1937. He accidentally discovered the healing powers of essential oils when he burned his hand and plunged it into a bucket of lavender oil. He was amazed by how quickly and painlessly the burn healed.

How it works Essential plant oils are used in various ways, including massage, inhalation, baths, cold compresses, and vaporizers. The smell of the oils is thought to affect the part of the brain that controls emotions, mood, and memory. It may have a calming or an invigorating effect, depending on the aromas used.

Is it harmful? It should be used with caution in pregnancy and in conditions such as high blood pressure, epilepsy, and skin conditions. There may be hypersensitive reactions to sunlight. The oils should never be ingested and should always be kept out of the way of children.

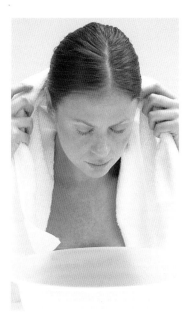

▽ Steam inhalation of certain aromatic oils can soothe anxiety and tension.

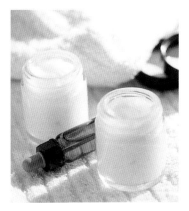

△ Essential oils can be used in many different forms – added to moisturizer, for example.

HERBALISM

Almost all drugs used to be derived from plant parts. Many people like the idea of using herbal remedies, because they feel that they are safer and more natural than conventional drugs.

What is it? Herbalists believe that stress, pollution, poor lifestyle, and a bad diet lead to a draining of our life force. They feel that the body's battle to maintain a harmonious balance creates illness. Many people also use herbs to prevent disease by bolstering their immune systems and detoxifying the body.

How are they used? Herbs can be infused, made into tinctures, teas, capsules, creams, compresses, and bath products. They can be effective for treating problems such as irritable bowel syndrome, urinary problems, eczema, and indigestion.

ACUPUNCTURE/ACUPRESSURE

An ancient Chinese treatment, used for thousands of years, acupuncture involves the insertion of thin needles under the skin at specific points. The points are located along energy channels or "meridians". Acupressure massages these points instead of using needles. No one is certain how this approach works, but it may increase secretions of the body's natural painkillers – endorphins and serotonin.

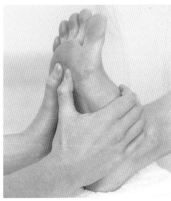

△ Reflexology may prove to be very effective in relieving problems such as back injury.

REFLEXOLOGY

This therapy involves massaging certain areas of the feet and the hands that correspond to different parts of the body and to specific organs.

HOMEOPATHY

Homeopathy fights disease by treating "like with like". In other words, elements that can cause the symptoms of a particular illness can be used to cure it. However, these elements are used in minute doses, to the point where the prescribed substance is so diluted that it is undetectable.

▽ Try "Rescue remedy" and *Arnica* to help recovery from minor bruises and shock.

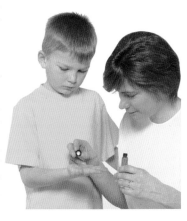

Complementary first-aid kit

SEE ALSO

➤ Understanding
complementary
therapies, p210

➤ Using therapies 1
and 2, p214, p216

You can obtain many essential oils and herbs, as well as homeopathic remedies, from local drugstores. Choose those that you find appealing or maybe select the remedies that cover most of the common everyday injuries and the aches and pains that may affect us all from time to time – such as headaches, co[ ] sore throat, arthritis, insomnia, depression, [ ] anxiety. Always check the sell-by dates [ ] bear in mind that it is good to buy in sm[ ] quantities, until you have established that [ ] find the remedies useful, to avoid wastage.

Recently, a study showed that burning aromatherapy oils on a psychiatric ward had a significant calming effect on the often disturbed patients. Different oils, homeopathic remedies, and herbs work on different ailments, and you could make up a useful first-aid kit of these to use alongside more conventional remedies.

As with many drugs, there are really only a small number of complementary therapies that are definitely safe in pregnancy. It is a good idea to check with an aromatherapist, homeopath, or herbalist before trying any therapies – a therapist will be able to advise you on the remedies that will be most useful for you.

PEPPERMINT

Used as an oil or herb, peppermint has active ingredients that are effective at clearing the upper respiratory tract of mucus, so it is useful as a decongestant in colds and nasal blockage. It is an invigorating herb that can be chosen when you want to feel more awake and alive. Taken as a tea or in capsule form, it is excellent at calming digestive problems, especially trapped wind, heartburn, and indigestion. Diluted peppermint oil can also be rubbed into the temples at each side of the forehead and the neck muscles at the top of the spine and around the shoulders to relieve stress headaches.

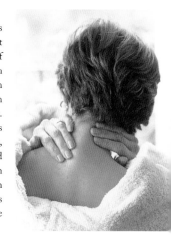

△ Gently massage diluted peppermint oil in the neck muscles to relieve tension headach[ ]

▷ Herbal and homeopathic remedies should be stored away from direct sunlight, in dark glass bottles.

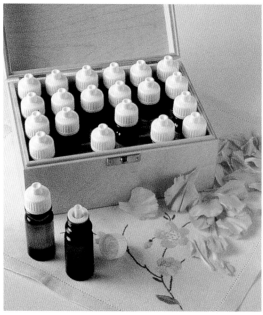

GINGER

This plant is very soothing for diges[ ] disorders and appetite loss. Ginger ro[ ] commonly drunk as a tea to ease tr[ ] sickness, and it can be used, if advised alleviate morning sickness. Effective [ ] muscle spasms and pains, ginger is [ ] useful in rheumatism and arthritis.

CLOVE

Extract of clove is a well-known p[ ] reliever, and a small amount of clove applied to a sore tooth will ease the pai[ ] toothache (note: avoid contact, especi[ ] prolonged, with gums or skin, as this [ ] cause some irritation). Clove is also a g[ ] insect repellent, so a few drops placed[ ] clothing or bedding will help keep bi[ ] insects and mosquitoes away.

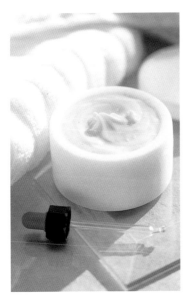

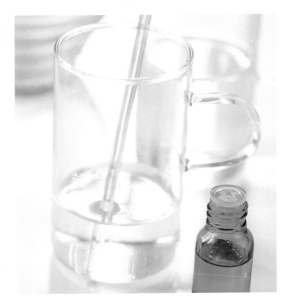

◁ Always check before using essential oils or adding them to your favorite lotions and creams. Some oils are very potent, and must be used in a certain way, or avoided if you have a particular health condition or are pregnant.

▷ If using oils diluted in water, stir very thoroughly.

ARNICA

This flowering herb is poisonous when taken internally, so should be used only in creams and oils topically, or internally as a homeopathic remedy. *Arnica* is useful for bruises, muscle soreness, shock, and to promote wound-healing.

LAVENDER

Used as an essential oil, lavender is highly antiseptic and effective when used as a compress for superficial burns, blisters, and

▽ Sniff a tissue containing a few drops of lavender oil to relieve insomnia.

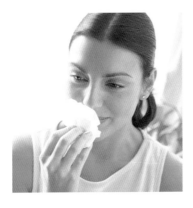

bites. It can be used to help ease depression and insomnia – simply add a few drops to a tissue and sniff, or place the tissue inside your pillowcase, to help you get off to sleep and enjoy a refreshing rest.

TEA TREE

The essential oil of tea tree is used topically as an antibacterial, antiseptic remedy. Diluted in water, a tea tree spray can ease the pain of a sore throat.

CHAMOMILE

Made up as a tea, chamomile is extremely calming and soothing, and is good for insomnia, depression, and anxiety. A few drops of the oil in a bedtime bath will also aid peaceful sleep.

GERANIUM

This is a very effective herb when used to treat psychological problems such as anxiety or panic attacks.

CLARY SAGE

This is a useful essential oil for dealing with depression, anxiety, and frayed nerves. It can be added, diluted, to a bath, or dispersed in an oil burner.

SOME OTHER IDEAS FOR YOUR NATURAL KIT

➤ Tincture of *Calendula* (pot marigold) – minor burns and scalds.

➤ Comfrey oil/ointment – bruises and sprains. Never use any oil/ointment on open wounds (it encourages infection).

➤ Witch hazel – insect bites and stings, sprains, bruises, mild sunburn.

▽ Oil from geranium leaves is a calming and cooling remedy, ideal for easing anxieties.

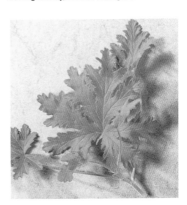

Using complementary therapies 1

SEE ALSO

➤ Refer to index for all other references to these conditions throughout book

Accidents, injuries, and trauma may produce a wide range of associated conditions, ranging from nausea and constipation to cramp. These kinds of symptoms can often be eased by complementary therapies. Psychological after-shock and tension are also natural reactions to injury and accident, and you might find that complementary approaches can be effective in these cases, too. However, always remember that your first priority must be to arrange for conventional medical treatment for an individual's injuries.

NAUSEA AND VOMITING

There are many causes of nausea and vomiting. Most of them will be "self-limiting", which means they will settle without the need for further treatment or investigation. It is recommended that you should seek conventional advice first when tackling health conditions, but mild nausea can usually be treated safely with natural remedies. However, as with diarrhea, if the symptoms are not settling in 1–2 days and dehydration is developing, or the symptoms are mild but persistent, medical help must be sought.

Herbal remedies An infusion of ginger root may settle nausea. Also try chamomile or black horehound (but always avoid the latter in pregnancy).

Acupuncture/acupressure Use the anti-nausea point that is two thumb widths above the wrist crease, between the two prominent tendons passing to the hand. A therapist can treat this area with a needle, or you can use firm pressure at this point for

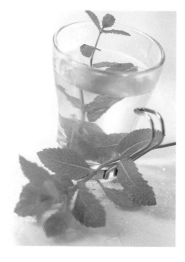

△ A peppermint infusion is a highly effective remedy for nausea and indigestion – and also useful as a general pick-me-up.

one minute. There are also wristbands for sale that exert pressure, and can be used in pregnancy. For travel sickness, press your index finger into the hollow at the back of the jawline for a minute.

Homeopathy *Ipecac* and *Nux Vomica* are useful for nausea. Take up to 12 doses every 2 hours until the symptoms settle.

DIARRHEA

Herbal remedies Geranium, peppermint, and chamomile infusions are effective in settling diarrhea if taken as 3–4 tbsp of tea three times a day.

Acupressure Use firm pressure four thumb widths above the inside of the ankle just behind the shin bone.

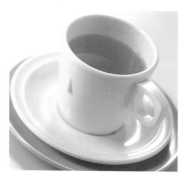

△ Chamomile-containing herbal teas are excellent for soothing anxiety.

Reflexology Apply pressure to the point for the small intestine (which is located between the arch and the heel of the foot) and then the large intestine points on either side.

Homeopathy *Arsenicum album* is the recommended remedy for diarrhea.

CONSTIPATION

Aromatherapy Gently massage a diluted mixture of rosemary, marjoram, and chamomile into the area around the navel.

Herbal remedies Dandelion leaves are a gentle laxative.

Acupressure Place a finger four thumb widths up from the back of the wrist crease. Bend the arm and press the opposite thumb into the outer edge of the elbow crease for a minute, then repeat on the other arm.

Reflexology Use the large intestine pressure point (see picture for exact location). Press firmly and then massage for 10 minutes.

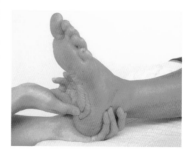

△ A reflexologist is able to massage the large intestine pressure point (the relevant area is drawn on the foot in this photograph) in order to relieve constipation.

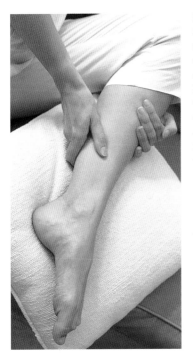

△ Massage cramp with a blend of basil and marjoram diluted in almond oil.

CRAMP

This is when a muscle goes into a painful spasm and feels rock-hard. It occurs most often after exercise, when you are dehydrated, and also often strikes in the middle of the night. Initial measures should involve using the muscle by walking around or stretching and massaging it, and drinking plenty of water every day – at least 3 ½ pints.

Aromatherapy Massage with basil and marjoram diluted in almond oil.

Herbal remedies Ginkgo infusion helps ease intractable cramp.

Acupressure Press into the bottom of the calf muscle for 5 minutes.

Homeopathy *Caprum metallicum* tablets may help to ease a cramp-like ache.

▷ Irritability and anxiety are often relieved by massage. Massage is straightforward to learn and easy to do to yourself.

HEADACHE

Stress and tension, which are commonly associated with the trauma of injuries and accidents, may manifest themselves in different ways. One of the most common is headache. The person may complain of tightness in the muscles at the back of the scalp and neck.

Aromatherapy Diluted lavender oil rubbed into the temples is wonderful for a tension headache. Inhaling eucalyptus is also very effective for sinus headaches.

Herbal remedies Feverfew may help with a migrainous headache, but should not be taken in pregnancy.

Acupressure Apply pressure to a point between the eyebrows at the bridge of the nose, and on either side of the neck at the base of the back of the skull.

Reflexology Press a thumb firmly to the base of the big toe for 10–20 seconds.

Homeopathy *Kali bichromicum* 6c is good for sinus headache, and *Bryonia* can help a general headache.

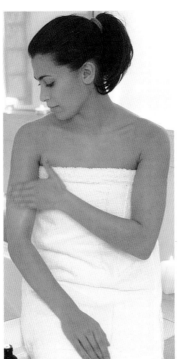

△ Try relieving stress headaches by applying gentle pressure to the area around the temples.

SHOCK

Aromatherapy Neroli and lavender oils are known for their relaxing and calming properties.

Herbal remedies Chamomile and lemon balm combine well to make a tea to calm and soothe agitation, and encourage peaceful rest and sleep.

Homeopathy *Arnica* tablets are effective after a bad fall for bruising and shock. Aconite may also be helpful for treating the symptoms of shock.

SOOTHING STRESS AND TENSION

Once any injuries have been treated by a medical practitioner, massage with soothing oils and relaxation exercises can be helpful for easing the stress and tension associated with any accident.

Using complementary therapies 2

SEE ALSO

➤ Refer to index for all other references to these conditions throughout book

Some relatively minor injuries can be treated effectively with one of the complementary therapies. There are often a number of options, from which you may choose the one you prefer. For example, to treat bruises you can use *Arnica*, lavender oil or rosemary oil; sunburn can be treated with lavender oil, *Hypericum* (St John's wort), aloe vera or *Calendula*. "Rescue Remedy" combines five of the Bach flower remedies and can be bought as a tincture or a cream – it is useful for reducing the effects of trauma or shock.

There are all kinds of scenarios that respond well to complementary treatments, either used alone or in tandem with conventional first aid treatment. Complementary means exactly that – these treatments are not necessarily an alternative to a more traditional medical approach, and the two approaches should complement each other.

BITES AND STINGS

Aromatherapy Add a few drops of lavender or tea tree oil to a little iced water and apply it to the area. Soak a cloth in the water and place that on the sting, or use a cotton pad and apply some of the water every 10 minutes until the pain subsides.

Herbal remedies Fresh onion on an insect bite may take the pain out of the area. Useful herbs for making into an infusion and applying to a burn or sting are chamomile, elderflower, or red clover (the latter is also a proven natural alternative to hormone replacement therapy). Fresh leaves of lemon balm, plantain, and yellow dock applied to the damaged skin may be soothing and speed up pain relief.

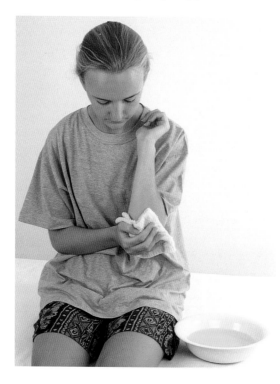

▷ For soothing sore bites and stings, wring a cloth out in iced water or an iced herbal infusion and hold it over the affected area.

BRUISES

Bruising happens because the blood vessels beneath the skin break and the blood escapes. This is usually after a traumatic event, and it is painful. However, certain people may bruise virtually without injury, perhaps if they are on anticoagulant treatment such as warfarin or have problems with their blood-clotting abilities. This last group of people should always seek medical help.

Aromatherapy Lavender oil made up as a cold compress is very good at reducing swelling and bruising after injury. Diluted rosemary oil massaged into the tissues is also soothing and may speed up healing.

Homeopathy Use *Arnica* on unbroken skin in ointment form or as a bath lotion; the latter is very soothing when suffering from general aching – after an unaccustomed horse ride or aerobics class, for example.

BURNS

Before you do anything to any type of burn you should cool it down. If the burn is bigger than the palm of the victim's hand, they must get medical advice.

Aromatherapy Lavender essential oil is good for numbing the pain of a burn, which can be excruciating. It promotes healing and reduces scarring. Use neat on small areas, or on sterile gauze for larger areas.

Herbal remedies Fresh gel from the aloe vera plant is very effective – simply snap off part of a leaf and apply the plant gel directly.

SPRAINS AND STRAINS

Aromatherapy/herbal remedies It can be useful to add some lavender oil or chamomile to water and store them in a

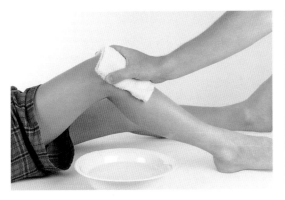

△ Lay a person flat to apply a cold compress to sprains and strains.

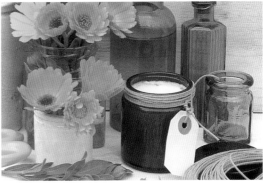

△ *Calendula* (pot marigold) remedies are ideal for healing cuts and grazes.

bottle in the refrigerator so that you have something at hand for soothing sprains and strains. A comfrey or marigold leaf infusion applied ice-cold is also good. Comfrey ointment is effective when applied for a few days after a strain has occurred, or to aching muscles.

Homeopathy Homeopathic remedies include *Arnica*, *Rhus tox*. and *Ruta grav*.

SUNBURN

Aromatherapy For widespread sunburn, add some drops of diluted lavender oil to a tepid bath. Lavender oil can also be applied directly to the skin, especially if the sunburn is severe. The blood-red oil of St John's wort or aloe vera juice are highly soothing, cooling and healing.

Homeopathy Homeopathic options include *Cantharis* and *Urtica urens*, especially if the pain of the sunburn is intense and persistent. *Hypericum* or *Calendula* cream is also good.

NOSEBLEED

Aromatherapy A pad of cotton soaked in cold water to which a few drops of lemon oil have been added is good at slowing down a nosebleed when placed across the bridge of the nose.

Herbal remedies A cotton pad soaked in an infusion of yarrow and then squeezed at the end of the nose for a few minutes may prove effective in stopping a nosebleed.

CUTS AND GRAZES

Aromatherapy Lavender and tea tree can be used neat on small cuts and scratches, added to a bowl of water for cleaning the wound, or used on a dressing applied over the injury. These oils have a disinfectant effect so may well reduce the chances of infection settling into the wound.

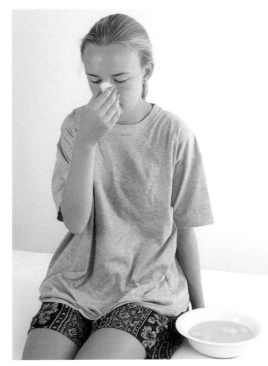

Herbal remedies Witch hazel can be used directly on small wounds or on a dressing, as can tinctures of marigold or myrrh. Comfrey is also a powerful tissue-healer.

Homeopathy A homeopathic compress of *Hypericum* (St Johns wort) or *Calendula* can be used direct on dressings, or in ointment form once the skin has healed over.

◁ To stop nosebleeds, try applying a pad of cotton wool soaked in a cooled yarrow infusion over the soft part of the nose.

SKILLS CHECKLIST FOR
COMPLEMENTARY THERAPIES

KEY POINTS

- The remedies described in this chapter are intended to be complementary or additional rather than alternatives ☐

- Always seek qualified medical assistance initially ☐

SKILLS LEARNED

- How to treat minor injuries with natural, complementary treatments ☐

- Recognizing that complementary treatments may be effective in the aftermath of injury, trauma, or accident, for treating anxiety, insomnia, depression, and stress ☐

- Recognizing that complementary treatments can have side-effects just as conventional medical treatments do ☐

15

KEEPING SAFE

Safety in the home, safety in the garden, and safety on the road are supremely important considerations in the prevention of accidents. The great majority of accidents are preventable. This chapter looks at the hazards to be encountered both in the home, especially in the kitchen and the bathroom, and outside it. Being aware and taking sensible precautions will help you to minimize the chances of an accident befalling either you or a member of your family. When accidents do occur, coping with them quickly and effectively can do much to mitigate the effects and prevent further injury.

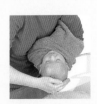

CONTENTS

Keeping yourself safe 220–221

Safety on the road 222–223

Safety in the home 224–225

Safety in the kitchen 226–227

Safety in the bathroom 228–229

Safety in the garden 230–231

Dealing with fire 232

Avoiding electrical accidents 233

Safe home for infants 234

Avoiding sudden infant death 235

Skills checklist 236

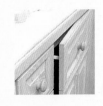

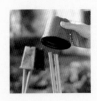

Keeping yourself safe

SEE ALSO
➤ Drowning: what to do, p60
➤ Safety on the road, p222
➤ Dealing with fire, p232

Most people do not give enough thought to their own safety when they spot someone in danger and in need of assistance. However, you must do everything you can to protect yourself while helping an accident victim. Taking time to survey the scene and think through your actions is essential. You should not, for example, rush in to rescue someone from a burning building. Without the right training, you are likely to become a victim yourself and may hinder a rescue operation. It is wiser to wait for the professionals.

The first rule of first aid is not to put yourself in any danger. You may make matters worse if you jump into the scene without first standing back and assessing the situation. You should be aware of your limitations and training. For example, even a strong swimmer should be wary of diving into the water to help someone struggling. You should always consider safer ways to help first, such as throwing in a rope and life ring or an inflatable ball. Rescue attempts often end in a double tragedy that could have been avoided had more time been taken to survey the scene. Always take a few moments to look for danger – there may be flammable chemicals, electric cables, or other hazards present.

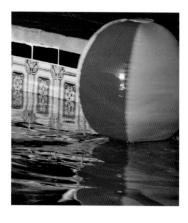

△ Throw an inflatable ball or rope to someone who is having difficulties in deep water rather than jumping in yourself.

CARE WITH BODY FLUIDS

Helping someone may involve coming into contact with body fluids. There has never been a recorded case of anyone catching HIV or hepatitis from mouth-to-mouth, but this should not lead to complacency.

Generally, HIV needs contact with fresh blood or semen to be dangerous. It is a relatively fragile virus that does not survive outside the body for long. Hepatitis B, on the other hand, can still be active in dried blood, even when it is several days old. It is also possible to contract tuberculosis (TB) and meningitis from body fluids.

To protect yourself, use a mouth shield when giving mouth-to-mouth, or place a handkerchief across the person's mouth. This gives you some protection while still allowing air to pass into their lungs.

AGGRESSIVENESS

You should never underestimate how violent a person might be, particularly if they appear to be drunk or on drugs. If in any doubt about your own safety, wait for the emergency services to arrive and keep away, especially if you suspect that the person might be carrying a weapon.

Sick people may become aggressive for many reasons, including low blood sugar as a result of diabetes or lack of oxygen. If you are worried about getting hurt, it is best to leave them until someone from the emergency services arrives and is able to give them appropriate treatment.

AVOIDING INFECTION FROM BLOOD AND OTHER BODY FLUIDS

The best way to guard against infection is to avoid another person's body fluids altogether. However, if that is not possible, there are several ways to minimize the risk.

➤ Wear disposable gloves and wash your hands after contact with blood or other body fluids.

➤ Protect any wounds on your own body from infection by covering them with waterproof dressings.

➤ Wear plastic goggles or plastic glasses to protect your eyes from splashes.

➤ If body fluids come into contact with your mouth, eyes, or nose, wash the area thoroughly for 10 minutes under briskly running water.

➤ If you receive an injury that comes into contact with body fluids, see a doctor. It is possible to detect infection with hepatitis B early on, and to reduce the risk of contracting the disease.

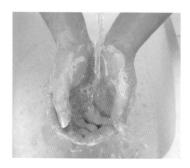

△ Wash your hands thoroughly under running water if you come into contact with body fluids such as blood or semen.

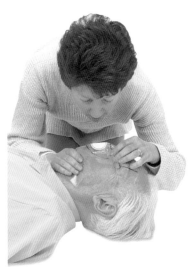

△ Use a mouth shield if you are giving mouth-to-mouth resuscitation. If you do not have one placing a handkerchief over the person's mouth gives some protection.

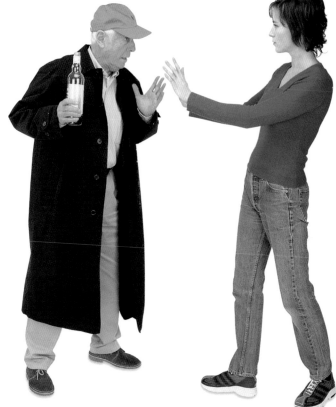

▷ Be wary of approaching anyone who is drunk or aggressive. You do not know whether they may lash out or if they have a weapon.

PSYCHOLOGICAL STRESS

It can be exhilarating and rewarding to help someone who is injured or in danger, but it can also be upsetting and disturbing however psychologically strong you are.

You may have witnessed scenes that you find difficult to get out of your mind, even weeks, months, or years after the event. You may have disturbing dreams that disrupt your sleep even when you thought you had forgotten the incident. Talking to other people about the event or speaking to a trained counselor may help you come to terms with the trauma.

Life-threatening emergencies can be frightening affairs, and if death is involved you may feel guilty that you did not do enough to help. You should accept that you may need support to help you to get back to normal.

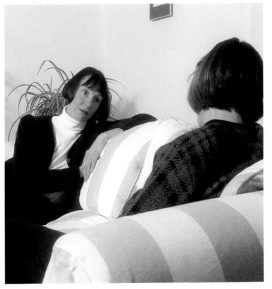

◁ Following a serious accident, bystanders, helpers, and paramedics risk developing post-traumatic stress disorder. If you feel agitated or you are sleeping badly after witnessing a trauma, ask your doctor to refer you to a trained counselor for help.

Safety on the road

SEE ALSO

➤ What is first aid?, p12
➤ Cardiac compressions, p32
➤ Full resuscitation sequence, p34

The most common site for people to have a road accident is within 2 miles of their own home – perhaps because of fatigue or because drivers exercise less care when on their home ground. Other common causes of motor vehicle accidents include inexperience and carelessness by young and newly qualified drivers, being distracted by children and driving while under the influence of alcohol. The best way to avoid accidents is to drive not only safely but also watchfully, so that you can compensate for the mistakes of others.

Roads around the world are becoming increasingly busy. Although there are stringent laws governing road safety in many countries, most motor vehicle accidents are caused by human error – 95 percent are somebody's fault, rather than simply being due to an unlucky twist of fate. Perhaps surprisingly, most road traffic accidents happen in daylight; less surprisingly, these often occur in the rush hours: 7–9 a.m. and 3–7 p.m.

WHY ACCIDENTS HAPPEN

Alcohol is a big factor in many accidents. It affects multiple aspects of driving ability – decision-making, self-criticism, balance, coordination, touch, sight, hearing, and judgment, to name a few. It is best not to drink at all if you are planning on driving rather than trying to stick to a general "safe limit" that may not be safe for a particular individual at all.

Inexperienced and young drivers, especially men, often drive without enough thought for road safety or their responsibility as drivers. This is why those under 20 years old have to pay large amounts for their car insurance – and can then be a hazard on the road.

Older drivers can be a danger to themselves and others if their eyesight and reaction speeds are failing, particularly if they do not have any insight into the problem. Lack of concentration caused by

WARNING
You should never use cellphones when driving – neither hand-held nor hands-free models.

chatting to others in the car, turning to reprimand children, or talking on a cellphone can also cause an accident.

Tiredness is a major killer. Its incidence is probably underestimated because no one can know the exact details of what has gone on before a fatal car crash. Planning regular breaks, being aware of times when you are likely to feel drowsy (for example, just after lunch or between

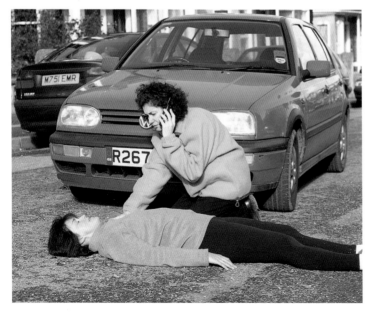

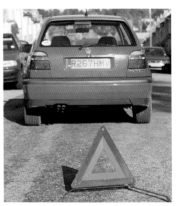

△ Always carry a warning triangle in your car. Place this near the stationary vehicle to warn approaching drivers of an accident.

◁ Make sure that an injured person is in a safe place – move them if absolutely necessary – then call the emergency services for help.

the hours of 2 a.m. and 6 a.m.) and stopping for a nap or a coffee if tiredness hits can all help to prevent a tragedy.

Motorways are particularly hazardous because the monotony of driving on long, straight roads and the lack of gear changing can cause the driver to feel tired or be inattentive. But fatigue and lack of concentration can also cause accidents on urban and suburban roads just as easily. Most road accidents occur within 2 miles of the driver's own home.

WHAT TO DO IN A CAR ACCIDENT

If you witness a motor vehicle accident, be aware that stopping could jeopardize your own safety. Check all your mirrors before pulling up at the scene. Stay calm and ensure that your car is visible and that the accident scene is protected from oncoming traffic. Switch on your hazard lights as soon as you have stopped.

If the accident has happened on a bend, try to warn approaching drivers by using a hazard warning triangle or asking another driver to flag the cars down. Watch out for broken glass and metal. Make sure that your handbrake is on and that your car is safe to leave.

On motorways, the speed that vehicles travel at may well make stopping to help too hazardous. If this is the case, drive on and use a telephone to summon help.

TO REDUCE THE RISK OF FIRE

Turn off the damaged car's engine and, if possible, disconnect the car battery. Stop people from smoking at the scene, and cover any fuel spillage with soil or sand.

FIRST AID FOR TRAFFIC ACCIDENT VICTIMS

People are often trapped in cars after accidents. This should not stop you from initiating first-aid measures. You can still protect and open the airway of a person in an upright position.

Make the area safe. Move people to safety if possible. But do not move anyone who is injured unless they are in further danger.

Telephone the emergency services with precise details of your location.

Stop heavy bleeding.

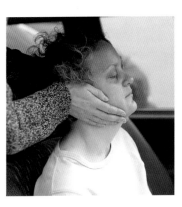

Instigate CPR if needed.

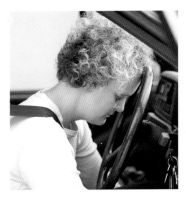

△ An accident victim slumped forward in the driver's seat should be moved so their airway is opened, even if spinal injury is a possibility.

▽ To clear the airway of someone who is still in the car, tilt their jaw slightly upward and remove any blood or vomit. Then use the resuscitation techniques.

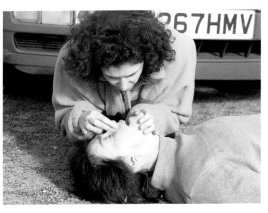

◁ When dealing with any roadside accident victim, assume that there may be a neck/spinal injury and handle with great care. Wherever possible, treat the person in the position found.

Safety in the home

SEE ALSO
➤ Safety in the kitchen, p226
➤ Safety in the bathroom, p228
➤ Dealing with fire, p232

One in three of all accidents happen in our own homes, the place where we feel safest and at our most comfortable. Our houses are filled with hazards – from faulty electrical appliances to ill-fitting carpets or prominent nails in the floorboards. Even a hot pan of soup can cause a serious injury. Most of these accidents are preventable, so making our homes safe must be a prime consideration. The majority of home accidents involve children. So, if you have children of your own, or if children visit your house, home safety is all the more important.

Most of us love our homes, and we feel secure and safe when we are in them. However, although we may feel protected from the dangers of the outside world, our home environments are actually filled with potential hazards.

Domestic accidents are what keep the country's emergency rooms busy. On average, more people are killed every week in domestic accidents than die in motor vehicle accidents. Many of these accidents are due to a combination of carelessness, ignorance, and human frailty – and most of them are preventable.

HOME HAZARDS

Almost anything has the potential to be a hazard. For example, accidents suffered by elderly people are most commonly a result of them putting their slippers onto the wrong feet and then attempting to walk in them. Pants are another unsuspected hazard, especially in the elderly and less physically able. Simply sitting down before attempting to put on a pair of pants cuts down the chance of an accident. Naked feet are also vulnerable – stepping on broken glass or dropping something on your foot can cause a nasty injury.

AVOIDING ACCIDENTS

Most accidents can be prevented by taking a few simple precautions.

➤ Don't leave toys lying around.

➤ Don't leave plastic bags within easy reach of children.

➤ Don't smoke in bed.

➤ Don't leave shoes in people's way.

➤ Don't leave flexes trailing or hanging.

➤ Don't allow pets to play on the stairs.

➤ Don't ever put a mat at the top or bottom of stairs.

➤ Don't place anything on a table covered with an overhanging cloth if you have children.

➤ Don't hang a mirror or toys over a fire.

➤ Don't put plants on the television – it is hazardous when you water them.

➤ Repair or throw away rickety ladders.

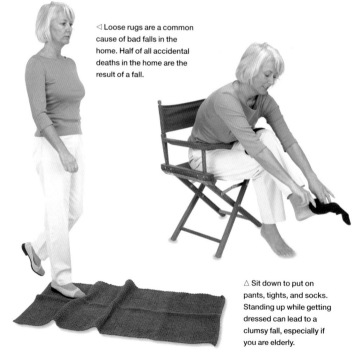

◁ Loose rugs are a common cause of bad falls in the home. Half of all accidental deaths in the home are the result of a fall.

△ Sit down to put on pants, tights, and socks. Standing up while getting dressed can lead to a clumsy fall, especially if you are elderly.

A TIDY HOME

Messy houses are without a doubt more dangerous than immaculate ones. Falls – the number one killer in the home – are much more likely to occur if the floor is covered with clutter. Glossy magazines strewn across a floor can be as slippery as a sheet of ice, and a bean bag in a hallway is difficult not to trip over. Children's toys left scattered across the floor are another major source of accidents.

Keeping a house clear of hazards is obviously a good idea, but this can be difficult when you are busy. The best policy

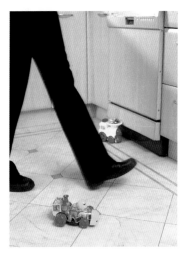

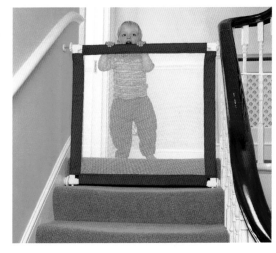

◁ Never leave toys or shoes lying around on the floor because they are a common cause of falls.

▷ Protect toddlers from falling down stairs by fitting gates at the top and bottom of each flight.

is to have a place for everything and to make sure that all walkways are kept as free of clutter as possible.

gates helps to protect children from falls. These gates need to be at the top and bottom of the stairs.

SAFE STAIRWAYS

It is particularly important to keep the stairs absolutely clear. Leaving objects on the stairs to be taken up (or down) later on, when you get around to it, is a major hazard. A vacuum cleaner left at the top of the stairs while you are dusting a room, for example, is easily tripped over.

Stair carpets wear out quickly and may develop lethal holes or tags. Repair any damage as soon as possible. Fitting stair

PREVENTING FIRE HAZARDS

Cracked plugs, loose flexes, old wiring, furniture placed too close to the fire and unguarded fires are all common factors in domestic fires. Fire is one of the most serious hazards in the home, and yet one of the most preventable. Smoke alarms cut deaths from fires by 60–80 percent, but even people who install smoke detectors often fail to maintain them by ensuring the batteries they contain are in working order.

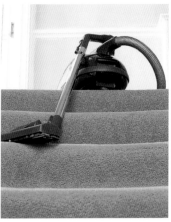

△ Always keep the stairs free of appliances, cables, toys, and pets to reduce the chance of an accidental fall.

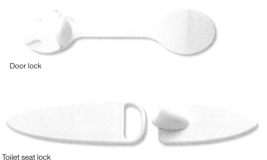

Door lock

Toilet seat lock

Table corner protectors

△ Child-safety gadgets such as these are a worthwhile investment for your home. Other items include covers for electrical sockets.

CAUSES OF ACCIDENTS IN THE HOME

➤ Falls – 50 percent.

➤ Accidental poisoning from taking medicines – 20 percent.

➤ Fires – 10 percent.

➤ Other, miscellaneous causes, including repair projects – 20 percent.

Safety in the kitchen

SEE ALSO

➤ Safety in the home, p224

➤ Dealing with fire, p232

➤ Avoiding electrical accidents, p233

Hundreds of thousands of accidents occur in kitchens every year. This is not surprising since many of us spend a lot of time in the kitchen, where we come into contact with many potential hazards from sharp knives to hot surfaces and electrical appliances. The kitchen is also a place where we use both water and electricity, which must be kept separate. As well as making the kitchen as safe as possible, you should keep a fire extinguisher, a fire blanket, and a sturdy pair of oven gloves always within sight, in case an accident does occur.

A few simple precautions taken when planning and designing a kitchen will prevent a lot of the problems that occur in this part of the home. In addition, laying down some basic kitchen rules may serve a useful purpose in protecting everyone in the home from avoidable accidents.

CLEAR UP CLUTTER

It is impossible to stop children bringing toys into the kitchen, but having to dodge dolls, small metal cars or a farmyard on your way to the sink is an obvious and avoidable hazard. Take special care to clear toys from the floor.

You should also keep counters and tabletops clear of appliances unless they are in daily use. Even then, it may be much safer to put them away.

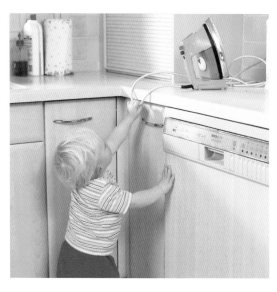

◁ Ensure that flexes and cables are kept to the back of kitchen worktops to prevent a child from pulling down a heavy appliance.

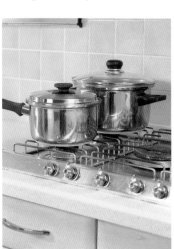

△ Use the back burners in preference to the front ones and turn handles away from the edge.

GUARD AGAINST BURNS

• Toddlers are at a perfect height for grabbing and yanking things off kitchen surfaces. If what they reach for is attached to a kettle or an iron, they could be badly hurt. Put irons away when you have finished with them, and never leave an iron unattended on the ironing board.

• Buy appliances with coiled flexes since these are neater and more difficult to catch hold of by accident. Don't choose appliances with long flexes.

• Remember that tablecloths have dangling edges that are very tempting to small children wandering past.

• Use mugs for hot drinks. As civilized as it is to drink out of cups and saucers, they are much more likely to be tipped over than mugs.

• Don't try to drink coffee or tea with a small child in your lap; they may wriggle and cause you to spill it.

• Make a habit of always using the back rings on the hob, and of turning the handles of pots and pans away from the edge of the cooker. Cooker guards are not a great idea – they can get very hot, they make it awkward to cook and lift pans off the hob, and they don't stop a child from poking their fingers through and burning them on the gas flame.

• Oven doors can get very hot. The time around opening the oven door and getting the food out can be an especially dangerous one. Your attention may be on ensuring that you get the food onto the kitchen surface in one piece, and not on the small child heading for the oven.

- Burning oil is one of the biggest hazards in a kitchen. If you deep-fat fry a lot, you should seriously consider buying an electric fryer.
- Putting a shelf above your cooker is never a good idea. As you stretch over the cooker to reach it, you may burn yourself. If the shelf is made of wood or contains flammable objects, it will also increase your chances of setting the kitchen on fire.
- Leaving the gas on and unlit for more than 10–15 seconds can result in a fireball, which will burn you and anyone else who is near you. If you can smell gas, but cannot see anything left on that is causing it, get out of the house immediately and call the emergency number for your local gas authority. They are available 24 hours a day.

PREVENT SKIDS AND FALLS
- Try to wash the floor in the evening when everyone is settled and out of the kitchen.
- Keep drawers and doors closed when not in use – when open, they are an obstacle.
- Baby chairs that screw onto kitchen tables are dangerous. Avoid them.
- Always wipe up immediately any grease and food spills, and wipe the patch with a dry cloth afterward.
- Keep the floor clear of obstacles.

◁ A wet floor can be as slippery as an ice rink – and a fall could put out someone's back for weeks.

MINIMIZE HAZARDS
- Most people store their bleach, cleaning fluids, and dishwasher powder under the sink. Although they are fiddly to fit, cupboard locks prevent a child gaining access to these harmful substances.
- Never leave wiring exposed; if wiring starts to fray, stop using the appliance until it is repaired. Every power socket should be at least 3ft from any water supply, so that there is no chance of someone having one hand on an electric source and the other in water.

- Lacerations from careless chopping account for a lot of kitchen injuries. Keep knives sharp as blunt ones are more likely to slip. Use a proper chopping board and cut with all your fingers above the blade of the knife.
- Beware of searching for broken glass in a sink full of water. Let the water drain out and then clear up the glass.
- Do not use broken crockery and glasses; throw them away.
- Store plastic bags, knives, and matches out of sight and reach of children.

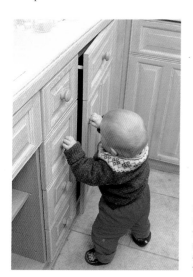

◁ Fit all low-level cupboards and drawers with childproof catches to stop an inquisitive toddler from pulling out heavy objects.

▷ The curious toddler must be protected from toxic cleaning products by means of a childproof catch on the door.

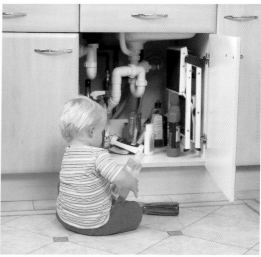

Safety in the bathroom

SEE ALSO
➤ Dealing with shock, p68
➤ Safety in the home, p224
➤ Avoiding electrical accidents, p233

Some 90 percent of accidents in the home that involve electricity happen in the bathroom. The chief hazards here are the combination of water and electricity, the water itself, and medicines left within reach of young children. Getting in or out of the bath is another hazard.

It is a common cause of falls, particularly among the old, but these can be minimized by choosing a bathtub with side grips and placing a non-slip mat on the base. Children love bathtime but need to be supervised – leaving them alone in the tub could have fatal results.

The two big dangers that come together in the bathroom are water and electricity. Together they form a lethal combination that, if not treated with the greatest care, may lead to tragedy. Water alone is a particular hazard to children, making careful supervision during bathtime essential. Electrical equipment – unless designed to be used in a bathroom – should be avoided at all cost. You should not, for example, take a mains-operated sound system into the bathroom.

All medicines should be kept in a medicine cabinet – this is particularly important if children live in the house or are likely to come to visit. The cabinet should be safely screwed to a wall, well out of the reach of children.

BABIES AND YOUNG CHILDREN

Bathing babies and children up to the age of 5 years should always be supervised by an adult. Young babies should always be bathed in a baby bath or on a specially shaped foam insert for a normal bathtub. For toddlers and older children, make sure you do not overfill the bath and avoid using slippery bath foams.

It is essential that you test the temperature of the water before the baby or child is immersed. For a baby, use your elbow – the water should feel just warm.

TEENAGERS

Favorite teenage pursuits usually include soaking in the tub for several hours at a time, and bathing by candlelight and while

SAFETY IN THE BATHROOM

➤ Turn down the hot water thermostat to 130°F.

➤ Make sure that all bathroom lights have pull-cord switches; do not use wall-mounted switches.

➤ Have a non-slip floor. Avoid using rugs and mats in the bathroom.

listening to music. Make sure they know the dangers of dragging a sound system into the bathroom using an extension lead. Water is a great conductor of electricity, so electric shocks in the bath are usually fatal.

Teenagers should also be made aware that falling asleep in the bath and bathing after they have consumed alcohol or illegal drugs is potentially very dangerous.

OLDER PEOPLE

Fatigue, reduced mobility and lapses in concentration or memory can lead to the elderly having accidents in the bathroom. They may run a bath that is too hot and scald themselves. They may slip and have a nasty fall. They may fall asleep in the bath making drowning a real possibility.

Make sure that the bathroom of an elderly person is as safe as possible. You should install a bath with hand grips in the sides and place a non-slip mat in the bath, to reduce the risk of a fall when getting in and out of the bath. Elderly people should carry a call alarm to enable them to contact the emergency services in the event of an accident.

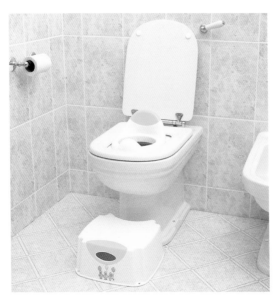

▷ The bathroom should be kept completely clear of obstacles. Invest in special lavatory stools and seats for infants and toddlers so that they can learn to use the toilet without any danger of accidents.

BATHING A BABY

Until your baby starts to demand the right to sit up and play, this is the way to hold them safely in the bath so that they cannot slip or roll over. Always remember to check that the water is not too hot before you begin bathing.

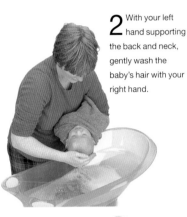

1 Hold the baby cradled in your left arm (right arm if left-handed).

2 With your left hand supporting the back and neck, gently wash the baby's hair with your right hand.

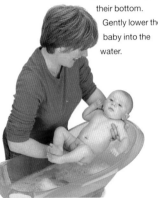

3 Hold high up under the baby's left arm and use your right hand to support their bottom. Gently lower the baby into the water.

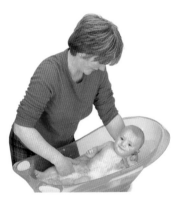

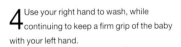

4 Use your right hand to wash, while continuing to keep a firm grip of the baby with your left hand.

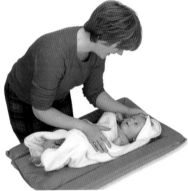

5 Once you've finished bathing the baby, wrap their head and body in a towel and dry thoroughly.

TIPS FOR BATHING BABIES

➤ Never leave a baby (or child) unattended in the bathtub.

➤ Be wary of leaving bathing duty to someone who is not familiar with bathing children. Drowning accidents happen most often when the bathing is carried out by someone who does not realize the dangers.

➤ Even if the baby is in a baby bath seat, do not leave them unattended.

➤ Ignore a ringing telephone or doorbell – or get your child out of the bath before you answer it.

TIPS FOR BATHING CHILDREN

➤ Always run the cold water into the bathtub before the hot. This avoids any risk of the child scalding themselves if they get into the water unaided.

➤ Never leave a step or chair near or next to the tub. Toddlers are fearless, and if they see a toy floating invitingly on the surface of the water they will reach for it.

➤ Don't ask an older child to watch your toddler while bathing. They are unlikely to exercise the same care as an adult.

➤ Don't give children baths in shifts if it means leaving in the bath water with no adult in attendance. Empty the bath while you put small children to bed, and refill it for the older children later.

➤ Be aware that a razor looks like a toothbrush to a toddler, so they might try to use it like one. Keep all sharp objects out of their way.

➤ Bathroom doors should be impossible for a child to lock. The easiest way to achieve this is to place the lock high up out of small children's reach.

Safety in the garden

SEE ALSO

➤ Drowning: what to do, p60

➤ BURNS AND SCALDS, p173

➤ Avoiding electrical accidents, p233

The garden can be an oasis of calm in a busy life. However, ponds, bonfires, barbecues, and even plants can all present hazards, particularly if children are around. To ensure your garden is a safe haven for everyone, you'll need to take a few sensible precautions. Choose water features that are child-friendly, fence off a swimming pool, and make sure that paths are easy to negotiate. Check that children and pets are out of the way before you start to mow, and store garden tools and implements in a locked shed together with all garden chemicals.

A little forward planning and good sense will go a long way toward preventing accidents in the garden. Many accidents happen when a child or elderly person is visiting a garden that has not been made safe for them. Small children, including those from neighboring houses, often go wandering. Your elegant ornamental pond with its shimmering goldfish may be a fatal attraction for them.

CARE WITH CHEMICALS

Lock away garden chemicals in a dark, dry and cool place, out of reach of children and animals. Follow the instructions for use exactly and do not decant chemicals into other bottles; keep them in their original containers so you know what they are. Minimize chemicals in the garden: for example, rather than using slug pellets, use environmentally-friendly methods such as dishes of beer sunk into the soil.

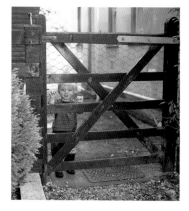

◁ Do not underestimate the climbing abilities of a toddler; this type of gate has been designed to keep out horses, not children.

Covering the water with wire netting can give a false sense of security since they could still fall in if they landed on top of it. Placing a sturdy cover over the pond is the safest option. If you really want a water feature but have children, install one in which the water cascades out of a container to drain into a bed of stones rather than into a pool of water. All swimming pools should be fenced off.

WATER SAFETY

Garden ponds are a major hazard for children. They have interesting things floating on the surface that invite curious children to lean over and grab at them. They are also usually placed at ground level, so are easy for a toddler to fall into.

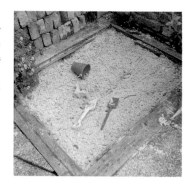

▷▽ A pond can be converted into a sandpit to provide children with an extra play area. When not in use, a sturdy cover will help to keep the sand clean.

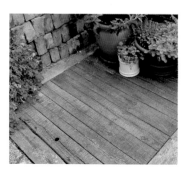

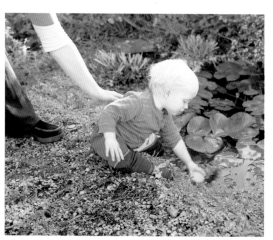

◁ Children are curious to explore their environment through taste and touch. A pond is particularly inviting – but is a potentially fatal hazard.

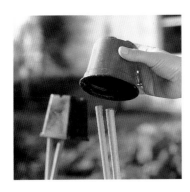

△ Place plastic containers or flowerpots on top of your garden canes, to protect your eyes when you are bending down near them.

ELECTRICITY IN THE GARDEN

- All electric garden tools should be plugged into residual current circuit breakers, so that the current switches off instantly if there is an accident.
- When using electric tools, keep the cable over your shoulder and well away from lawnmower blades and hedge trimmers.
- Keep children out of the garden when you are mowing the lawn or using anything electrical in the garden.
- Water conducts electricity, so great care should be taken when using the two together in a water feature. Many of the pumps available for water features are completely sealed and will automatically switch off if the system fails in any way.
- Exterior lights are designed to be used safely in the garden. If you are unsure, get an electrician to install or check them.

USING LADDERS SAFELY

Accidents on ladders are common but almost entirely avoidable. Make sure that all the rungs are safe before climbing up a ladder. Do not place it so that you have to lean over or stretch up to do the job – move the ladder or use a taller one if necessary. When pruning trees, use two ladders with a plank between them. If you are using a ladder up against the side of the house, ask someone to stand at the foot to secure it; or if it is a long job, put up scaffolding.

MAKING YOUR GARDEN SAFE

➤ Steps should be well lit. They should have a handrail if elderly people are to use them.

➤ Moss gathers on patios and can be slippery. Wash surfaces with diluted bleach to get rid of it.

➤ Nylon line trimmers throw up stones and other potentially dangerous things, including irritants from plant sap. Wear goggles, long-sleeved shirts and pants when using them.

CHILDREN AND PLANTS

Few children die from eating poisonous garden plants. However, they can become ill with stomachache and diarrhea. It is best to discourage young children from eating any flowers, fruit, or foliage, rather than teach them which ones to avoid.

Certain toxic plants are best kept out of the garden altogether since they are very poisonous in small amounts. These include laburnum, foxgloves, monkshood, woody nightshade, and deadly nightshade. Others, such as yew, could be fenced off. Cut back trailing plants, such as thorny brambles and roses, if they could catch a child across their face.

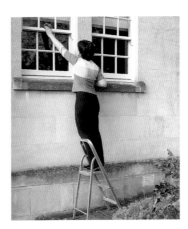

△ The golden rule of home safety is to be on top of the job – these steps are too low.

➤ Get into the habit of wearing heavy boots and thick gloves when you are working in the garden.

➤ To stop canes from poking your eyes, place film canisters, plastic bottles, or flowerpots over the top of them.

➤ Keep all garden tools tidy and store them in a locked shed. Lock away gasoline, kerosene, and chemicals.

➤ Ensure that a clothesline is not positioned at children's neck level.

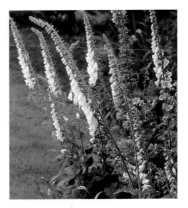

△ Foxgloves are poisonous and have no place in a garden where young children play.

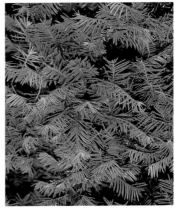

△ Yew is a common toxic plant. To protect children, fence off dangerous plants and trees.

Dealing with fire

SEE ALSO
➤ Tackling fume inhalation, p58
➤ BURNS AND SCALDS, p173
➤ Avoiding electrical accidents, p233

Fires in buildings produce invisible toxic fumes that kill in a few minutes. It is the suffocating effect of these as much as the flames that kill. No one should enter a burning building unless they are trained to do so. Oxygen feeds the flames, and if a door is opened into a burning room, the effect will be a massive explosion. Even a small amount of smoke should be a warning to keep out. Fire may be hidden behind walls, under floors, and above ceilings. The most useful thing an untrained witness to a fire can do is to call the emergency services.

An untrained person is easily able to put out small fires, such as one in a frying pan (see Warning box) or in a wastepaper bin. However, once fire starts to spread, expert help is needed and the best thing you can do is to get away from the flames.

FIRE IN A BUILDING

- Try to stay calm, and if you are at work or in a public building follow the evacuation protocol. Walk to the nearest fire exit quickly and calmly. Do not go back for a bag, coat, or any other possessions.
- Don't use elevators. Some have heat-activated panels that prevent them stopping at the fire floor, but if the electricity fails you may be trapped in the elevator. The elevator shaft can act like a chimney, sucking up flames and fumes.
- If you find yourself in smoke, stay close to the floor. If possible, cover your mouth and nose with a damp cloth or towel.

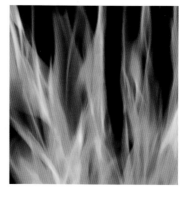

△ Fire is unpredictable and you should not underestimate how quickly it can spread.

- Close doors on the fire as you leave the building, thus starving it of oxygen.
- Never open a door that feels hot or has hot door handles – this suggests that there is a fire raging behind.
- If you cannot find an escape route, find a fire-free room with a window, shut the door, open the window and shout for help. Keep close to the floor.
- Don't turn on a light even if it is dark, since this may cause an explosion.
- Breathing in toxic fumes quickly leads to disorientation and confusion. If you have to enter a smoky area keep to the walls to guide you in and out.
- Remember that children may hide away from fumes in places such as wardrobes and cupboards.

What to do when clothing is on fire
Remember to STOP, DROP, and ROLL. STOP the victim from running around.

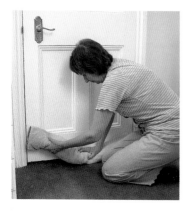

△ Blocking a door helps to keep fumes out of the room you are in and may deprive a fire of oxygen.

WARNING

Deep-frying pans are a very common cause of fires in the kitchen. Never put water anywhere near a burning oil pan. Water will feed the flames and cause a massive flare-up. Cover the flames with a pan lid or blanket to deprive them of the oxygen they need.

This fans the flames. DROP them to the ground. Having them lie horizontally stops the flames rising to their face. ROLL them on the ground to put out the flames, ideally after wrapping them in non-flammable material such as a curtain or a winter coat.

Once the flames are extinguished, you should assess the victim's airway, breathing and circulation. Start resuscitating if necessary. Carry out first aid on burns.

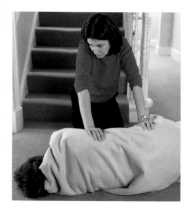

△ Stop, drop, and roll someone whose clothing is on fire. Place them in the recovery position.

Avoiding electrical accidents

SEE ALSO
➤ Safety in the home, p224
➤ Safety in the kitchen, p226
➤ Safety in the bathroom, p228

The danger of electricity is that it surrounds us in our everyday lives, and it is easy to become complacent about it. The fraying plug on the iron, the bare wires on the vacuum flex, and the gaping power sockets left uncovered with a toddler in the house are all electric shocks waiting to happen. Electricity harms because it can cause the heart to beat irregularly and then stop; the muscles, nerves and blood vessels to fry; and the skin to burn. One-third of all victims of electrical accidents are children, and 20 percent of those children die as a result.

One of the main causes of electric shock is contact with faulty electrical appliances or exposed wiring. Children poking sharp objects into sockets or chewing on electrical cords are other hazards, as is flashing from high-voltage power lines.

LIGHTNING INJURIES

The severity of an injury due to lightning depends on several factors:

• How long the victim is in contact with the electric current – the longer the contact, the greater the damage.

• The type of current – Alternating Current (AC) is used in mains electricity and power cables, because it allows greater amounts of electricity to be sent down the power lines. It is more likely to cause cardiac arrest at lower voltages than Direct Current (DC), which is what batteries produce. AC may also cause muscle spasms, with the result

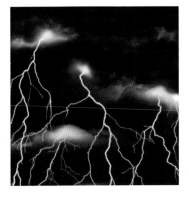

△ Keep away from metal, from cars, from trees, and from power cables during a lightning strike.

that the victim cannot let go of the electrical source.

• The size of the current – overhead power cables and lightning are more damaging than the home power supply or batteries.

ELECTRICAL ACCIDENTS

If you touch someone who is still in contact with a live circuit, they may electrocute you. Make sure that the power source is turned off at the main switch, or the appliance is unplugged. Simply turning off the appliance will not work.

If you cannot turn off the power at source or unplug the appliance, try to separate the victim from the power using a non-conducting object, such as a wooden or plastic broom handle or chair, or a rubber doormat. Try to do this while standing on something dry and non-conducting such as dry newspapers, a telephone directory or a wooden board.

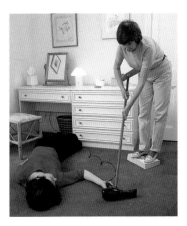

△ Separate the victim from the source of electricity using a wooden or plastic object.

If the source is a high-voltage current from a power line, be aware that the current can jump a considerable distance. Do not approach the victim until the power lines are disconnected. Once they are free of the current, check if the victim is breathing. If not, begin CPR.

Treating the injured person

Once you have excluded any further danger to yourself, approach the victim and assess them. If you are alone, call the emergency services now. Otherwise get someone else to do it for you.

Open the person's airway, being aware that if they have fallen or been thrown, they may have cervical spine damage. Avoid moving the head and neck, particularly if they are unconscious. If they are not breathing, begin to do mouth-to-mouth. Start to give cardiac compressions if they are not trying to breathe or move.

Be alert to other injuries if they have been thrown, and treat if necessary. If they have obvious burns, remove any clothing and rinse the burn under cool, running water. Apply a sterile dressing.

PREVENTING ACCIDENTS

➤ Cover sockets with childproof guards.

➤ Never use electrical appliances when you are wet, or if there is any water on crucial parts of the appliances.

➤ Teach children about electrical dangers.

➤ Never place a socket less than 3ft away from a water source.

Safe home for infants

SEE ALSO
➤ Safety in the kitchen, p226
➤ Safety in the bathroom, p228
➤ Safety in the garden, p230

When safety-proofing your home for a new baby, be at your most paranoid and suspicious. Accidents happen in seconds, and most of them are preventable. It helps if you crawl around at your baby's level, seeing what looks interesting, what dangles enticingly, and what might be eaten, opened, poked, or climbed. But remember that children grow fast, and their safety needs change just as quickly. In trying to make your home safe, you must be prepared to keep re-evaluating the potential hazards in the light of your child's development.

There is a wide range of dangers for babies and young children in the home, and they will vary depending on the child's age. For example, an 18-month-old may have neither the interest nor the dexterity to do any damage with your lighter, whereas a 2-year-old could burn the house down. Don't forget that an older child could potentially harm a baby, and their age and sense of mischief should be taken into account. Another possible hazard is a grandparent or person who is not tuned into children – they may keep medication where a child can reach it or forget to empty the bath.

CHILDHOOD ACCIDENTS

Accidents involving children happen more often when there are more than two adults in the house, probably because the carers are distracted by their guests. Try to get a child used to a playpen at a young age, so that you can use this to keep them safe when your attention is elsewhere.

Protection from falls and crushing

• Avoid using baby walkers – the baby may walk over steps, off landings, or into burning fireplaces.
• Use stair gates at the top and foot of stairs. For older children, make sure all stairs have handrails and are well lit.
• Keep beds, cupboards, and toy boxes away from windows, and make sure all windows have locks on them.
• Use seating appropriate to the child's age and strap them in at all times.
• Make sure that bookshelves and other pieces of furniture are screwed to the wall in case your infant tries to climb up them.
• Place safety catches on toy boxes or the lid may crush their fingers.

CRIB SAFETY

Make sure that your baby's crib is a safe place for them to sleep.

➤ The crib bars should be no more than 2⅜in apart

➤ The top rail should be at least 26in higher than the lowest level of the mattress support.

➤ The mattress should be the correct size for the crib, with no gaps.

➤ Do not place the crib next to a radiator or in a draughty place.

➤ Avoid any soft, squashy bedding such as pillows or duvets.

Avoiding poisoning and choking

• Lock up all potential poisons and do not take medication in front of children.
• Remember that some plants are toxic.
• Avoid toys with buttons or removable small pieces, or breakable toys.

Preventing burns and drowning

• Put away hairdryers, irons, and toasters.
• Use the back burners on your hob and turn handles to the back.
• Cover all electric outlets.
• Cover hot pipes and radiators.
• Use a fixed fireguard in front of the fire.
• Do not leave the bathwater unattended or leave a child alone in the bathtub.
• Cover fish-tanks with a fixed top.

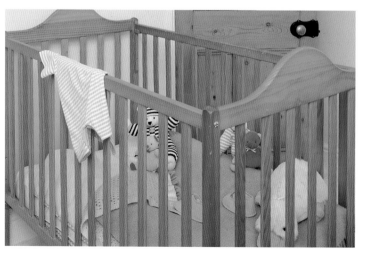

◁ Choose a good crib with a well-fitting mattress and high sides.

Avoiding sudden infant death

SEE ALSO
➤ Resuscitating a baby or child p46
➤ Recognizing childhood illness p110

Most crib deaths occur quickly and while the baby is asleep, with no outward signs of suffering. Any child's death is a tragedy for the parents, but sudden infant deaths are particularly traumatic because they are unexpected and sudden and may be treated as suspicious by the police. Crib deaths are most likely to occur in babies aged between 1 and 4 months. Nobody knows exactly why they happen, but there are certain risk factors that make them more likely. Protecting your baby from these reduces the chance of crib death.

There are many theories about why sudden infant death occurs, but the causes are still unknown. Some of the known risk factors, such as smoking around the baby, can be avoided; and others, such as prematurity and poverty, cannot. Sudden infant death is known to be more common in the winter months and in male babies.

REDUCING THE RISK

- Do not smoke while pregnant or if you have a baby. It is also advisable to discourage anyone living in your home from smoking, too. The risk of crib death is higher in families where a smoker lives.
- It is also best to prevent visitors smoking in the house, and avoid taking the baby into smoky areas.
- Place the baby on their back to sleep. Babies lose heat from their faces and if they lie prone they may overheat. They are no more likely to choke if they sleep on their backs.

- Do not overheat the baby. Try to keep the bedroom at about 60–68°F. Avoid heaters, hot-water bottles, placing the baby in direct sunshine to sleep, and electric blankets. If the baby's stomach feels hot to touch or they are sweating, take off the blankets. If they have a fever, take off blankets.
- Never put a baby to bed with a hat on, as they lose a lot of heat through their heads.
- Never sleep on a sofa with the baby. Avoid sleeping in the same bed with a baby if you smoke, have drunk alcohol, are excessively tired, or have taken sedatives.
- Do not use duvets until a baby is over 1 year old.

BREATHING MONITORS

Some parents buy breathing monitors for their babies. These have not been shown to prevent crib death, but they do create anxiety as they are prone to false alarms and may go off several times in a night.

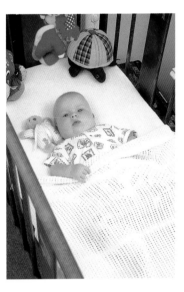

△ Make sure that your baby does not get overheated when asleep; don't use too many blankets, keep the room cool, and do not cover the baby's head.

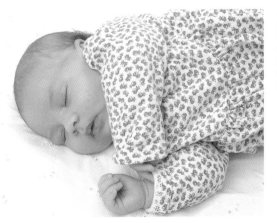

◁ A baby should initially be placed on their back to sleep, but it is quite normal for them to move on to their side as they nap.

WARNING

You should seek urgent medical attention if the baby:

➤ Stops breathing or turns blue.

➤ Is unresponsive and shows no awareness of what is going on.

➤ Has glazed eyes and does not focus on anything.

➤ Cannot be woken up.

➤ Has a fit.

SKILLS CHECKLIST FOR
KEEPING SAFE

KEY POINTS

- Most motor vehicle accidents occur within 2 miles of the driver's own home ☐

- Keep your stairway clear ☐

- The kitchen is the most hazardous area of the home ☐

- Never leave a young child unattended in the bathtub – even for a moment ☐

SKILLS LEARNED

- Making your kitchen a safe place to be ☐

- How to bathe babies and children ☐

- Using common sense to make your garden a less hazardous place ☐

- Putting out a deep-fat fire ☐

- STOP, DROP and ROLL to put out burning clothing ☐

- Making your home safe for babies and young children ☐

OUTDOOR SAFETY

Outdoor pursuits offer a wide variety of hazards for which the sensible person must be fully prepared and properly informed. Appropriate clothing, footwear, and equipment, together with a basic first-aid kit, are essential to enjoy your chosen sport or activity without unnecessary risk. Always be on the alert for changing environmental conditions (such as weather and tides) and for warning notices by oceans, rivers, and lakes. When traveling, be as informed as possible about your surroundings and about issues such as the safety of local drinking water and where to contact a doctor who speaks your language.

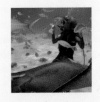

CONTENTS

Safety in sport 238–239

Safety in land sports 240–241

Safety in water sports 242–243

Safety in snow sports 244–245

Traveling safely 246–247

Skills checklist 248

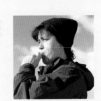

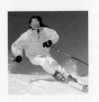

Safety in sport

SEE ALSO

➤ What is first aid?, p12

➤ Managing heat and cold disorders, p106

➤ Assembling a first-aid kit, p198

The thrills of outdoor sports are great, but sometimes the risks can be even greater. Being aware of potential risks is vital and taking appropriate actions to avoid accidents in the first place is a much better approach than just learning how to deal with an emergency. Safety is the key word, and this doesn't take away all the fun. So, if you're undertaking an outdoor sport in a new location, be prepared – even find out where the nearest hospital is. On the subject of having fun, it goes without saying that alcohol and sporting pursuits never mix.

Adventure sports have never been as popular or as accessible as they are today, each new one a little more dangerous and thrilling than the last – whitewater rafting, bungee jumping, and abseiling down mountains are all possible, even for the novice. But all such activities have strict safety guidelines and provisions to ensure your safety at all times.

Even though some outdoor sports require a certain level of training, it is surprising that many people embark on outdoor pursuits, such as mountain or hill climbing, with little or no training and little or no thought to safety issues at all. It's a good idea when setting out on an outdoor activity to be prepared for the worst-case scenario – in that way, you'll be alert to potential hazards and be able to avoid them, if possible, and if not, then be best placed to deal with them.

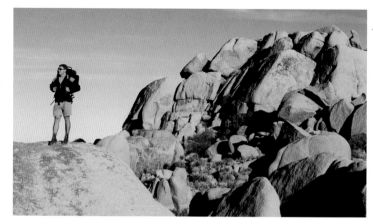

HIDDEN PERILS

It is not always amateurs that come to grief, but inexperience and ignorance of a sport's risks and dangers inevitably increase the chances of mishaps and accidents. Most problems can be traced back to poor training, a lack of fitness or poorly maintained equipment. While a certain amount of risk adds to the enjoyment and attraction of some sports, prevention of accidents through awareness of the safety aspects is the best course of action when considering engaging in any outdoor pursuit. Initial training is a good way to find out about risks, and practicing with experienced people reinforces this.

△ Weather can change without warning so be prepared with waterproofs and extra layers.

UNPREDICTABLE WEATHER

All outdoor pursuits have one thing in common – exposure to the elements. Weather in cities and towns is often a minor irritation that happens high above the rooftops, but in isolated situations a sudden and unexpected change in the weather can make the difference between

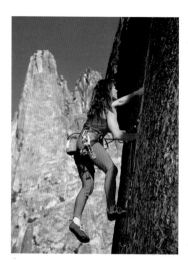

◁ Never climb alone. Climbing as part of a team means that a rescue and first aid can be easily organized if necessary.

▷ Weather at sea is notoriously changeable. Be sure to carry flares, a cellphone, and warm clothing and always wear a life jacket.

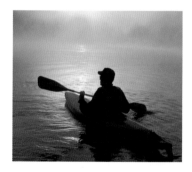

life and death if you are unprepared. Certain areas of the world are renowned for their sudden and unpredictable changes in weather, but it's a good idea to be prepared for the worst wherever you are and whatever you are doing.

PEER PRESSURE

Although it is certainly safer to perform many outdoor sports in a group, there is sometimes a herd mentality at work in group activities, particularly when there is a physical challenge such as climbing up a mountain. It's easy to be spurred on by the group to do things that you know are unwise and possibly beyond your level of skill and stamina. In such circumstances, try to hold on to your common sense and resist the urge to undertake a challenge to be "part of the group". You'll probably know instinctively if an activity is one step beyond your capabilities or confidence.

It is also worth remembering that many people view extreme sports as the ultimate challenge, a way of proving something to themselves and others. They may not be willing or able to accept their limitations until it is too late and they are in trouble.

FIRST AID – BACK TO BASICS

All of the principles of first aid are as applicable out in the wilds of a windswept mountain as they are in a domestic or workplace setting. The main difference is that the victim may be isolated and a long way from any rescue center or hospital, and may have to wait some time for treatment in the case of illness or accidental injury.

Keeping a clear head (and making sensible, safe decisions) is just as important as knowing the correct first-aid approach for a particular condition. Applying the perfect leg splint, for example, is a useless skill if you then abandon the injured person with little protection against the elements and/or equipment to continue to call for help while you go for assistance.

Try to remember that first aid is often about knowing what not to do, just as much as it is about knowing what to do.

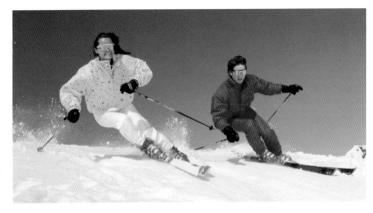

△ Skiing off-piste is the ultimate challenge, but carry a bleeper or cellphone in case of snow drifts or avalanches.

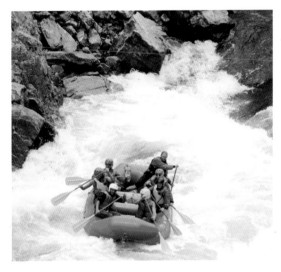

◁ Check that adventure sports organizers are qualified and experienced before you set out on an activity with them.

A BASIC SURVIVAL FIRST-AID KIT

Whatever your choice of outdoor activity, always carry a basic first-aid kit with you. A suitable kit need not be heavy or widely comprehensive but should contain the following items:

➤ An assortment of adhesive dressings.

➤ Sterile dressings in various sizes.

➤ A couple of triangular bandages.

➤ A lightweight foil survival blanket, cellphone, whistle, and flashlight are other recommended items.

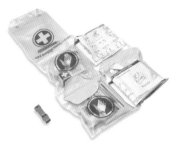

△ A basic first-aid kit is an essential part of any outdoor-based pursuit.

Safety in land sports

SEE ALSO

➤ What is first aid?, p12

➤ Dealing with shock, p68

➤ Dealing with broken bones, p150

Mountaineering, walking, cycling, and trekking all have hazards as well as presenting exciting and tremendous challenges. As well as being alert to potential dangers of the activity itself, remember to be aware of the possibility of changes in your environment and the havoc these can wreak – sunburn, heatstroke and frostbite, to name a few. Always carry maps of the area you're exploring and make sure you're well equipped regarding footwear and clothing. Also, tell someone where you're going and never go alone – there's safety in numbers.

Like many people, you probably love to escape civilization once in a while. Putting on a pair of walking boots or getting on a bike are two of the most accessible and popular leisure activities. What's more, they are also fantastic ways of getting fit.

But any outdoor activity comes with its own hazards and it's a good idea to know what these are so that you can avoid them or, in the worst cases, have some idea what first aid you might need to give.

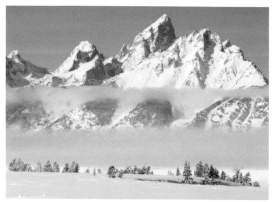

◁ Weather in mountainous regions is unpredictable, so be aware that loss of visibility and drops in temperature can be amazingly sudden.

CYCLING IN SAFETY

Almost 75 percent of cyclists killed in accidents die from injuries to the head. So no wonder safety pundits recommend that all cyclists – whether in cities or the countryside – wear a cycle helmet. Such safety helmets reduce the chances of death from a head injury by 80 percent.

On the roads, most cycling accidents happen at junctions, but cycle-related injuries don't just happen on roads. With the ever-increasing popularity of mountain biking, a growing number of accidents take place on hills and mountains well away from traffic. As with other pursuits, it is important not to push yourself too far too soon on rough terrain, and to always cycle as part of a group. Make sure at least one person has a first-aid kit and a cellphone. Many mountain bikers carry water reservoir rucksacks on their back. Having plenty of water is vital to avoid dehydration – a condition that could lead to dizziness, fatigue, and ultimately to an accident while cycling.

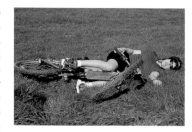

△ Do not move an injured person if you suspect a neck or spine injury. Call for help immediately on your cellphone.

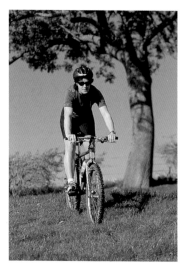

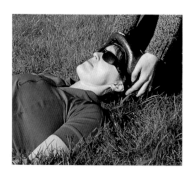

◁ Always wear a well-fitting helmet and appropriate footwear for safety's sake. And a padded pair of shorts will cushion your ride.

▷ Reassure the injured person and try to obtain some information about the accident so that you can give this to the emergency services.

Common causes of biking accidents are:
- Wet surfaces, leading to loss of control (wet bike brakes).
- Traveling too fast downhill or around corners.
- Mechanical bike failure.
- Hitting an animal or pedestrian.

HAZARDS WHEN WALKING

Most of the following hazards are avoidable by being aware and taking adequate precautions before you set out on a trek.

Blisters

Some people are prone to getting blisters, but commonly they develop in those with ill-fitting boots and in those who don't undertake such walking very often. Make sure your boots are comfortable, you wear natural-fiber socks and your boots are not too loose nor too tight. If you get a blister, stick an adhesive dressing over the area; never pop it as it could become infected.

Heat exhaustion

To avoid heat exhaustion, make an early start when hiking so that most of the walk is done in the cool of the morning.

WHAT TO TAKE WALKING

Even a short day walk in the hills may lead to problems if weather conditions deteriorate or if there is an accident. It is best to take the following equipment:

- ➤ Waterproof clothing.
- ➤ Strong footwear.
- ➤ Spare dry inner clothing – in the summer one other warm article will do.
- ➤ Map and compass.
- ➤ Whistle.
- ➤ Flashlight.
- ➤ First-aid kit.
- ➤ Reserve food and drink.
- ➤ Sunglasses.
- ➤ Pocket knife and matches.

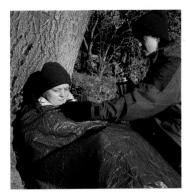

△ Prevent someone with hypothermia from losing more heat and rewarm them slowly.

Hypothermia

Walking in cold conditions requires a serious approach to the risks of such extreme low temperatures. If a person appears confused, quiet, or is stumbling a lot, they could have hypothermia. In such instances, get them into some shelter and wrap them in spare clothes, sleeping bags or anything warm and dry. Then, give them something warm to drink, avoiding caffeine- and alcohol-containing drinks.

Soft-tissue injuries

Sprains and strains are common injuries and are difficult to prevent. As anywhere, the basic RICE (rest, ice, compression, elevation) first-aid techniques apply.

Sunburn

Always wear sunscreen of at least 15SPF, and sunblock on the lips and eye area. Remember to reapply every few hours.

MOUNTAINEERING SAFETY

Mountains should be treated with great respect. Demanding climbing combined with unpredictable weather can make accidents more likely. Any mountain rescue can be difficult, especially when changing weather causes loss of visibility and plummeting temperatures.

In cases of serious injury or in severe cold, use a cellphone to alert the mountain

SIGNS AND SYMPTOMS OF MOUNTAIN SICKNESS

This is one of the most serious problems that can hit anyone climbing above 8,000ft. It is usually caused by ascending a mountain too fast and is due to reduced atmospheric pressure and oxygen levels at high altitudes – it can be fatal if urgent action is not taken. Early symptoms include increasing fatigue, breathlessness that is unrelieved by rest, headache, and vomiting.

If the person continues to climb, they may develop:

- ➤ Confusion, unsteadiness, and lassitude.
- ➤ Pulmonary edema, in which the lungs fill with fluid.
- ➤ Cerebral edema, in which the brain swells.

The golden rule is that if the mild symptoms do not settle after a day of rest and plentiful fluids, or if they worsen, the person must descend at least 1,000ft until they recover.

rescue team; or send one or two people from your party to get help. If you have to leave an injured person, protect them from the elements, leave them a flashlight and whistle, mark the site and note local landmarks. Learn the international distress signal: six successive whistle blasts or light flashes, repeated after a 1-minute pause.

▽ Acknowledge a distress signal by blasting three times, repeating after 1 minute.

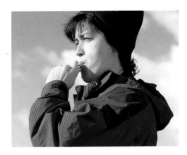

Safety in water sports

SEE ALSO

➤ Understanding resuscitation, p26

➤ Drowning: what to do, p60

➤ Managing heat and cold disorders, p106

Splashing about at the seaside, zooming about on jet-skis or windsurfers, or skimming the waves in a motorboat are just a few of the ways we enjoy the water. Like other sports, all water sports come with their own hazards and a watery environment poses its own unique risks too. To be safe in the water, you must be a proficient swimmer and be aware of the power of the sea and the dangers of animals and plants that live beneath the water's surface. Also, bear in mind that many water-related accidents happen when people have been drinking.

Both salty and fresh water areas provide chances for recreational activities. Like any outdoor pursuit, water sports should be treated with great respect. It is vital to be aware at the outset of the possible hazards involved – many people underestimate water-related dangers.

Bodies lose heat more quickly in the water than on land, even in warm tropical waters, so it's advisable to wear a wet suit for sports such as scuba diving or windsurfing. A full wet suit, or what's called a dry suit, with head and hand gear, is required during the colder months.

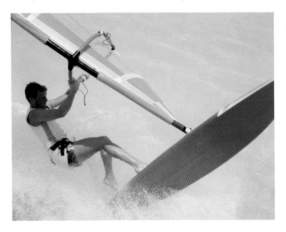

◁ Windsurfers should beware of spring tides and rip tides pushing them far out of their depth.

WEATHER AND THE WATER

Waterskiing on all but the calmest waters is ill-advised, but sailing in high winds and choppy seas is what experienced sailors thrive on (although it is not advisable for a novice). Always check the weather forecast to ensure that it suits your plans and that you are prepared. Sunglasses are vital in most water sports as the water increases the sun's glare, which can burn the eyes' cornea, causing temporary or even permanent damage. Don't forget that you can still get sunburn when you are in the water so it is vital to wear waterproof sunscreen lotion and replenish it regularly.

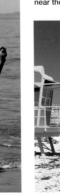

◁ Children should always be supervised when near the water's edge.

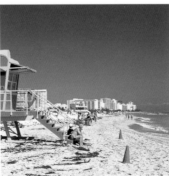

SWIMMING SAFELY IN THE OCEAN

Some beaches are patrolled by lifeguards and are safer than others. These beaches are usually marked by flags and sealed by joined floats to keep watercraft out of the area. If conditions are dangerous, the lifeguards will fly warning flags, which you should check before setting off for the water. Know what the different flags mean: local codes may vary but should be displayed at the approaches to the beach.

• Green flag – It's safe to swim.
• Red/yellow flag – Lifeguards are on patrol and you should swim only in the area between the flags.
• Red flag – Dangerous to swim. You should not enter the water.
• Black/white check flag – Area is zoned for surfboards and not safe for swimmers.
• Blue/white flag – Divers in the area.

◁ If you have young children it is a good idea to choose a beach that is patrolled by lifeguards.

Any non-swimming child, or child under 12, should be supervised near the water's edge, especially if wading or swimming. Keep clear of rocks when swimming and keep an eye out for animals in the water such as sea urchins and jellyfish. In tropical waters, avoid swimming near the beautiful but dangerously sharp coral.

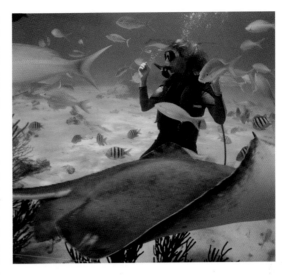

◁ The world beneath the ocean's surface can be exciting to explore, but you should be aware of potential dangers. For example, if coral grazes the skin it can lead to infection.

TIDES AND RIP TIDES

A large part of the ocean's danger lies in the tides. Sands seemingly miles away from the shore can be covered by an incoming tide in seconds. Rip tides are narrow bands of current that create a powerful force in the water, often pulling swimmers or surfers out to sea. Swimming against these forces is pointless; it rapidly leads to exhaustion and the risk of drowning. The simplest way to safety is to work out the direction the rip tide is taking you and swim at right angles (90°) to this for about 30–60ft, and then swim toward the shore.

SCUBA DIVING

Anyone taking part in scuba diving has to undergo rigorous training in the use of equipment, signaling between divers and how diving affects the body. Even so, accidents can happen, such as near drowning, decompression ("the bends"), and ruptured eardrum and/or lung.

▽ Diseases like bilharzia are carried by blood flukes like these. People can become infected by bathing or swimming in contaminated water.

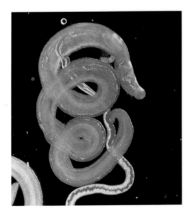

HAZARDS IN FRESH WATER

Most water-related accidents involve swimming in strong currents or cold water. Ponds, rivers, lakes, and reservoirs can be extremely cold and pose a serious threat to life from drowning and hypothermia.

Deep rivers and lakes often have dangerous debris hidden beneath the surface. Pollution can cause skin reactions and infections such as Weil's disease. Getting in and out of the water can be tricky, and slimy banks with reeds and grasses can be hazardous.

▽ Avoid fast-flowing water and be aware that sharp branches and other hazards may be hidden in deep water.

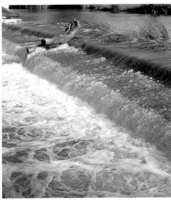

MAKING A WATER RESCUE

Giving first aid while in the water is extremely difficult, so unless you have proper training get the person to dry land before resuscitating them.

Avoid getting into the water: use a branch to pull them in or throw a float.

Once out of the water, protect them from the wind and lay them on their back.

Open their airway and check breathing. Be prepared to start resuscitation.

Remove any wet clothing and wrap in warm blankets to avoid hypothermia.

Safety in snow sports

SEE ALSO
➤ Managing heat and cold disorders, p106
➤ Handling lower-leg injuries, p164
➤ Managing sprains and strains, p168

Having a good attitude toward safety will mean that snow sports are enjoyable rather than dangerous. Your first considerations should be clothing and footwear. Make sure you've got enough warm layers on and a waterproof jacket. A hat will keep you cosy as a huge amount of heat is normally lost through your head. Gloves are a must, as are ski goggles or sunglasses. Boots need a good grip and should be roomy enough for thick, warm socks. Once properly kitted out, you can concentrate on having fun in the snow.

People who live where there is rarely much snow sometimes seem to go slightly mad when the first snowflakes fall. They seize any item they can sit on – plastic bags, trays, plastic crates – and hurl themselves down the nearest snow-covered hillside. It's not surprising that many injuries occur in this way, from a bruised back and ribs to fractured ankles and limbs.

With the increasing popularity of snow sport holidays, such injuries are becoming more common as people spend only a week a year on the slopes and underestimate the level of fitness and skill required.

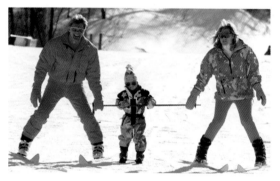

◁ Help your child to learn properly on lower slopes before taking them on steeper slopes.

AVOID INJURIES ON THE SLOPES

• Ski in control. Some people seem to delight in skiing or snowboarding on slopes beyond their level, but they risk injuring others as well as themselves.
• Train beforehand. Snowboarding and skiing are arduous sports. Make sure you build stamina, strengthen leg muscles, and improve flexibility before you go.
• Use properly maintained equipment. Wearing someone else's ski boots and an old pair of skis is just asking for trouble.
• Stop as soon as you feel tired or cold, because this is when injuries happen.

If you fall while skiing, try to keep your knees flexed and do not try to get up until you have stopped moving or sliding. Ski patrols regularly check the slopes and are trained in first aid. To warn others that you are injured, get someone to plant your skis in an X pattern just uphill from where you're lying. Stay calm until help arrives.

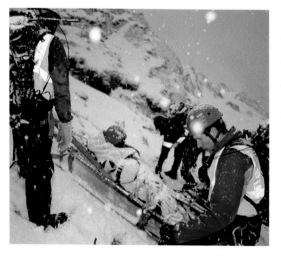

◁ This mountain rescue team have wrapped the injured person in a waterproof covering to protect him from the cold. The team paramedic assesses his injuries before they transport him down the mountain.

SIGNS AND SYMPTOMS OF FROSTBITE

➤ The affected area of skin goes white and is painful – the sensation is similar to pins and needles.

➤ Sensation is gradually lost and the skin feels numb. The color changes from white to blotchy.

➤ The skin and underlying tissue start to feel hard and stiff.

➤ The affected skin turns blue.

If the skin tissue color then changes from blue to black it means that gangrene has set in.

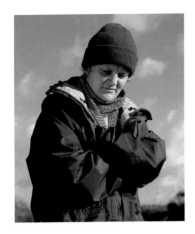

◁ If you suspect you have frost-bitten fingers, warm your hands under your armpits.

DEALING WITH FROSTBITE

In temperatures below freezing, the body diverts blood to the vital organs and away from the ears, nose, hands, and feet. If tissues freeze, the condition is known as frostbite. Freezing temperatures or cold and windy conditions can cause frostbite, which often occurs with hypothermia.

If you suspect someone has frostbite, it is essential that you try to warm them up slowly and arrange to get them to hospital.

• Initially, get them out of the cold, replace any wet clothes and warm their hands by placing in your hands or lap or under their armpits, after removing rings and any other constricting objects.
• Once in the warm, put the frostbitten part in a sink or bowl of warm (never hot) water and dry it without rubbing.
• Elevate the affected limbs and support them to reduce any tissue swelling.
• Arrange transport to hospital.

COMMON INJURIES

Propelling yourself at high speed down the rough terrain of a mountainside is bound to entail the risk of falling. Most injuries on the slopes are sprains and strains, and so you should follow the RICE (rest, ice, compression, elevation) first-aid guidelines.

Knee injury

There are several ligaments in the knee. The one that is most commonly damaged in skiing is the anterior cruciate ligament. If a skier straightens their leg at the knee, often while still in motion, and a ski edge catches, the knee twists nastily. The knee does not always swell, but it is extremely painful and may give way suddenly.

Skier's thumb

If the thumb becomes jammed by the ski poles in a fall, a small ligament in the lower part of the thumb (the ulnar collateral ligament) may become sprained or even completely ruptured.

Snowboarder's wrist

Injuries to the wrist and bones in the hand are common in snowboarding where people use their hand to steady themselves and land on it outstretched.

SNOW BLINDNESS

The sun reflects off the snow, thus doubling its harmful effects. Without sunglasses or ski goggles, the sun may burn the layer of cells covering the eyeball (the cornea). This causes temporary blindness and great pain. As a first-aider, cover their eyes and get them to medical help.

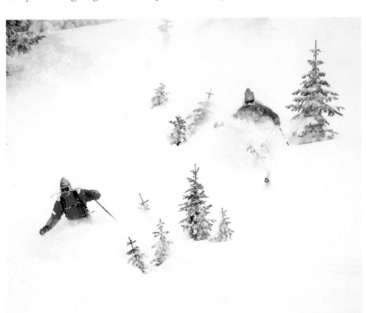

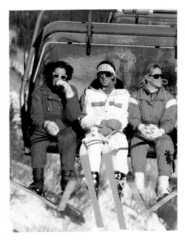

△ Ensure that your skis are always lifted well off the ground when you are traveling back up the mountain.

◁ Only ski off-piste if you are very experienced and have checked conditions before leaving.

Traveling safely

SEE ALSO
➤ Dealing with vomiting and diarrhea, p115
➤ Tackling sunburn, p183
➤ Keeping yourself safe, p220

Whether you are going to France or Fiji, it pays to prepare for the trip. As airfares become cheaper, people travel to more and more exotic destinations. With far-flung places come new and sometimes deadly hazards. But, by following a few simple guidelines, you can ensure that your trip will be as safe as possible. Even the journey can be hazardous – so stretch your legs, drink plenty of water, and avoid alcohol. And don't forget to take out travel insurance; if you do have an accident abroad it is vital for prompt medical assistance.

If you are heading somewhere off your usual beaten track, it's advisable to visit your doctor or healthcare provider for travel advice at least 6 weeks before you leave. You may need to have certain immunizations or start a course of antimalarial tablets in advance of your departure date.

DO YOU NEED ANY JABS?
Immunization offers protection against particular diseases. Some immunizations, such as that against yellow fever, are mandatory, and a certificate dated with the time and place of immunization is an entry requirement for some countries.

Even if you're heading for places such as Europe, Australia or New Zealand, you need to be up-to-date on tetanus and polio (though no other immunizations are required at the time of writing). Common conditions to be immunized against include hepatitis A and typhoid. Which immunizations are needed for which countries varies over time, so always check in plenty of time.

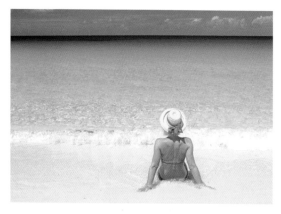

◁ The sun's rays are intensified as they are reflected off the water. Protect yourself by wearing a wide-brimmed hat, sunscreen, and sunglasses.

TRAVELER'S DIARRHEA
This common condition usually strikes in the first 2 weeks of a visit; most often it's due to bacteria or viruses in the food and/or local water. Follow these simple prevention tips, and you will stand a good chance of avoiding the problem:
• Wash hands before you eat anything.
• Wash all fruits, vegetables and salad leaves in purified water, or peel if possible.
• Avoid eating undercooked shellfish, meat and fish.
• Buy bottled water or purify local water using iodine, puritabs, or a water-purifying pump.
• Avoid uncooked foods or cold drinks that may have been in contact with local water (and therefore possibly loaded with germs) – drinks with ice cubes, ice cream, salads, fresh fruit and vegetables.
• Use bottled water (check the seal is intact) to rinse your teeth after brushing and for any washing of fruit or vegetables that you prepare yourself.

PROTECTING YOURSELF AGAINST MALARIA
Certain areas of the world put the traveler at risk of catching malaria through mosquito bites. The actual tablets that protect against malaria vary with the country being visited. Check with your doctor which tablets you need to take; they can be bought from any drugstore and the course should be started a few weeks before you depart for your trip.

Follow these simple guidelines for a malaria-free trip:

➤ Keep arms and legs fully covered after dusk and when trekking through forested areas.

➤ Use an insecticide (ideally one containing the chemical DEET) to keep mosquitoes away at night; they come in coils, mats and vaporized forms.

➤ If you're staying in jungle areas, take an insecticide-impregnated mosquito net with you. (Staying in an air-conditioned hotel room cuts down on exposure to mosquitoes.)

➤ Bear in mind that mosquitoes are most common in country areas near water and that they are more active at night.

➤ Apply mosquito-repellent cream for added protection – day or night.

What to do if you have diarrhea

The main concern when suffering from diarrhea is to prevent dehydration, so drink plenty of fluids. Oral rehydration salts are an excellent remedy for dehydration. These can be bought from a drugstore – ready-made in individual sachets – before your trip, and then made up as and when needed. If you don't have any such salts, you can easily make some from water, salt, and sugar. Use 1 level tsp of salt and 8 level tsp of sugar and add these to 1¾ pints of boiled, purified or bottled water.

For each loose stool passed give a quarter of a mug to babies (but seek medical help as soon as possible), half a mug to small children, a mug to older children and two mugs to adults, plus plenty of bottled or boiled water.

If you need to travel or don't have time for the rehydration salts to work, then you could take one of the following medicines:
- The antidiarrheal drug loperamide will help to "dry up" the diarrhea.
- An antibiotic called ciprofloxacin taken after the first loose stool will cut the duration of uncomplicated watery diarrhea down to a day.

In any case, if you are suffering from a high fever, there is blood in your stools, or the diarrhea persists for more than 4 days, then it is advisable to seek medical help as soon as you can.

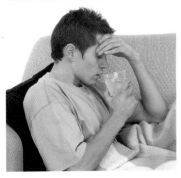

▽ Drink plenty of fluids; rehydration fluids are best for relief from diarrhea.

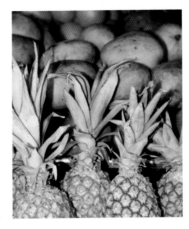

△ If you buy fruit from a stall make sure that you peel it or wash it with bottled water.

THE RISK OF BLOOD CLOTS

Reduce the risk of clots on long-haul flights by following these tips:
- Drink plenty of non-alcoholic fluid.
- Wear elasticated stockings to thigh level.
- Walk up and down the aisle for a few minutes at least once every 2 hours.
- Be aware that pregnancy, recent operations, obesity, and the contraceptive pill can all increase the risk.
- Take aspirin (a 75–150mg tablet) on the day of the flight (or clopidogrel if allergic).

PRACTISE SAFE SEX

Many sexually transmitted infections are contracted on holidays or trips abroad. The best form of protection against diseases such as hepatitis B, HIV and gonorrhea are condoms, although they cannot protect against all of them 100 percent. Take plenty of condoms with you if you think you're going to be sexually active while away; in some countries, condoms are not as reliably made or are not as easy to buy.

DEALING WITH TRAVEL SICKNESS

Some people are prone to motion or travel sickness regardless of the mode of travel, but boats are particular culprits. If you suffer regularly from motion sickness, there are drugs to prevent it. Acupressure

bands (also suitable for children), may help to quell nausea. Try these tips, too:
- Keeping your eyes on the horizon or on a fixed point.
- Keeping your head still by lying down or leaning upright against a pillar or wall.
- Staying in the fresh air, rather than cooped up indoors.
- Sitting in the front passenger seat of a car rather than the rear seat.

GETTING THROUGH JET LAG

When flying across time zones, your natural body clock can find it difficult to readjust to the local time. This jet lag is a common problem. Symptoms of jet lag include: tiredness, difficulty concentrating, loss of appetite, and constipation. It can take several days to adjust, and it's a good idea not to do too much initially. Try to fit in with local times but rest when you need to.

USEFUL MEDICINES FOR A TRAVEL FIRST-AID KIT

The following suggestions for travel medicines are given only as a guide. If traveling to a remote area, it is wise to discuss malaria treatment and antibiotics for traveler's diarrhea with your doctor before you leave.

➤ Antihistamines are useful for insect bites and itchy rashes. They are also useful in travel sickness.

➤ Hydrocortisone cream (1 percent) can be bought over the counter in many drugstores – it is good for allergic skin rashes, insect bites, and sunburn.

➤ Antifungal creams are good for itchy rashes (which are often due to a fungus) in hot sweaty places, such as between the toes or in the armpits.

➤ Antidiarrheal tablets help prevent and control diarrhea.

➤ Painkillers – such as acetaminophen or ibuprofen – always come in handy for quelling headaches and toothache or for bringing down a fever.

SKILLS CHECKLIST FOR
OUTDOOR SAFETY

KEY POINTS

- Prevention is far preferable to cure, especially in outdoor activities when it may take considerable time to obtain assistance ☐

- Don't be tempted to push yourself beyond your abilities ☐

- Always supervise children in hazardous situations ☐

- Always carry a basic first-aid kit and a cellphone ☐

- Get as much information as possible before you set out ☐

- Move about regularly when flying in a plane ☐

SKILLS LEARNED

- How to have fun while minimizing risk ☐

- Recognizing the value of researching your sport or activity and location ☐

- Checking out your equipment, first-aid kit, and maps ☐

- Obtaining in advance specific medications for various medical complaints ☐

- How to avoid a bout of diarrhea – the most common travelers' complaint ☐

USEFUL
INFORMATION

CONTENTS

Useful addresses 250–252

Index 253–256

Acknowledgments 256

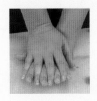

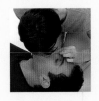

Useful addresses

USA

Agency for Healthcare Research and Quality
United States Preventive Services Task Force (USPSTF)
www.ahcpr.gov

AIDS Information Hotline
Public Health Service
(800) 342-AIDS
(800) 243-7889; Deaf and hearing impaired (TTY)
(800) 344-7432; Spanish-speaking

Al-Anon and Alateen
(800) 356-9996

Alcoholism and Drug Addiction Treatment Center
(800) 382-4357

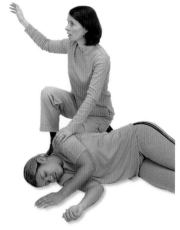

American Academy of
Family Physicians
11400 Tomahawk Creek Parkway
Leawood, Kansas 66211-2672
Tel: 1-800-274-2237
www.aafp.org; fp@aafp.org

American Diabetes Association
ATTN: National Call Center
1701 North Beauregard Street
Alexandria VA 22311
Tel: 1-800-342-2383
www.diabetes.org

American Diabetes Association
(800) 232-3472
(703) 549-1500 in Virginia and the
District of Columbia metropolitan area

American Heart Association
7272 Greenville Avenue
Dallas, Texas 75231
Tel: 1-800-242-8721
www.americanheart.org

American Lung Association
61 Broadway, 6th Floor
New York 10006
Tel: 212-315-8700
www.lungusa.org
info@lungusa.org

American Red Cross
National Headquarters
431, 18th Street NW
Washington DC 20006
Tel: 0202 639 3520
www.redcross.org

American Trauma Society (ATS)
(800) 556-7890

Child Family Health International
953 Mission Street, Suite 220
San Francisco, California 94103
Tel: 415-957-9000
www.cfhi.org; cfhi@cfhi.org

Centers for Disease Control and Prevention
1600 Clifton Road
Atlanta, GA 30333
Tel: 404-639-3311
National Immunization Hotline:
1-800-342-2437
National Immunization Hotline
(Spanish): 1-800-232-0233
www.cdc.gov

Epilepsy Foundation
4531 Garden City Drive
Landover MD 20785-7223
Tel: 1-800-332-1000
www.epilepsyfoundation.org

Heartline: (804) 965-6464

Juvenile Diabetes Foundation
International Hotline: (800) 223-1138
(212) 889-7575 in New York

Lung Line, National Asthma Center
(800) 222-5864
(303) 355-LUNG in Denver

National Clearinghouse for Alcohol and
Drug Information: (800) 729-6688

National Cocaine Hotline
(800) COCAINE

National Council on Alcoholism and
Drug Dependence
(Hope)line; (800) NCA-CALL

National Institute on Drug Abuse
Helpline: (800) 662-HELP

National Institutes of Health
9000 Rockville Pike
Bethseda, Maryland 20892
Tel: 301-496-4000
Email: NIHinfo; www.nih.gov
Other toll-free NIH telephone numbers
can be found at:
http://www.nih.gov/health/infoline

National Pesticide Telecommunications
Network Hotline
(800) 858-PEST
(806) 743-3091 in Texas

National Safety Council
1121 Spring Lake Drive
Itasca
Illinois 60143-3201
Tel: 0630 285 1121
www.nsc.org

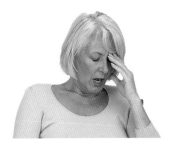

Occupational Safety and Health
Administration
US Department of Labor
200 Constitution Avenue NW
Washington DC 20210
Tel: 1-800 321 6742
www.osha.gov

National Safekids Campaign
1301 Pennsylvania Avenue NW
Suite 1000
Washington DC 20004
Tel: 0202 662 0600
www.safekids.org

United States Department of
Health and Human Services
200 Independence Avenue, SW
Washington DC 20201
Tel: 202-619-0257
Toll free: 1-877-696-6775
www.os.dhhs.gov

CANADA

Asthma Society of Canada
130 Bridgeland Avenue
Suite 425
Toronto
Ontario M6A 1Z4
Tel: 1-800-787-3880
www.asthma.ca
info@asthma.ca

Canadian Diabetes Association
Tel: 1-800-226-8464
Email: info@diabetes.ca
www.diabetes.ca

Canadian Health Services
Research Foundation
1565 Carling Avenue
Suite 700, Ottawa
Ontario K1Z 8R1
Tel: 613-728-2238
www.chsrf.ca

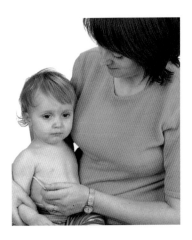

Canadian Immunization
Awareness Program
Canadian Public Health Association
400-1565 Carling Avenue
Ottawa, ON K1Z 8R1
Tel: 613 725-3769
Email: immunize@cpha.ca
www.immunize.cpha.ca

Canadian Institute of Child Health
Suite 300, 384 Bank Street
Ottawa, Ontario K2P 1Y4
Tel: 613-230-8838
www.cich.ca

Canadian Red Cross
National Office
170 Metcalfe Street
Suite 300, Ottawa
Ontario K2P 2P2
Tel: 0613 740 1900
www.redcross.ca

Epilepsy Canada National Office
1470 Peel Street
Suite 745
Montreal QC H3A 1T1
Tel: 514-845-7855
Toll-free: 1-877-734-0873
Email: epilepsy@epilepsy.ca
www.epilepsy.ca

Heart and Stroke Foundation
of Canada
222 Queen Street
Suite 1402
Ottawa
Ontario
K1P 5V9
Tel: 613-569-4361
www.heartandstroke.ca

St John Ambulance Canada
1900 City Park Drive
Suite 400
Ottawa
Ontario K1J 1A3
Tel: 0613 236 7461
www.sja.ca

Canada Safety Council
1020 Thomas Spratt Place
Ottawa
ON K1G 5L5
Tel: 0613 739 153
www.safety-council.org

Safe Kids Canada
180 Dundas Street West
Toronto
ON M5G 1Z8
1-888-SAFE-TIPS
www.safekidscanada.ca

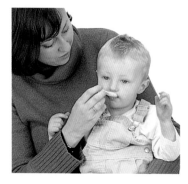

AUSTRALIA

Australian Red Cross
155 Pelham Street
Carlton
Victoria 3053
Tel: 03 9345 1800
www.redcross.org.au

St John Ambulance Australia
PO Box 3895
Manuka ACT 2603
Tel: 02 6295 3777
www.stjohn.org.au

National Safety Council of Australia
322 Glenferrie Road
Malvern
Victoria 3144
Tel: 03 9832 1555
www.safetynews.com

Kidsafe Australia
Kidsafe House
50 Bramston Terrace
Herston
Queensland 4029
Tel: 07 3854 1829
www.kidsafe.com.au

NEW ZEALAND

New Zealand Red Cross
PO Box 12–140
Thorndon
Wellington 6038
Tel: 04 472 3750
www.redcross.org.nz

St John Ambulance National Office
Level 11, St John House
114 The Terrace
PO Box 10 043
Wellington
Tel: 04 472 3600
www.stjohn.org.nz

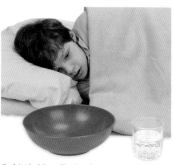

Safekids New Zealand
162 Blockhouse Bay Rd
PO Box 19544
Avondale
Auckland 7
Tel: 09 820 1190
www.safekids.org.nz

SOUTH AFRICA

The South African Red Cross
PO Box 50696
Waterfront, Cape Town 8002
Tel: 021 418 6640
www.redcross.org.za

St John Ambulance
The Order of St John
PO Box 7137
2000 Johannesburg
Tel: 011 646 5520
www.stjohn.org.za

The KidSafe Project
c/o PASASA, Suite 10
10 Pepper St.
PO Box 16225
Vlaeberg 8018
Cape Town
Tel: 021 424 3473
www.pasasa.org

*Note: all address details pages 250–252
correct at time of going to press.*

Index

A

abdomen
  pain 100-101, child 116-117
  wounds 135
acetaminophen, overdosage 188
acupressure/acupuncture 211
aggressiveness, encountering in
  an emergency 220
alcohol
  intoxication 190
  poisoning 190, in child 194
  road accidents 222
allergy 102-103
  anaphylactic shock 70-71
amputation 126, 136
anaphylactic shock 70-71
aneurysm 84
angina pectoris 73
animal bites 104, 127
ankle injuries 165
  sprained 165, 169
antenatal emergencies 92-93
antidepressants, overdosage 189
appendicitis, child 117
arm
  fractures 158-159
  slings 206-207
aromatherapy 210, 211, 212
arrhythmia 74
aspirin, overdosage 188
asthma 56-57
  child 119
atherosclerosis 84
AVPU code 28

B

babies
  bathing 228, 229
  choking 50
  colic 113
  crying 112
  diarrhea 115
  home safety 234
  rashes 113
  resuscitation 44-46, 49
  sudden infant death 235
  teething 113

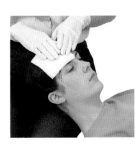

vomiting 115
back pain 170-171
bandaging 200, 201
  applying 202-205
  roller bandage 202
bathroom safety 228-229
bee stings 104
bites 104-105, 126, 127
  complementary therapies 216
bleeding
  control of severe 138-139
  ear 143
  internal 140-141
  mouth 143
  nose 143, 217
  pregnancy 92-93
  rectum 142
  vagina 142
blisters 241
blood 67
  circulation 26, 66-67
  clots, travel risk 247
  coughing up 142
  vessels 66
  vomiting 142
body fluids, avoidance of
  infection in an
  emergency 220
bones 148
  needs 148
  skeleton 148
  see also fractures
brain 78-79
  epilepsy 82-83
  injury 80-81
  stroke 84-85
breathing 54-55

child 118-119
  difficulties 55, 56-57
  mouth-to-mouth rescue
    30-31
bruises 126, 127
  complementary therapies 216
burns 174-177
  chemical 180-181
  complementary therapies 216
  electrical 181
  facial 182
  inhalation 181
  kitchen safety 226-227
  sunburn 183, 217, 241
  treatment of 178-179
  types 174

C

car accidents 222-223
carbon monoxide poisoning 59
cardiac arrest 74-75
cardiac compressions 32-33
cardiopulmonary resuscitation
  (CPR) 26-27
  baby and child 44-45
cardiovascular system 66-67
cheekbone fractures 153
chemicals
  burns 180-181
  garden safety 230
  poisoning, first aid for
    child 195
chest wound 135, 161
childbirth, emergency 94-95
childhood problems 110-123
  abdominal pain 116
  alcohol poisoning 194
  appendicitis 117
  asthma 119
  breathing difficulty 118-119
  chemical poisoning 195
  choking 50, 51
  constipation 117
  coughing 118
  diarrhea 115
  drug poisoning 195
  earache 122

fever 114
  headaches 120-121
  intussusception 117
  meningitis 121
  plant poisoning 195, 231
  poisoning in 194-195
  pulled elbow 167
  rashes 121
  recognizing 110
  resuscitation 44-45, 47-49
  seriously ill child 111
  solvent abuse 191
  sore throat 123
  swallowed objects 144
  toothache 123
  urinary tract infections 123
  vomiting 115
choking 38-41
  baby 50
  child 51
circulation of blood 26, 66-67
clothing
  burns 179
  removal in an emergency
    18-19
cold disorders 106
colic 113
collarbone fracture 158
complementary therapies
  210-211
  first-aid kit 212-213
  using 214-217
concussion 80
confusion 80-81
constipation

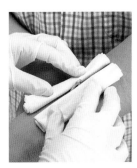

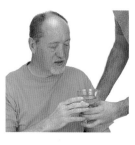

child 117
complementary therapies 214
coughing
  blood 142
  child 118
cramp 99, 107
  complementary therapies 215
crib death 235
crying, baby's 112
cuts 126
  complementary therapies 217
cycling safety 240

D
diabetes 96-97
diaper rash 113
diarrhea 99
  child 115
  complementary therapies 214
  traveler's 246-247
dislocations 166-167
dizziness 88-89
dressings 200-201
drowning 60-61
DRSABC code 12-13, 14
drugs
  first aid for child 195
  illicit 191
  medical, overdosage 188-189

E
ear
  bleeding 143
  earache, child 122
  foreign bodies in 145
elbow
  bandaging 203

injury 159
  pulled, child 167
electricity
  accidents 233
  burns 181
  garden safety 231
embedded objects 130-131
embolism 84
emergency action 12-23
  DRSABC code 12-13, 14
  examination of injured person
    16-17
  first principles 8-9
  gathering information 14-15
  identification devices 15
  information for the
    emergency services 13
  moving and handling
    20-23, 29
  personal safety 220
  psychological stress 221
  removal of clothing and
    helmets 18-19
  signs and symptoms 15
epilepsy 82-83
eyes
  burns 182
  foreign bodies in 144-145

F
face
  burns 182
  fractures 152-153
fainting 88-89
fever 99
  child 114
finger
  bandaging 204
  fractures 159
fire, dealing with 232
first-aid kit 198-199
  complementary 212-213
  outdoor activities 239
  travel 247
fish hooks 130
food poisoning 192-193
foot

bandaging 203
  fracture 165
foreign bodies 130-131, 144-145
fractures 149, 150-151
  arm 158-159
  closed 149, care of 150
  collarbone 158
  dealing with 150-151
  facial 152-153
  fingers 159
  foot 165
  hand 159
  healing 149
  leg 164-165
  open 149, care of 151
  pelvic region 162-163
  rib 160-161
  skull 152
  thighbone 163
  wrist 159
frostbite 244, 245
fume inhalation 58-59
  burns 181
  child, first aid for 195

G
garden safety 230-231
genitals, foreign bodies in 144

H
hand
  bandaging 203
  dislocation 167

fractures 159
hanging 62-63
head
  bandaging 205
  injury 80-81
headache 86
  child 120-121
  complementary therapies 215
heart 66
  arrhythmia 74
  attack 72-73
  cardiac arrest 74-75
  cardiopulmonary resuscitation
    (CPR) 26-27
  failure 73
  palpitations 75
  rate 74
heat disorders 106-107
  cramps 107
  exhaustion 106-107
  heatstroke 107
helmet, removal in emergency 19
herbalism 210, 211, 212, 213
hip dislocation 167
home safety 59, 224-225
  baby 234
  bathroom 228-229
  house-dust mites 103
  kitchen 226-227
  poison-proof 194
homeopathy 211, 212
hyperglycemia 97
hyperventilation 57

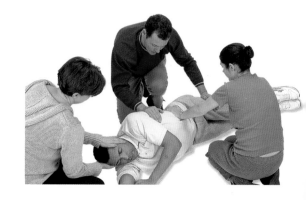

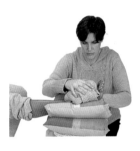

hypoglycemia 97
hypothermia 106, 241

I
immunization for travel 246
infection of wounds 132-133
injuries
    ankle 165, 169
    brain 80-81
    crush 137
    elbow 159
    facial 152-153
    head 80-81
    knee 164
    lightning 233
    neck 156-157
    snow sports 244-245
    soft-tissue 168, 241
    spinal 154-155
    teeth 153
    thigh 139
    see also fractures, wounds
intussusception 117
iron supplements,
    overdosage 189

J
jaw
    dislocation 167
    fractures 153
jet lag 247

K
kitchen safety 226-227
knee
    bandaging joint 203
    injuries 164

L
labor 94-95
leg fractures 164-165
lightning injuries 233
"log roll" technique 157
lungs 54-55

M
malaria, protection against 246
marine stings 105
meningitis 121
migraine 87
milia 113
miscarriage 92-93
mites 103
mountaineering safety 241
mouth bleeding 143
mouth-to-mouth rescue
    breathing 30-31
moving an injured person 20-23,
    29
    "log roll" technique 157
mushroom poisoning 192-193

N
nausea 98
    complementary therapies 214
neck injuries 156-157
nervous system 78-79
nose
    bleeds 143
    complementary therapies 217
    foreign bodies 144
    fractures 153

P
palpitations 75
pancreas 96
pelvic region 162
    fractures 162-163
plants
    complementary first-aid kit
    212-213
    garden safety 231
    poisoning 192-193, first aid
    for child 195

poisoning 186-195
    alcohol 190
    carbon monoxide 59
    children 194-195
    drug 188-89, illicit 191
    effect on body 187
    food and plant 192-193
    solvent abuse 191
pregnancy, antenatal
    emergencies 92-93
psychological stress following
    an emergency 221
pulse 67

R
rashes
    baby 113
    child 121
rectum
    bleeding 142
    foreign bodies in 144
reflexology 211
respiratory system 54-55
resuscitation 26-37
    airway 29
    baby 44-46, 49
    cardiac compressions 32-33
    cardiopulmonary resuscitation
    (CPR) 26-27
    child 44-45, 47-49
    full sequence 34-35
    mouth-to-mouth rescue
    breathing 30-31
    recovery position 36-37
    responsiveness assessment 28
rib fractures 160-161
RICE guidelines 169
road accidents 222-223

S
safety
    garden 230-231
    home 59, 194, 224-229
    personal in an emergency 220
    road 222-223
    sport 238-245
    travel 246-247

scalds 178-179
scuba diving safety 243
seizures 82-83
sex on holiday, safety 247
shock, circulatory 68-69
    anaphylactic 70-71
    complementary therapies 215
shoulder dislocation 166
skeleton 148
skiing
    injuries 245
    safety 244
skin
    burns 174-183
    structure 174
skull
    fractures 152
    injuries 80-81
slings 206-207
snake bites 105
snow sports safety 244-245
soft-tissue injury 168, 241
solvent abuse poisoning 191
sore throat, child 123
spine 154
    injury 154-155
splinters 130
sport safety 238-239
    land 240-241
    snow 244-245
    water 242-243
sprains 168-169
    ankle 165, 169
    complementary therapies

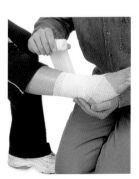

216-217
stings 104-105
  complementary therapies 216
strains 168-169
  complementary therapies
    216-217
strangulation 62
stroke 84-85
sunburn 183, 241
  complementary therapies 217
swallowed objects 144
swimming safety 242-243

T
teeth
  injuries 153
  teething 113
  toothache, child 123
tetanus 133
thigh injury 139

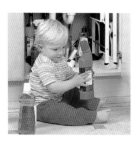

thighbone fracture 163
toothache, child 123
tourniquets 136, 139
tranquilizers, overdosage 189
transient ischemic attacks
  (TIAs) 85
travel safety 246-247
  sickness 247
triaging 8

U
urinary tract infections, child
  123

V
vaginal bleeding 142
vertebral column, see spine
vertigo 88
vomiting 98
  blood 142
  child 115
  complementary therapies 214

W
walking hazards 241
wasp stings 104
water sports safety 242-243
wounds
  abdominal 135
  amputation 126, 136

bleeding, control 138-139
chest 135, 161
cleaning and dressing 129
embedded objects 130-131
healing process 128
infected 132-133
major 134-135
types 126-127
wrist fracture 159

Acknowledgements

The publishers would like to thank the following people for their assistance in the making of this book:

The models:
Peter Akinola, Neil Barnes, Sue Barraclough, Heather Batchelor and Angus (18 months), Aaron Beha-Parks, Lesley Betts, Neil Bradbury, Jim Britton, Natasha Brown, Iva Buckova, Matthew Charlton, Rachel Chilcott and Tabitha (18 months), Valerie Ferguson, Jack France, John France, Tom France, Irene Halton, Jane Harris, Hannah Higgins, Lydia Hitchings, Simona Hill, Oliver Hitchings, Louise Hughes, Brian Jackson, Emma Jackson, Sam Jones, Pippa Keech and William (aged 7), Dallas Kidman, Ralph Leming, Helen Lowe, Debra Mayhew and Jamie Austin (18 months), Emily MacQueen, Denise Olive, Alan Powell, Joanne Rippin, David Spicer, Helen Sudell, Vivien Tobies, Melanie Ward, Evie Wyld. Thanks to Dammers Model and Promotion Agency, Bristol, for providing some of the models listed above.

Others:
Two Wheels Service, Bath, for the loan of a crash helmet. Pat Coward, for compiling the index.

Photographic acknowledgements

The publishers would like to thank the agencies listed below for their kind permission to reproduce the following images in this book:

l=left; r=right; t=top; b=bottom; c=centre

p67bc Medical-On-Line/Mediscan; p71t Garry Watson/Science Photo Library; p121t image courtesy of Meningitis Trust © 2003; p133b Jim Selby/Science Photo Library; p137b Marcelo Brodsky/Latin Stock/Science Photo Library; p242br Robert Harding Picture Library Ltd; p243bl Sinclair Stammers/Science Photo Library; p244b Robert Harding Picture Library Ltd.

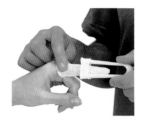

NOTES

NOTES

NOTES

NOTES

NOTES

NOTES